OXFORD MEDICAL PUBLICATIONS

Oxford Handbook of
Nutrition
and
Dietetics

Published and forthcoming Oxford Handbooks

Oxford Handbook of
Nutrition and Dietetics

Joan Webster-Gandy

Angela Madden

Michelle Holdsworth

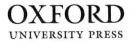

OXFORD
UNIVERSITY PRESS

OXFORD
UNIVERSITY PRESS

Great Clarendon Street, Oxford OX2 6DP

Oxford University Press is a department of the University of Oxford.
It furthers the University's objective of excellence in research, scholarship,
and education by publishing worldwide in

Oxford New York

Auckland Cape Town Dar es Salaam Hong Kong Karachi
Kuala Lumpur Madrid Melbourne Mexico City Nairobi
New Delhi Shanghai Taipei Toronto

With offices in

Argentina Austria Brazil Chile Czech Republic France Greece
Guatemala Hungary Italy Japan Poland Portugal Singapore
South Korea Switzerland Thailand Turkey Ukraine Vietnam

Oxford is a registered trade mark of Oxford University Press
in the UK and in certain other countries

Published in the United States
by Oxford University Press, Inc., New York

British Library Cataloguing in Publication Data
Data available

Library of Congress Cataloging in Publication Data
Data available

Typeset by Newgen Imaging Systems (P) Ltd., Chennai, India
Printed in Italy
on acid-free paper by LegoPrint S.p.A.

ISBN 0–19–856725–1 978–0–19–856725–7 (flexicover)

10 9 8 7 6 5 4 3 2 1

Preface

When we were approached to write this handbook the original idea was to write a book for general practice. However, we all remember being student dietitians and all created our own handbook of useful information that we carried around with us and were totally lost without. On reflection of what text books are now available in nutrition or dietetics, it became clear that although there are now concise pocket books written for dietitians working predominantly in a clinical setting, there was a need for a user friendly handbook of nutrition and dietetics for a wider audience that included doctors, nurses, nutritionists and other health care professionals. The available textbooks are, by necessity, large tomes or series that are unlikely to adorn the shelves of many doctors or nurses whether in primary or secondary care.

As a result, we have tried to present nutritional science, therapeutics and community public health nutrition in a concise and integrated manner. While writing the text we have tried to identify what information would be useful to different professionals in a variety of settings. For example a doctor or nurse may want information on obesity and will find a ready reckoner for the calculation of BMI, information on associated problems and treatment options. Dietitians working in the community or public health will have this information but will find the sections on the measurements of obesity or nutrition interventions more informative. How well we have achieved this is for the reader to decide.

Nutrition is fascinating for many reasons, one of which is the fact that it is a very dynamic discipline. We have tried very hard to be contemporary but there will inevitably be changes in basic science, practice and policy as the discipline continues to evolve. Major developments and changes will be posted on the relevant page of the OUP web site. For us it has been a very enjoyable, if at times rather demanding, process and we hope that this book is useful to all health care professionals.

J.W-G.
A.M.M.
M.H.

Foreword

Both health professionals and the general public now realize that good nutrition is essential for good health. Indeed, nutrition is the health topic on which the lay public receives the most advice from popular books and magazines, but often this advice is unsound. It is therefore essential that health-carers have readily available reliable information about all aspects of nutrition. This includes nutritional science, public health nutrition, and therapeutic nutrition.

This handbook provides, in concise format, the information about nutrition needed by those training to be dietitians (RD), nutritionists (RNutr), public health nutritionists (RPHNutr), or doctors or nurses either in hospital or primary care. It will continue to be a valuable resource after graduation, since the scope of modern nutrition is so large that a specialist in one field (say, public health nutrition) cannot hope to have instantly accessible all the necessary information about therapeutic diets, or nutritional sciences, and *vice versa*.

The three authors of this Handbook are all registered dietitians, each of whom has a solid research record as well as extensive experience of the nutritional problems that dietitians, hospital doctors, general practitioners, and specialist nurses will encounter. I am confident that readers will be thankful to have this book in their pocket to guide them to the correct immediate response to a nutritional problem, even if later they have to consult a senior dietitian or textbook for more detailed advice.

John Garrow MD PhD FRCP
Emeritus Professor of Human Nutrition
University of London.

Acknowledgements

Special thanks go to everyone who has helped and supported us during the production of this book. We are particularly grateful to: Julie Beckerson, Alison Culkin, George Grimble, Michelle Harvie, Catherine Hodgson, Catherine Humphries, Tom Humphries, Jamie Hustler, Cathy Mooney, Gail Rees, Alan Rio, Ann Van Duzer, and Liz Weekes.

Finally, thanks to the medical division at OUP for all the encouragement and support.

Dedication

To Beth, Didier, Catherine, Matthew, Milo, Paula, and Will, with much love.

Contents

Detailed contents

List of contributors

Janice Barratt,
Trust Lead for Dietetics,
Derbyshire Mental Health
Services NHS Trust, Derby, UK

Luci Daniels,
Dietetic and Nutrition
Consultant, London, UK

Dr Francis Delpeuch,
Research Director,UR106
Nutrition, Alimentation et
Sociétés,WHO collaborating
centre in Human Nutrition,
Institut de Recherche pour le
Développement- IRD, France

Ruby Dillon,
Food project Co-ordinator/
Public Health Nutritionist,
Fernbank Medical Centre, UK

Marjorie Dixon,
Specialist Metabolic Dietitian,
Great Ormond Street Hospital for
Children NHS Trust, London, UK

Dr Alizon Draper,
Principal Lecturer in Public Health
Nutrition, School of Integrated
Health, University of Westminster,
London, UK

Barbara Engel,
School of Biomedical and
Biomolecular Sciences, University
of Surrey, Guildford, UK

Dr John Garrow,
Emeritus Professor of Human
Nutrition, University of London, UK

Catherine Hodgson,
Senior Lecturer in Nutrition and
Dietetics, London Metropolitan
University, London, UK

Dr Michelle Holdsworth,
Associate Professor in Human
Nutrition and Dietetics,
Division of Nutritional Science,
University of Nottingham, UK

Lynne Hubbard,
Nutrition & Dietetic
Department, Selly Oak
Hospital, UK

Dr Angela M. Madden,
Principal Lecturer in
Dietetics, University of
Hertfordshire, UK

Fiona Moor,
Head of Dietetic Services,
Derby Hospitals NHS Foundation
Trust, Derby, UK

Elizabeth Neal,
Research Dietitian,
Institute of Child Health,
London, UK

Dympna Pearson,
Freelance Dietitian,
Quorn, UK

Dr Michael D. Randall,
Reader in Cardiovascular
Pharmacology,
University of Nottingham
Medical School, UK

Isabel Skypala,
Director of Rehabilitation and
Therapies, Royal Borompton &
Harefield NHS Trust, UK

Clare Soulsby,
Nutrition and Dietetic
Department, Barts and
the London NHS Trust,
London

Nicki Stewart,
Chief Dietitian, Nutrition &
Dietetic Department,
Lister Hospital, UK

Helen Storer,
Community Dietetic Services
Manager, Nottingham City
PCT, UK

Dr Lisa Waddell,
Community Paediatric Dietitian,
Nottingham City PCT, UK

Dr Joan Webster-Gandy,
Reader in Nutrition, Research
Centre for Health Studies,
Buckinghamshire Chilterns
University College, UK

Abbreviations and medical shorthands

Contains abbreviations for organizations that are no longer in existence but may be referred to in the literature.

#	fracture
#NOF	fractured neck of femur
µg	micrograms
µmol	micromoles
A & W	alive and well
A2RB	angiotensin II receptor blocker
AA ($\alpha\alpha$)	amino acid
ABV	percentage alcohol by volume
AC	before meals
ACBS	Advisory Committee on Borderline Substances
ACE	angiotensin-converting enzyme
ACNFP	Advisory Committee on Novel Foods and Processes
ACTH	adrenocorticotrophic hormone
ADA	American Dietetic Association
ADH	antidiuretic hormone/alcohol dehydrogenase
ADI	acceptable daily intake
ADL	activities of daily living
AF	atrial fibrillation
AHP	allied health professional
AIDS	acquired immune defeciency syndrome
Al	aluminium
ALDH	aldehyde dehydrogenase
AMA	American Medical Association
AN	anorexia nervosa
ANF	anti-nuclear factor
APIT	activate partial thromboplastin time
ARF	acute renal failure
ASCVD	arteriosclerotic heart disease
ATN	acute tubular neurosis
ATP	adenosine triphosphate

AV	arteriovenous
AXR	abdominal X-ray
AZT	azidothymidine
BaE	barium enema
BAPEN	British Association of Parenteral and Enteral Nutrition
BBSRC	Biotechnology and Biological Sciences Research Council
BCAA	branched chain amino acids
bd	twice a day
BDA	British Dietetic Association
BHA	butylated hydroxyanisole
BHF	better hospital food
BHT	butylated hydroxytoluene
BIA	bioelectrical analysis
BIBRA	British Industrial Biological Research Association
BM	bowel movement
BMA	British Medical Association
BMI	body mass index (weight (kg)/height (m)^2)
BMJ	British Medical Journal
BMR	basal metabolic rate
BMT	bone marrow transplant
BNF	British Nutrition Foundation/ British National Formulary
BNO	bowels not open
BOR	bowels open regularly
BP units	British Pharmacopoeia units
BP	blood pressure/ British Pharmacopoeia
BS	blood sugar/bowel sounds
Bx	biopsy
Ca	calcium
CA	carcinoma
Ca:P	calcium: phosphorus ratio
Cap	Capsule
CAPD	continuous ambulatory peritoneal dialysis
CAT/CT	computer assisted tomography
CBC	complete blood count
CBT	cognitive behavioural therapy
CC	critical care
CCF	chronic cardiac failure
CCPD	continuous cyclic peritoneal dialysis

CD	Crohn's disease
CD4	cluster of differentiation 4
CDC	Center for Disease Control (USA)
CF	cystic fibrosis
CHD	coronary heart disease
CHO	carbohydrate
CI	confidence interval
CJD	Creutzfeldt–Jakob disease
Cl	chlorine/chloride
cm	centimetres
CNG	Community Nutrition Group
CNS	central nervous system
Co	cobalt
CoE	Council of Europe
COMA	Committee on Medical Aspects of Food Policy
COPD	chronic obstructive pulmonary disease
CPAG	Child Poverty Action Group
CPN	community psychiatric nurse
CPR	cardiopulmonary resuscitation
Cr	chromium
CRF	chronic renal failure
CRP	C-reactive protein
CRRT	continuous renal replacement therapy
CSF	cerebrospinal fluid
CT	computer-assisted tomography
Cu	copper
CV	coefficient of variance
CVA	cerebrovascular accident
CVD	cardiovascular disease
CVP	central venous pressure
CVS	cardiovascular system
CXR	chest X-ray
CyA	cyclosporin A
D	diagnosis
D&V	diarrhoea and vomiting
D_2	ergocalciferol
D_3	cholecalciferol
D4T	di-dehydro-deoxythymidine
DA	dietetic assistant

DAFNE	Dose Adjustment For Normal Eating (programme)
DBP	diastolic blood pressure
DD	differential diagnosis
DEFRA	Department for Environment, Food, and Rural Affairs
DES	dietary energy supply
DESMOND	Diabetes Education Self-Managed Ongoing and Newly Diagnosed (programme)
DEXA	dual energy X–ray absorptiometry
DFES	Department for Education and Skills
DHA	docosahexaenoic acid
DIT	dietary induced thermogenesis
dl	decilitre (100 ml)
DM	diabetes mellitus
DNA	deoxyribonucleic acid/ did not attend
DoH/DH	Department of Health
DRV	dietary reference value
DSM	Diagnostic and Statistical Manual of Mental Disorders
dsp	level dessertspoonful
DTs	delirium tremors
DU	duodenal ulcer
EAA	essential amino acids
EAR	estimated average requirement
EC	European Community
ECF	extracellular fluid
ECG	electrocardiogram
ECT	electroconvulsive therapy
EDTA	European Dialysis and Transplant Association
EE	energy expenditure
EEG	electroencephalogram
EFA	essential fatty acids
EFAD	European Federation of the Associations of Dietitians
EGR	erythrocyte glutathione reductase
EGRA	erythrocyte glutathione reductase activity coefficient
EPA	eicosapentaenoic acid
ER	emergency regimen
ERCP	endoscopic retrograde cholangiopancreatography
ESPEN	European Society of Parenteral and Enteral Nutrition
ESRC	Economic and Social Research Council
ESRF	end-stage renal failure

EU	European Union
F	fluorine
FAD	Flavin adenine dinucleotide
FAO	Food & Agriculture Organisation (UN)
FBC	full blood count
FBDG	food-based dietary guidelines
FBS	fasting blood sugar
FDA	Food & Drug Administration (USA)
Fe	iron
FFM	fat-free mass
FFQ/FAQ	food frequency/amount questionnaire
FH	family history
fl oz	fluid ounce
FM	fat mass
FMN	flavin mononucleotide
FOS	fructo-oligosaccharides
FP 10	form used for the prescription of medicines in the UK
FSA	Food Standards Agency
FSGS	focal segmental glomerulosclerosis
FSH	follicle stimulating hormone
Fx	fracture
G	grams
GBM	glomerular basement membrane
GDA	guideline daily amount
GDM	gestational diabetes
GF	gluten-free
GFR	glomerular filtration rate
GI	glycaemic index/ gastrointestinal
GL	glycaemic load
gln	glutamine
GMO	genetically modified organism
GN	glomerulonephritis
GORD	gastro-oesophageal reflux disease
GP	general practitioner
GTN	glyceryl trinitrate
GTT	glucose tolerance test
GU	genitourinary
GVHD	graft versus host disease
HAART	highly active antiretroviral therapy

Hb	haemoglobin
HbA1$_c$	glycosylated haemoglobin
HBV	high biological value
Hct	haematocrit
HD	haemodialysis
HDA	Health Development Agency
HDL	high density lipoprotein
HF	haemofiltration
hGH	human growth hormone
HIV	human immunodeficiency virus
HLA	human lymphocyte antigen
HMG-CoA	3-hydroxy-3-methyl-glutaryl coenzyme A
HO	house officer
HPC	Health Professions Council
HT	hypertension
I	iodine
IBD	inflammatory bowel disease
IBS	irritable bowel syndrome
IBW	ideal body weight
ICD	International Classification of Diseases
ICF	intracellular Fluid
Id	intradermal
IDA	iron deficiency anaemia
IDD	iodine deficiency disorder
IDL	intermediate density lipoproteins
IDPN	intradialytic parenteral nutrition
IF	intestinal failure
IgA	immunoglobulin A
IgE	immunoglobulin E
IgG	immunoglobulin G
IgM	immunoglobulin M
IGTT	impaired glucose tolerance test
IM	intramuscular
IMD	inherited metabolic diseases
INS	International Numbering System (for Food additives)
IPD	intermittent peritoneal dialysis
ITU	intensive therapy unit
IU	international units
IV	intravenous

IVHP	intravenous high potency
IVNAA	*in-vivo* neutron activation analysis
JHCI	Joint Health Claims Initiative
JVP	jugular venous pressure
K	potassium
KDOQI	Kidney Disease Outcomes Quality Initiative
kcal	kilocalories
KD	ketogenic diet
kg	kilograms
kJ	kilojoules
l	litre
lb	pound
LBM	lean body mass
LBV	low biological value
LBW	low birth weight
L-CAT	lecithin-cholesterol acyl transferase
LCFA	long chain fatty acids
LCMG	long chain monoglycerides
LCP	long chain polyunsaturated fatty acid
LCT	long chain triglycerides
LDL	low density lipoprotein
LFT	liver function tests
LRNI	lower reference nutrient intake
LVF	left ventricular failure
m	metres
MAC	midarm circumference
MAFF	Ministry of Agriculture, Fisheries, and Food (superseded by DEFRA)
MAMC	mid arm muscle circumference
MAOI	monoamine oxidase inhibitors
MAS	milk alkali syndrome
MCH	mean cell haemoglobin
MCHC	mean cell haemoglobin concentration
MCN	minimal change nephropathy
MCT	medium chain triglycerides
MCV	mean cell volume
MEOS	microsomal ethanol-oxidizing system
mEq	milliequivalents
Mg	magnesium

mg	milligrams
MI	myocardial infarction
MIMS	Monthly Index of Medical Specialities
MJ	megajoules
ml	millilitres
mm	millimetres
mmol	millimoles
MN	membranous nephropathy
Mn	manganese
MND	motor neurone disease
Mo	molybdenum
mosmol	milliosmoles
MRC	Medical Research Council
MRI	magnetic resonance imaging
MS	multiple sclerosis
MSG	monosodium glutamate
MSU	mid stream urine
MSUD	maple syrup urine disease
MUAC	mid upper arm circumference
MUFA	mono unsaturated fatty acid
MUST	Malnutrition Universal Screening Tool
N	nitrogen
N&V	nausea and vomiting
Na	sodium
NAD	nothing abnormal detected/ no apparent disease/ nicotinamide adenine dinucleotide
NADP	nicotinamide adenine dinucleotide phosphate
NAMCW	National Association for Maternal and Child Welfare
NAS	no added salt
NASH	nonalcoholic steatohepatitis
NCD	nutrition-related chronic disease
NCHS	National Centre for Health Statistics (see CDC)
NCT	National Childbirth Trust
NDNS	National Diet & Nutrition Survey
NMC	Nursing and Midwifery Council
NFS	National Food Survey
NG	nasogastric
NGO	non-governmental agency
NHANES	National Health and Nutrition Examination Survey

NHS	National Health Service
Ni	nickel
NICE	National Institute for Health and Clinical Evidence
NJ	nasojejunal
NKF	National Kidney Foundation
NMN	N^1-methylnicotinamide
nPCR	normalized protein catabolic rate
NPE:N	non-protein energy: nitrogen ratio
NS	nephrotic syndrome
NSAID	nonsteroidal anti-inflammatory drug
NSF	National Service Framework
NSP	non-starch polysaccharides
NTD	neural tube defect
OA	osteoarthritis
OAS	oral allergy syndrome
od	everyday/ once daily
Osmol	osmoles
OTC	over-the-counter
oz	ounce
P	phosphorus
P/S ratio	polyunsaturated fatty acids: saturated fatty ratio
PA	physical activity
PABA	para-amino benzoic acid
PAL	physical activity level
PAR	physical activity ratio
Pb	lead
PC	after meals
PCHR	personal child health record
PCK	polycystic disease of the kidney
PCOS	polycystic ovary syndrome
PCR	protein catabolic rate
PCT	primary case trust
PD	peritoneal dialysis
PDis	Parkinson's disease
PDUO	previous day's urine output
PEG	percutaneous endoscopic gastrostomy
PEJ	percutaneous endoscopic jejunostomy
PEM	protein energy malnutrition
PERT	pancreatic enzyme replacement therapy

PF	peak flow
PG	prostaglandin
PGV	proximal gastric vagotomy
PHCT	primary health care trust
phe	phenylalanine
PICC	peripherally inserted central catheter
PKU	phenylketonuria
PMH	past medical history
PN	parenteral nutrition
PO_4	phosphate
Post op	post-operative
PPF	plasma protein fraction
ppm	parts per million
PR	per rectum
PRG	percutaneous radiological gastrostomy
PSE	portal systemic encephalopathy
PT	prothrombin time
pt(s)	pint(s)
PTA	prior to admission
PTH	parathyroid hormone
PUFA	polyunsaturated fatty acids
PWS	Prader–Willi syndrome
Qd	every day
Qh	every hour
Qid or Qds	4 times daily
Qod	every other day
QUID	Quantitative Ingredient Declaration
RA	rheumatoid arthritis
RAST	radioallergosorbent test
RBC	red blood count/cell
RCGP	Royal College of General Practitioners
RCN	Royal College of Nursing
RCP	Royal College of Physicians
RCPCH	Royal College of Paediatrics and Child Health
RCS	Royal College of Surgeons
RCT	randomized controlled trial
RD	registered dietitian
RDA	recommended dietary allowance/recommended daily amount

RDI	recommended daily intake
RDis	Refsum's disease
RDS	rapidly digestible starch
REE	resting energy expenditure
RGN	registered general nurse
RIG	radiologically inserted gastrostomy
RMR	resting metabolic rate
RNA	ribonucleic acid
RNI	reference nutrient intake
RQ	respiratory quotient
RR	relative risk
RS	re-feeding syndrome/resistant starch
RTA	renal tubular acidosis
SACN	Scientific Advisory Committee on Nutrition
SBP	systolic blood pressure
SBS	short bowel syndrome
SCF	Scientific Committee for Food (European)
SCI	spinal cord injury
sd	standard deviation
SDS	slowly digestible starch
Se	selenium
se	standard error
SFA	saturated fatty acid
SFGA	small-for-gestational age
SGOT	serum glutamic-oxaloacetic transaminase activity
SGPT	serum glutamic-pyruvic transaminase activity
SH	social history
SHA	Strategic Health Authority
SHO	senior house officer
SHS	Scientific Hospital Supplies
SI	statutory instrument/Système internationale
SLE	systemic lupus erythematosus
SOB	shortness of breath
SPT	skin prick test
SRD	state registered dietitian (this has been superseded by RD)
STP	standard temperature and pressure
T12	12th thoracic vertebra
T3	triiodothyronine
T4	thyroxine

Tab	tablet
TB	tuberculosis
TBK	total body potassium
tbs	level tablespoonful
TBW	total body water
TCI	to come in
tds	three times daily
TEE	total energy expenditure
TF	transferrin
TIBC	total iron binding capacity
Tid or tds	3 times a day
TLC	total lymphocyte count/ tender loving care
TOBEC	total body electrical conductivity
TPN	total parenteral nutrition
TPP	thiamine pyrophosphate
TSF	triceps skin fold thickness
TSH	thyroid stimulating hormone
tsp	level teaspoonful
TST	triceps skinfold thickness
TT	thrombin time
U&E	urea and electrolytes
UC	ulcerative colitis
UHT	ultra-heat treatment
UTI	urinary tract infections
VLCD	very low calorie diet
VLDL	very low density lipoproteins
VMA	vanillylmandelic acid
W	watt
WBC	white blood cells
WCC	white call count
WHO	World Health Organisation
WRVS	Women's Royal Voluntary Service
Wt	weight
Z	diagnosis
Zn	zinc
Δ	diagnosis
#	Fracture

Introduction to nutrition

Definitions and titles

Nutrition

'Nutrition is the branch of science that studies the process by which living organisms take in and use food for the maintenance of life, growth, reproduction, the functioning of organs and tissues, and the production of energy.'[1]

Dietitian (dietician)

The titles dietitian (UK) and dietician (US) are protected by law in the UK; anyone using these titles must be registered with the Health Professions Council (HPC). Anyone using these titles without registration is liable to prosecution and may be fined. Registered dietitians are also able to use the post-nominal letters SRD and RD (UK) or RD (US). The European Federation of the Associations of Dietitians (EFAD) has defined the role of the dietitian as follows.

- A dietitian is a person with a qualification in nutrition and dietetics recognized by national authority(s). The dietitian applies the science of nutrition to the feeding and education of groups of people and individuals in health and disease.
- The scope of dietetic practice is such that dietitians may work in a variety of settings and have a variety of work functions.

European academic and practitioner standards for dietetics can be found on the EFAD web site (www.efad.org).

Many dietitians work in the NHS and may specialize, e.g. oncology, renal disease. They are employed in primary and secondary care and are a key part of the health-care team. Dietitians also work outside the NHS in areas such as industry, sport, education, journalism, and research.

Health Professions Council (HPC)   More information about HPC is available at www.hpc-uk.org.

British Dietetic Association (BDA)

The BDA is the professional body representing dietitians and was established in 1936 in order to:

- advance the science and practice of dietetics and associated subjects;
- promote training and education in the science and practice of dietetics and associated subjects;
- regulate the relations between dietitians and their employer through the BDA trade union.

Specialist groups within the BDA cover areas of specialist interest, e.g. Paediatrics Group, Community Nutrition Group (CNG). Full membership is available to RDs; other membership categories are available for dietetic assistants, students, and affiliates. More information about the BDA is available at www.bda.uk.org.

[1] Bender, A.E. and Bender, D.A. (1995). *Oxford dictionary of food and nutrition.* Oxford University press, Oxford.

Nutritionist

The title 'nutritionist' has no legal standing and no educational requirements are necessary for a person to be called 'nutritionist'. The Nutrition Society is endeavouring to regulate the field of nutrition and protection of the title 'nutritionist', possibly in collaboration with the Health Professions Council.

The Nutrition Society

The Nutrition Society was established in 1941 'to advance the scientific study of nutrition and its application to the maintenance of human and animal health'. The society covers 4 key areas:

• promotion of professional study;
• promotion of high standards in professional practice;
• promotion of professional careers;
• public protection through professional registration.

The Nutrition Society holds registers of nutritionists and registrants are bound by the Society's code of ethics and its statement of professional conduct. To register with the Nutrition Society it is necessary to demonstrate preset qualifications and experience in nutrition; the society awards the titles associate nutritionist (Assoc Nutr.), registered nutritionist (R Nutr.) and registered public health nutritionist (R PHNutr.). Further details can be obtained at www.nutritionsociety.org.uk.

Dietetic assistants (DA)

DAs work under the direct supervision of a RD who has a minimum of 12 months' experience. Their roles include administration and tasks as delegated by the RD. Within a hospital setting these may include assisting patients requiring special diets to choose from the hospital menu and collecting and recording information regarding the patient's consumption and weight. In primary care they may include providing dietary consultation, under the direction of the dietitian and liaising with the RD regarding the patient's progress. Within a community setting they may include assisting the dietitian to assess the food and health needs of local residents and enabling people to eat a healthier diet to prevent disease, offering guidance in relation to food selection and preparation, planning menus, standardizing recipes, and testing new products.

Components of the diet

Diet
Diet is what a person habitually eats and drinks, so everyone is always on a diet. When we speak of 'going on a diet' it usually means trying to follow a prescribed diet in order to lose weight. One of the most important, and difficult, tasks in nutritional medicine is to estimate accurately the habitual nutritional intake and diet of the patient. These difficulties arise because a person's diet may vary widely from day to day, food processing may greatly affect the nutrient content of foods s/he eats, and hardly anyone with a nutritional problem can accurately recall what s/he has eaten.

Dietary value
Dietary value is assessed by the measured energy and nutrient content of a particular diet and often in reference to dietary reference values (see Chapter 2, 'Dietary reference values') or recommendations. Foods and diets also have many other kinds of value including political, economic, social, and cultural values (see 'Influences on food choice', Chapter 14). In most societies where people live above starvation level effort is put into diversifying meals and the overall diet, e.g.
- use of food in rituals, e.g. the last supper, birthday and wedding cakes, also fasting (Ramadan and Lent);
- use of food to express values and social relationships, e.g. sharing food, preparing special foods as expression of love, etc.;
- prestige foods, e.g. champagne and caviar as symbols of wealth and privilege.

Components of the diet
Diets are composed of nutrients: macronutrients (protein, fats, carbohydrates, and alcohol) and the micronutrients (vitamins, minerals, and trace elements). Food also contains many non-nutritional, but biologically active substances. These include toxins and contaminants, such as alkaloids and aflatoxins, that are detrimental to health as well as constituents, such as phytochemicals, that may be health-promoting. As consumers we do not eat nutrients, but meals and foods. These are the components of diet most meaningful to the public and usually the basis of food choice.

Food groups
Foods vary in their energy and nutrient content. Food groups are a classification of foods on the basis of the nutrient profile sugar (see 'Balance of good health' in 'Food-based dietary guidelines', Chapter 2, and Table 1.1). Commonly used food groups are:
- high protein foods, e.g. meat, fish, eggs, dairy products, pulses/legumes;
- carbohydrate-rich foods, e.g. cereals, roots, and tubers;
- dairy foods;
- fruit and vegetables;
- foods rich in fat or oil.

Table 1.1 Nutrient profile of the main food groups

Food group	Fat	Carbo-hydrate	Protein	Fat-soluble vitamins	Water-soluble vitamins	Minerals
Cereals		+ + +	+ +		+ + (Bs) but variable	+
Roots & tubers		+ + +	+ but variable		+ + (C) but variable	
Legumes/ pulses	+ but variable		+ +		+ + (Bs)	+
Meat, fish, eggs	+		+ + +	+ +	+ (Bs)	+
Dairy products	+		+ +	+ +	+ (C)	++
Fruits		+			+ + + (C)	
Vegetables			++		+ + + (C, folate)	++
Sugar		+ + +				
Fats and oils	+ + +			+ + + but variable		

+, This food group is a source of the nutrient(s) in most human diets; ++, this food group is an important source of the nutrient(s) in most human diets; +++, this food group is a major source of the nutrient(s) in most human diets.

Food groups are widely used in the formulation of dietary guidelines and for nutrition education messages of various kinds, such as eat five portions of fruit and vegetables a day (a current UK health message). While useful, such classifications are also somewhat arbitrary; so some foods can be placed in more than one food group.

Staple foods
A staple food is one that forms the basis of the diet in terms of both quantity and frequency of consumption and that provides the highest proportion of energy. Staple foods vary with geographic region, but in global terms the most important staple foods are the following.
• Cereals; globally cereals supply approximately 51% of the world's dietary energy supply (DES) with rice, maize, and wheat the most important, although other cereals, such as millets and sorghum, are also important in some regions. Cereals are a good source of

carbohydrate, but also contain reasonable amounts of protein and, depending on variety and processing, some micronutrients, e.g. Fe and some B vitamins.

- Roots and tubers, and particularly cassava or manioc; in sub-Saharan Africa they supply 22% DES, with this figure rising to over 70% in individual countries, such as the Democratic Republic of Congo. Other important roots are potatoes, yams, sweet potatoes, and taro. They are high in carbohydrate, but low in fat, protein, and, with some important exceptions, e.g. sweet potatoes, micronutrients.

Other less common staple foods are sago eaten in parts of Malaysia and Indonesia and plantain and bananas in many tropical countries (sub-Saharan Africa, Asia, Caribbean, and South America. The importance of staple foods has declined in industrialized countries (e.g. in industrialized countries cereals only supply 26% DES), but they remain important in many low income countries. In Nepal 77% DES from cereals (predominantly rice) while in the USA only 23% DES derives from cereals (as mixture of rice, wheat, and maize).

Meals

Most foods are eaten as part of meals. Meals may differ in the following ways.

- The combination of foods eaten, e.g. the traditional British meal of 'meat and two veg'.
- How they are processed, prepared, and cooked. This can have an impact on the nutritional value of food, e.g. steaming rather than boiling vegetables reduces losses of water-soluble vitamins.
- The order in which particular items or dishes are consumed. In most European countries a formal meal is a three course sequence pattern of starter, main course, and pudding or dessert, whereas in Chinese banquets many dishes tend to be served at once.
- How food is eaten: with hands or implements, from separate dishes or a common bowl. This is largely a matter of social etiquette, but can be important in child feeding, e.g. if small children are fed from a common pot rather than given an individual serving.
- Who eats with whom and the allocation of food within the household. In some societies men and women eat separately and there is also an unequal division of food between the sexes, including children.

These meal patterns may impact upon the dietary intake of individuals within a household.

Snacks

Snacks are foods that are not eaten as part of meals. The place of snacks in peoples' diets and their contribution to overall dietary intake are variable.

Food composition tables

The food composition tables used in the UK are those of McCance and Widdowson. The 6th edition was published in 2002 by the Food Standards Agency in collaboration with the Royal Society of Chemistry (www.food.gov.uk).[1] Book and electronic versions are available. Food tables may be country-specific to account for country-specific food laws, e.g. fortification.

Food composition tables list the energy, macronutrient, and selected micronutrient content of selected foods. Mean values are derived from representative samples of each type of food and expressed in standard units of 100 g per food. Values are usually expressed in terms of the edible portion of the food although 'as purchased' values may be given. The contents are arranged by food groups: cereals and cereal products, dairy products, eggs, meat and meat products, etc. Foods are given an individual code. Supplements are available for specific foods, e.g. fish, fats, and oils.

Food composition tables are used to analyse the foods and diets of individuals and groups; the values obtained are often then compared with DRVs. Other uses of food composition tables include:
• the planning and assessment of food supplies, e.g. during famines or war;
• designing institutional and therapeutic diets, e.g. in schools or hospitals;
• prescription of diets in clinical practice;
• modifying diets to ↑ or ↓ particular nutrients;
• health promotion and teaching;
• nutrition labelling;
• food regulations and consumer protection;
• research on relationships between diet and disease.

Food composition tables are compiled by laboratory analyses of selected samples of foods and cooked recipe dishes. They may also be compiled from published results in the literature.

❶ Tables usually include an introduction explaining how they are compiled; it is important to read this section.

Calculation of energy values

The gross energies of foods are measured using a ballistic bomb calorimeter but the values used in the tables are the energy available for the body to metabolize—metabolizable energy. Metabolizable energy accounts for faecal and urinary losses. The difference between gross energy and metabolizable energy is about 5%. The direct measurement of metabolizable energy required human trials. Therefore, energy conversion factors, e.g., Atwater factors are used (see Table 1.2). These factors are derived from elaborate human studies.

[1] Food Standards Agency (2002). McCance and Widdowson's the composition of food, 6th summary edition. Royal Society of Chemistry, Cambridge.

Table 1.2 Energy conversion factors

Nutrient	kcal/g	kJ/g	Comments
Protein	4	17	
Fat	9	37	Original Atwater factor was 8.9 kcal, ∴ the lower kJ figure is preferable
Carbohydrate	3.75	16	Value is for available carbohydrate expressed as monosaccharides. If carbohydrate is expressed directly or by difference 4 kcal/g is used
Sugar alcohols	2.4	10	Mean value used in food labeling
Ethyl alcohol	7	29	
Glycerol	4.31	18	Assumes complete metabolism

Calculation of protein content

Most tables give protein and amino acid analyses. Protein content is usually derived from nitrogen content. It is assumed that on average protein is 16% nitrogen. Therefore the nitrogen content is multiplied by 6.25 (100/16) to derive protein content but there are limitations.
- The nitrogen content of food proteins varies.
- The nitrogen content varies with amino acid composition.
- Other food constituents contain nitrogen, e.g. purines, urea, pyrimidines, and dipeptides.

Calculation of fat content

Most tables give total fat and fatty acid analyses. Before determining the fat content of foods it is necessary to extract the fat with alcohol, which can be done by a variety of methods, e.g. Soxhlet extraction. Each method of extraction will vary in the extent to which different fats are extracted so introducing a possible error.

Calculation of carbohydrate content

Some tables report carbohydrate content by difference, i.e. carbohydrate = 100—amounts of protein, water, fat, and ash. This assumes that all carbohydrates have equal digestibility, which is not correct. Other tables sum measured values of total available carbohydrate (the sum of sugars and starches); this is usually reliable but the ↑ use of glucose and high fructose syrups may → overestimation of sucrose.

Dietary fibre is determined by one of two methods (Englyst and Southgate) and values from the methods should not be mixed. In the UK the Englyst method is used most widely and the 'fibre' content is described as 'non-starch polysaccharides' as this best describes biologically useful fibre.

Calculation of micronutrient content

There are many methods for measuring micronutrients and these have variable accuracy. Some micronutrients have a variety of forms that are biologically active, e.g. folate. No single assay gives total free folate activity in foods.

Limitations of food tables

Real variation in energy and nutrient content   All foods vary in energy and nutrient content because of many factors—variety or strain, sex and age of animals, agricultural processes, environmental factors, e.g. soil and climate, conditions and duration of storage, processing, and preparation. There is less variation in macronutrients than micronutrients with the exception of fat. The cut of meat will → a variation in fat content as will personal preference of the consumer.

Variation in water content   Water content is one of the most significant sources of variation in nutrients. Dry cereal grains have relatively little water but their content is variable and the amount of water absorbed in preparation is variable, e.g. cooked rice has a water content of between 65 and 80%.

Sampling errors   The sample analysed must be representative of the average composition of particular foods. This needs to take into account seasonal or regional variations. This is particularly true of processed foods where the recipe and process is variable. Different recipes will add another layer of inaccuracy. Recipes are often given in food composition tables or the recipe used should be calculated from raw ingredients.

Inappropriate methods   The choice of analytical method is important and should be reported. Some methods used for the determination of a nutrient may not be interchangeable, e.g. fibre.

Laboratory errors   Laboratories are standardized but errors may still occur.

Use of conversion factors   Conversion factors may introduce errors as described before.

Bioavailability   This is not an error but it is important to consider the bioavailability of specific nutrients.

Errors in coding and calculation   Calculation of the nutrient content of foods requires precise information on the amounts of food eaten. Often average portion sizes are used, which will introduce errors. Errors may also occur in the coding of foods and calculation of nutrient content.

Studies have compared values obtained directly and by using food tables and found that energy and protein values varied by 10–15% and that values for micronutrients varied by up to 50%. Provided the limitations of the use of food tables are understood they are invaluable tools for nutritionists and dietitians.

Food composition analysis programmes are now available that make the calculations less arduous, e.g. CompEat, Dietplan 6.

Digestion

Food is broken down by mechanical and chemical mechanisms in the gastrointestinal (GI) tract before nutrients can be absorbed into the body. The GI tract is a continuous tube from the mouth to the anus and is approximately 7 metres in length (Fig. 1.1). Food is transported through the lumen of the tract as it is digested.

The mouth and oesophagus

Food is chewed by teeth and mixed with saliva, which is produced by salivary glands (parotiod, submaxillary, and sublingual glands). Saliva contains the enzyme amylase, which starts the digestion of starch. The food is mixed with saliva, fluid, and mucus to form a bolus that is pushed into the pharynx by the tongue. The pharyngeal muscle contracts to swallow the bolus of food. The bolus is moved down the oesophagus into the stomach by peristalsis.

The stomach

The cardiac sphincter is found at the junction of the oesophagus and stomach and contracts to prevent food leaving the stomach and re-entering the oesophagus. The stomach is a muscular organ that further breaks down the bolus by mechanical, chemical, and enzymatic actions. Parietal glands in the stomach wall secrete hydrochloric acid, which helps break down the food, denatures protein, and converts the inactive pepsinogen into active pepsin. Pepsinogen is secreted by chief cells. Pepsin begins the breakdown of proteins. Renin and gastric lipase break down milk protein and fat respectively. Goblet cells secrete mucin, which protects the stomach from hydrochloric acid. The food is converted into chyme in the stomach, which then passes into the small intestine.

The small intestine

The pyloric sphincter is a circular muscle at the junction of the stomach and small intestine that controls the release of chyme into the small intestine. The small intestine consists of the duodenum, jejunum (approx. 20 ft in length), and the ileum. Chyme is transported along the small intestine by slow muscular contractions known as peristalsis. It can take up to 5 h to complete the movement through the small intestine; this slow transition aids absorption. The surface area of the small intestine is large to facilitate digestion and absorption. Villi and microvilli are finger-like projections lining the lumen. Enzymes lactase, maltase, and sucrase are secreted by the microvilli and complete carbohydrate digestion into monosaccharides. The villi have thin walls through which nutrients are absorbed into capillaries (carbohydrates and proteins) and lacteals (fat absorption) (Fig. 1.2). The lacteals connect with the lymphatic system. Proteins are further broken down in the small intestine into amino acids, which can be absorbed through the villi wall.

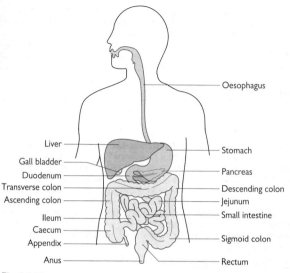

Fig. 1.1 The gastrointestinal tract.

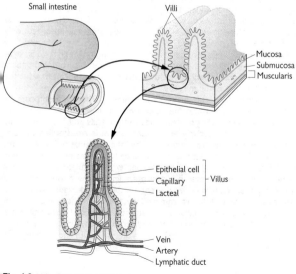

Fig. 1.2 Villi of the small intestine.

The pancreas secretes a mixture of enzymes that continue digestion; trypsinogen and carboxypeptidase break down proteins and polypeptides into amino acids and lipase breaks down fats into fatty acids. Bile is secreted by the liver and stored and concentrated by the gall bladder. Bile dilutes and buffers the chyme and emulsifies fat so enabling lipase to break it down. Water-soluble nutrients (amino acids, monosaccharides, and water-soluble micronutrients) and short and medium chain fatty acids are taken to the liver via the portal vein. Fat-soluble nutrients are transported in the lymphatic system and enter the blood system at the left subclavian vein.

The large intestine

The remaining chyme passes into the large intestine through the ileocaecal sphincter, a circular muscle that separates the small and large intestines. The large intestine consists of the caecum (and appendix), colon (ascending, transverse, descending, and sigmoid), rectum, and anus. <10 % digestion occurs in the large intestine. Water is reabsorbed to conserve water and to form faeces. Some vitamins including vitamin K and biotin are absorbed in the large intestine. Faeces consist of undigested food, particularly insoluble fibre, and is expelled from the rectum through the anus by powerful contractions. Defecation is controlled by the anal sphincter.

Fat digestion and absorption

Most dietary fat is in the form of triacylglycerides (triglycerides) and is digested by pancreatic lipase into non-esterified fatty acids and monoacylglycerides. Phospholipid digestion yields lysophosphoglyceride and a fatty acid. Cholesterol is hydrolysed before absorption. Triacylglyceride digestion is very efficient with 95% of fat being digested and absorbed; only 40% cholesterol is absorbed. The products of fat digestion pass into 'mixed micelles': large molecular aggregates of monoacylglycerides, large fatty acids, bile salts, and phospholipids. Cholesterol, carotenoids, tocopherols, and some undigested trigacylglycerides are taken into the hydrophobic core of the micelles.

Lipid absorption occurs mainly in the jejunum. The digestion products pass from the micelles into the enterocyte's membrane by passive diffusion. A fatty acid binding protein binds to fatty acids and they are rapidly re-esterified to monoaclyglycerides. Cholesterol is re esterified by acyl-CoA:cholesterol acyltransferase or by the reversal of cholesterol esterase. Cholesterol esterase is induced by high levels of dietary cholesterol. Fats are packaged into chylomicrons, which circulate and are mainly removed in adipose tissue by lipoprotein lipase. The chylomicrons are not completely consumed by the enzyme but are degraded to smaller particles, remnants that are removed by the liver. Short and medium chain fatty acids are directly absorbed into the portal vein. Lipids are synthesized in the liver and those delivered by chylomicron remnants are packaged into very low density lipoproteins (VLDL) and secreted into the blood.

Dietary reference values (DRVs) and food-based dietary guidelines

Dietary reference values (DRVs)

DRVs are established within a population as a measure of nutritional adequacy. The first DRVs were established in the late 19th century and international values were established by the League of Nations in 1936–1938 to prevent deficiencies in a population group. Many countries have their own values and international values have been published by FAO/WHO/UNU. DRVs for food, energy, and nutrients for the UK (report of the Panel on DRVs of the Committee on Medical Aspects of Food Policy (COMA) were last revised in 1991.[1] See OUP website for revisions since publication of this handbook (www.oup.com). Updates may be available from the Department of Health (www.dh.gov.uk) or the Food Standards Agency (www.food.gov.uk).

DRVs are based on the assumption that the individual requirements for a nutrient within a population or group are normally distributed and that 95% of the population will have requirements within 2 standard deviations of the mean as shown in Fig. 2.1. They assume that individuals are healthy and also consider gender, age, growth, and physiological status, i.e. pregnancy and lactation.

Limitations of DRVs

While DRVs can be useful, they can be misused and the inherent problems associated with making recommendations for the whole population should be appreciated.

- A standard distribution of nutrient requirements is assumed; the distribution may not be normal or insufficient data may be available to establish normality.
- Good data are required for the panel to evaluate requirements; these data may be derived from balance studies, tissue levels, pool size, etc., amount required to prevent symptoms of deficiency, or a measure of function of the nutrient. Such data are not always available and at times the panel has decided that the data are insufficient to set requirements and has ∴ recommended a 'safe level' of intake.

Factors affecting dietary requirements

- Metabolic requirement including:
  - age, gender, body size;
  - lifestyle (smoking, obesity, physical activity, etc.);
  - disease, e.g. fever, catabolism;
  - trauma;
  - growth.
- Bioavailability including:
  - altered absorption, e.g. milk Ca is better absorbed than non-milk Ca;
  - reduced utilization;

---

[1] Department of Health (1991). Dietary reference values for food and nutrients for the United Kingdom. HMSO, London.

- ↑ losses, e.g. diarrhoea, burns, renal disease;
- environment, e.g. heating of nutrients;
- drugs, e.g. diuretics;
- dietary concentration;
- dietary interactions;
- drug–nutrient interactions.

Uses of DRVs

- Dietary assessment of individuals, although it must be remembered that DRVs are based on populations and groups not individuals. Other factors may need to be considered.
- Dietary assessment of groups or populations; it is important that the population is comparable to that for which the recommendations are derived.
- Prescription of diets and provision of supplies, e.g. school meals.
- Food labelling.
- Food formulation.

Definitions

Dietary reference value (DRV)—a term used to cover LRNI, EAR, RNI, and safe intake.

Recommended daily amount (RDA)—'the average amount of the nutrient which should be provided per head in a group of people if needs of practically all members of the group are to be met'.*

Recommended Intakes—'the amounts sufficient, or more than sufficient, for the nutritional needs of practically all healthy persons in a population'.† 'Intake' emphasizes that the recommendations relate to food actually eaten.

Requirement—the amount of a nutrient that needs to be consumed in order to maintain normal nutritional status.

Estimated average requirement (EAR) (point y in Fig. 2.1)—is the mean requirement of a nutrient for a population or group of people. On average 50% will consume more than the EAR and 50% less.

Lower reference nutrient intake (LRNI) (point x in Fig. 2.1)—is the level at which only 2.5% of the population or group will have an adequate intake; it will not be enough for most people. An individual with this intake may be meeting his/her requirement but it is highly probable that he/she is not.

Reference nutrient intake (RNI) (point z in Fig. 2.1)—at this level intake will be adequate for 97.5% of the group or population. It is possible that an individual's intake will not meet his/her requirement at this level but is highly improbable. RNIs for micronutrients are given in Appendix 6 and as appropriate throughout the handbook.

Safe level   is given when insufficient information is available to derive requirements. It is an average requirement plus 20% and is believed to be adequate for most people's needs. The panel judges that there was no risk of deficiency at this level and that there is no risk of undesirable effects above this level.

* Department of Health and Social Security (1979). *Recommended daily amounts of food, energy and nutrients for groups of people in the United Kingdom*. Reports on health and social subjects no.15. HMSO, London.
† Department of Health and Social Security (1969). *Recommended daily amounts of nutrients for the United Kingdom*, Reports on health and social subjects no. 120. HMSO, London.

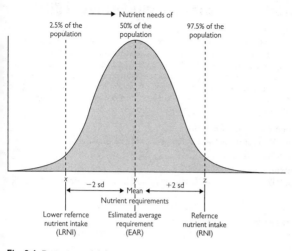

Fig. 2.1 Derivation and definition of dietary reference values.
(Modified with permission from Department of Health (1991). *Dietary reference values for food and nutrients for the United Kingdom*, London: Her Majesty's Stationary Office. Reprinted with Permission.)

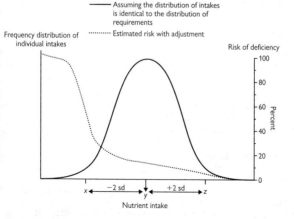

Fig. 2.2 Dietary intakes and risk of deficiency.
(Modified with permission from Department of Health (1991). *Dietary reference values for food and nutrients for the United Kingdom*, London: Her Majesty's Stationary Office. Reprinted with Permission.)

Food-based dietary guidelines (FBDG)

Historically, dietary guidelines were nutrient-based; FBDG were developed to facilitate the teaching of 'healthy eating' and nutrition to population groups. FBDG focus on foods, rather than nutrients, and are intended for use by the general public. They are designed to be understandable to most consumers. FBDG give practical information on 'healthy eating' and intakes of nutrients to meet DRVs of macro- and micronutrients (see Appendix 6). FBDG are designed to be appropriate to each population group; they may be country, age, or culturally specific.

Development of FBDG

The FAO report on the development of FBDG is available on the website (www.fao.org).

Key concepts

The following points should be considered in the development of FBDG.

Dietary patterns
- Total diet rather than nutrients.
- Reflect food patterns rather than numeric nutrient goals.
- Various dietary patterns can be compatible with health.

Practical considerations
- Food should be affordable, widely available, and accessible.
- FBDG should recognize social, environmental, and agricultural conditions affecting foods and eating patterns.
- They should be flexible such that they can be used by people with different lifestyles, ages, and physiological conditions, e.g. pregnancy.

Comprehensible
- Easily understood.
- Food groups should make sense.
- Visual representations.
- Testing is essential before dissemination.

Culturally acceptable
- Foods and colours should be culturally appropriate.
- Sensitive to cultural and religious considerations.
- Avoid racial changes in current practice.
- Use appropriate dialect or language.
- Positive and encourage enjoyment.

Underlying assumptions
- Foods are more than nutrients—food has cultural, social, ethnic, and family messages.
- Biological functions may not be fully elucidate. Foods may be more beneficial than nutrients alone.
- Combinations of nutrients in foods can have different metabolic effects.
- Food processing and preparation influence nutritional values.

- Specific dietary patterns can be associated with reduced risk of specific diseases.
- Science-based disciplines including:
  - nutrition;
  - food science;
  - behaviour;
  - communication;
  - agriculture.

Nutrition concepts
These concepts are generic and recommended by FAO. Country-specific concepts are developed.
❶ These concepts may be different to DRVs recommended for UK.
- Energy
  - Aims to prevent excess or deficiency.
  - Promotes appropriate energy intakes by encouraging appropriate food choices.
  - Physical activity is also encouraged.
- Protein
  - High quality protein: 8–10% total energy.
  - Vegetable-based mixed diet: 10–12% of total energy.
  - Elderly where energy intake low: 12–14% total energy.
- Fat
  - At least 15% energy from fats and oils.
  - Childbearing age women at least 20% to ensure adequate essential fatty acids.
  - Active non-obese <35% total energy (saturated fatty acids (SFA) <10%).
  - Sedentary <30% total energy.
  - SFA <10% total fat.
- Carbohydrate
  - Main energy source >50%.
  - Complex carbohydrate foods need to be cooked to be fully digestible.
  - Sugar usually ↑ acceptability and energy density. Inversely related to fat intake. Moderate intakes compatible with a varied nutritious diet. No specific limit to sugar consumption but usually <10% total energy. UK government recommends that no more than 10% of total energy should come from non-milk extrinsic sugars.
- Micronutrients
  - Compounds with different metabolic activities.
  - Essential for normal growth, development, and health.
  - Important in preventing infectious and chronic diseases.

Balance of good health

'The Balance of Good Health' (FSA) or plate model is the pictorial representation of FBDG in UK (Fig. 2.3). It is applicable to most people including minority ethnic groups, vegetarians, and people of all ages except children under 2 years. Between the ages of 2 and 5 years, children should make a gradual transition to family foods.

The 'Balance of Good Health' is based on 5 food groups.

1 Bread, other cereals, and potatoes.
2 Fruit and vegetables.
3 Meat, fish, and alternatives.
4 Milk and dairy foods.
5 Foods containing fat/foods containing sugar.

The FSA tips for healthy eating are as follows.
- Base your meals on starchy foods.
- Eat lots of fruit and vegetables.
- Eat more fish, include one portion of oily fish.
- Cut down on saturated fat and sugar.
- Try to eat less salt—no more than 6 g a day.
- Get active and try to be a healthy weight.
- Drink plenty of water.
- Don't skip breakfast.

A healthy diet should include:
- Meals based on starchy foods, such as bread, pasta, rice and potatoes—including high fibre varieties where possible.
- Plenty of fruit and vegetables—atleast 5 portions of a variety a day.
- Moderate amounts of milk and dairy products—choose low-fat options where possible.
- Moderate amounts of foods that are good sources of protien such as meat, fish, eggs, beans and lentils.
- Low amounts of foods that contain large amounts of fat or sugar.

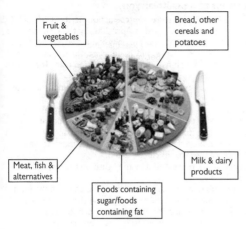

Fig. 2.3 The 'Balance of good health' plate model
(Reproduced with kind permission of the Food Standards Agency, UK.)

MyPyramid (steps to a healthier you)

MyPyramid (Fig. 2.4) is the pictorial representation of the USA FBDG (www.mypyramid.gov). It was released in April 2005 by the United States Department of Agriculture. It incorporates physical activity as an important part of good nutrition. Mypyramid is designed to be personalized and it is accompanied by a web-based personal nutrition plan. The design encompasses the following principles.

- **Activity**. The steps represent activity and the figure the importance of daily activity.
- **Moderation**. The bands represent moderation by narrowing as they reach the top. Foods with little or no fat and sugar are wider at the base and should be selected more frequently. Narrow bands represent foods with more fats and added sugars; the more active you are the more of these foods can be eaten.
- **Personalization**. This is represented by the figure on the steps, the slogan, and on the website.
- **Proportionality**. This is shown by the widths of the bands of the food groups. They are a guide as to how much a person should include in their diet. They are a general guide and not exact proportions.
- **Variety**. This is symbolized by the 6 bands that represent 5 food groups and oils. This shows that foods from each band are needed each day.
- **Gradual improvement**. This is shown by the slogan 'Steps to a healthier you'. Individuals are encouraged to take small steps each day to improve their diet and lifestyle.

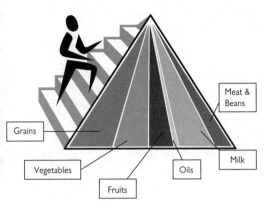

Fig. 2.4 MyPyramid food-based dietary guidance for USA (USDA center for nutrition policy and promotion).

Current dietary patterns in the UK

Current dietary patterns

Information on current dietary patterns in the UK is taken from the National Diet and Nutrition Survey (NDNS): adults aged 19 to 64 years. The survey was conducted between July 2000 and June 2001.

❶ Previous adult NDNS surveys have included 16–19 year old. ∴ be cautious when making comparisons.

Fruit and vegetable consumption

- The mean fruit and vegetable consumption (including composite foods) was 2.8 portions/d with women consuming slightly more than men (2.9 portions/day for women and 2.7 portions/d for men).
- Only 14% of adults eat the recommended intake of 5 portions/day.
- People in the age group 50–64 y consumed nearly 4 portions/d, with people in the younger age groups consuming decreasingly less with age.
- Households receiving state benefit consumed on average 1 less portion of fruit and vegetables/d.

Vegetarianism/veganism

- 5% reported being vegetarian or vegan; men were less likely to report being vegetarian or vegan—2% compared with 7% of women.
- It was particularly popular in women aged 10 to 34 years.
- All avoided red meat, 92% avoid white meat, 29% avoided all animal products.

Supplement usage and dieting for weight loss

- 35% reported taking supplements with more women (40%) than men (29%) taking them. In the 1986/87 adult survey 17% women and 9% men reported taking supplements.
- 10% men reported dieting to lose weight compared with 24% women.

Macronutrient and energy intakes (see Table 3.1)

- The mean daily energy intake was below EAR s for each sex and age group.
- Average protein intakes for all age and sex groups were above the RNI.
- The mean percentage energy derived from NMES was above DRV for all age and sex groups except women aged 50–64 y.
- The mean daily intake of NSP was below the recommended average intake of 18 g/d for all sex and age groups.
- The mean daily fat intake was 35%, the recommended intake.
- The mean energy derived from saturated fat was 13.3% which is above the recommended level of 11%.

Table 3.1 Average intake of macronutrients and energy* (2000/2001) compared with DRVs (NDNS)[†]

Energy/nutrient	Men	Women
Total energy intake		
(MJ)	9.72	6.87
(kcal)	2313	1632
%EAR	92%	85%
Protein (g)	88.2	63.7
% RNI	161%	140%
Total carbohydrate (g)	275	203
% food energy	47.7%	48.5%
NMES (g)	79	51
% food energy	13.6%	11.9%
NSP (g)	15.2	12.6
% intakes <18 g	72%	87%
Total fat (g)	86.5	61.4
% food energy	35.8%	34.9%
Saturated fatty acids (g)	32.5	23.3
% food energy	13.4%	13.2%

Abbreviations: EAR, estimated average requirement; RNI, recommended nutrient intake; NMES, Non-milk extrinsic sugars; NSP, Non-starch polysaccharides.
* Energy intake includes energy from alcohol.
[†] Source: Henderson, L., Gregory, J., and Irving, K. (2003). *The National Diet and Nutrition Survey: adults aged 19 to 64 years*. Vol. 2, *Energy, protein, carbohydrate, fat and alcohol intakes.* HMSO, London.

Alcohol consumption

- Men are more likely to consume alcohol than women in each age group.
- 38% men and 24% women exceeded the recommend maximum intakes of 4 units/d for men and 3 units/d for women.
- 20% men and 9% women drank heavily; >8 units/d for men and >6 units/day for women.
- Women aged 19–24 y drank more heavily than older women.
- Men aged 35–49 y drank the most heavily.

Vitamin and mineral intakes

- Both men and women aged 19–24 y had the lowest mineral and vitamin intakes.
- Mean intakes for all vitamins were close to RNI, except vitamin A in 19–24 y age group.
- Intakes of minerals were below the RNI for K and Mg in men aged 19–24 y.
- Mean intakes for all ages of women were below RNI for Mg, potassium, and Cu.
- Mean intake of Fe was below the RNI for all age groups of women except 50–64 y.
- Supplements ↑intake of vitamin A and Fe but intakes were still below RNIs.

Nutrition assessment

This chapter will consider nutrition assessment of the individual and dietary assessment of populations and groups.

Dietary assessment

Dietary assessment is an imprecise procedure; the imprecision can be minimized by using the appropriate technique and by an understanding of the errors implicit in the methodology. Dietary assessment is further hampered by the fact that in assessing diet it will change. Dietary assessment precision varies from very precise techniques such as metabolic balance studies to the broad estimates of population studies. The methodology chosen must be appropriate for the nutrient/s that are being assessed and for the individual or population being assessed. The timing of the assessment is also important and must consider cultural variations such as differences in the week (week day vs weekend day), seasons (wet vs dry season), and special occasions, e.g. Ramadan, Christmas.

This section gives a brief description of the methods used to assess diet; fuller descriptions and methods of assessing validity are described by Margetts and Nelson (1997).[1]

Country level assessment

Information is available on a national level on food production and agriculture; but this does not consider imports and exports. Food balance sheets (FBS), per country, are published annually by FAO (www.fao.org/es/ess/wfs.asp) and estimate a country's food supply (Table 4.1). Data are collated on domestic food production, food imports, and food taken from storage. Food per capita data can be derived as shown below and this can also be converted into nutrient values.

Per capita supply = total production + imports
+ adjustment for storage levels
− exports − animal use − seeds
− losses (storage, transport, and processing)

The information can be used to study the links between diet and disease and can aid the development of FBDG but the FBS only give information on availability not consumption. They give an estimate for the country as a whole and show no patterns of variation within the country.

[1] Margetts, B.M. and Nelson, M. (1997). *Concepts in nutritional epidemiology*, 2nd edn. Oxford University Press, Oxford.

Food balance sheets (FAO methodology)

Strengths
- Information available in 157 countries
- Data routinely collected in the countries
- Does not entail implementation of special surveys
- Assesses long-term trends
- Provides global information on undernourishment
- Provides information comparable across countries
- Is timely: estimates produced rapidly

Weaknesses
- Does not measure actual energy intake or utilization
- Inaccuracy of country food balance data
- In some countries estimates not consistent with socio-economic indicators
- In poor countries, underestimates actual energy needs
- Data on equality of food distribution not available
- No disaggregation at subnational level

Household–based surveys

Examples of this type of survey are conducted on a regular basis by the FSA in the UK (National Diet and Nutrition Survey (NDNS)) and dietary surveys that are part of the National Health and Nutrition Examination Surveys (NHNES). NHNES is conducted by the Center for Disease Control and Prevention (CDC), USA (www.cdc.gov). The limitations and strengths of each method are shown in Table 4.1.

Food account

The main respondent (often a housewife) notes all food that is purchased and all food grown or received as gifts. It assumes no change in stocks. Foods taken out of the household may be recorded. Waste is assumed to be between 5 and 10%. Records are usually kept for 1–2 weeks which may not reflect the full dietary cycle of the household. The degree of disaggregation of food codes affects the precision of the study, e.g. in Italy food is grouped into 46 groups which is less precise than in the Netherlands which uses 500 food groups for national surveys.

Inventory

This is similar to a food account with the addition of a larder inventory at the start and finish of the survey period. Over short periods the survey may be distorted as attention is drawn to larder items that would not normally be consumed.

Household record

Foods are weighed or estimated using household measures with an allowance for waste. An interviewer visits after breakfast and foods consumed at breakfast are recalled. Food for further meals is weighed or estimated. An afternoon or evening visit may be made to establish waste. This method is most useful in developing countries when most food is home produced and levels of literacy are low.

List recall

This survey is based on the recall of foods consumed in a household over a set period, usually 1 week. It does not estimate individual consumption.

Table 4.1 Strengths and limitations of household survey data*

Method	Strengths	Limitations
Food account	1. Cheap: data collected by government and readily available for analysis	i. Home foods only unless family members collect data.
	2. Representative: national sample	ii. Incomplete; may not include sweets, alcohol, soft drinks
	3. Possible subgroup analysis—by region, income, etc.	iii. No individual data
	4. Provides information on food consumption patterns	iv. Based on food composition tables see 'Food composition tables', Chapter 1
		v. No knowledge of change in food stocks
		vi. Bias of overpurchasing especially in elderly or low income households
Inventory	1–3 plus:	i–iv plus:
	5. Considers changes in larder stocks	v. Larder inventory may distort usual purchasing patterns
	6. Measures actual home food consumption	
Household record	3, 5, and 6 plus:	i, iii, and iv plus:
	7. Used in societies with low levels of literacy	vi. Observer presence may distort normal patterns
	8. Can be modified to measure individual consumption	vii. Seasonal variation in food availability may limit comparisons between groups
List-recall	1–3, and 6 plus:	i–iv plus:
	9. Based on single interview	viii. Memory errors
	10. Measures food use	ix. Observer presence may bias responses
	11. Retrospective; reflects actual patterns	

* Reproduced from *Human Nutrition and Dietetics*. Garrow JS, James WPT and Ralph A, table 17.1, p135. With permission from Elsevier.

Individual assessment

The assessment of an individual's diet is susceptible to many possible errors; these include under- or overreporting by subjects, recall difficulties, measurement errors, coding and calculation errors. Estimation of portion sizes may also introduce inaccuracies. Assessment may be prospective or retrospective; the strengths and limitations of each method are summarized in tables 4.2 and 4.3.

Duplicate diet

Subjects weigh and record their food at the time of consumption and a duplicate of the diet is weighed and stored for direct chemical analysis; this method does not require the use of food composition tables. This method is usually used in metabolic units so the onus of weighing, etc. is not on the subject. Aliquot sampling and equivalent composite are both duplicate diet methods. In aliquot sampling a sample, usually 10%, is taken rather than an exact duplicate. This is less wasteful but introduces possible sampling errors. In equivalent composite assessment an investigator prepares a duplicate diet from the list of ingredients used by the subjects.

Weighed inventory

This method is widely used: subjects weigh and record all food prepared and waste. The major advantage of this method is that it does not rely on assumptions of portion size. Food composition tables are used to estimate nutrient intake from the records.

Household measures

This method is similar to weighed inventory except that food portions are estimated. Photographs or household measures, e.g. spoons and cups, may be used to aid portion size estimation. This method requires less effort by the subject than the weighed inventory but is prone to more error.

24 hour recall

A trained interviewer guides the subject through food intake in the previous 24 hours. It is a quick method of dietary assessment but cannot be used to classify a subject's usual intake as it is not necessarily representative of the subject's normal eating pattern.

Diet history

A diet history is an extension of a 24 hour recall and gives more detailed information about the usual diet; it can typically take 2 hours. The reliability of the results is very dependent on the skills of the interviewer.

Steps and tips on choosing a dietary assessment method

Steps and tips on choosing a dietary assessment method

STEP 1 Defining the objective
The method is determined by the reason for the assessment—is it part of a research study or to clarify an individual 's deficiency?

⇓

STEP 2 Foods and/or nutrients?
Are data needed at the nutrient level or will a description of food patterns suffice?

⇓

STEP 3 Decide the conceptual timeframe of dietary intake
Past, present, usual?
Will a retrospective or prospective method be most applicable?

⇓

STEP 4 Decide the actual timeframe of dietary survey
Day, week, or year?
Number of interviews (e.g. multiple 24 hr recalls),
Consecutive days? Weekdays and/or weekends?
Account for seasonality?

⇓

STEP 5 Who will be interviewed and by whom?
e.g. children (interview parent or the child directly?)
Who will conduct the dietary assessment? Do they need training?
Who will record the information? (Interviewer or interviewee?)

⇓

STEP 6 What type of foods and drink need to be assessed?
If all, then a prescribed method like a FFQ may be inappropriate.
Is information needed on whether foods are raw or cooked and the cooking methods used?

⇓

STEP 7 Estimating how much is eaten and/or how often
Is frequency of intake enough to meet the objectives?
If the aim is to estimate nutrient intake then quantities will be needed. What method is best adapted to the context?

- Direct quantification: weigh, measure volume
- Indirect quantification: household measures, estimated with utensils and food containers
- Standard food portions
- Actual dimensions of the food
- Food models (2 or 3 dimensional)
- Photos of foods with a range of portion sizes
- A count of handfuls, e.g. with a shared dish
- Proportion of the prepared meal that was consumed, e.g. household intake

⇓

STEP 8 Comparing intake with recommendations
If data includes nutrient analysis: are all foods available in food composition tables? Which dietary analysis programme should be used? Dietary patterns could be explored or diet scores created to compare with FBDGs.

Food frequency (FFQ)

Printed questionnaires are used and subjects (or interviewer) tick the category that approximates to their usual consumption of a list of foods, i.e. never eaten, eaten once a month, eaten once a fortnight, number of times eaten per week. This is quantified and intake is estimated. FFQ can be interviewer led or self-administered (they can be conducted via post). The number of foods can vary from a few when assessing a food group or nutrient, e.g. fruit, and are sometimes called screeners. FFQ are often used in large surveys. It is necessary to validate FFQ against a more precise method such as weighed food intake. There are 3 main types of FFQ:

- Qualitative—no portion size;
- Semi-qualitative—standard portion size is used;
- Quantitative—subjects are asked to record data on portion size.

Table 4.2 Strengths and limitations of prospective measurements of individual food consumption*

Measurement	Strengths	Limitations
General features	Current diet	Labour–intensive
	Direct observation of what is eaten	Requires numeracy and literacy skills
	Duration may be varied to meet requirements of estimates of food consumption or nutrient intake	Subjects need to be well motivated
		Usual consumption may change due to:
		• inconvenience of recording • choice of foods that are easy to record • beliefs of which foods are healthy or unhealthy
		Overweight subjects tend to underreport
		Coding and data entry errors are common
Duplicate diet	Direct analysis of nutrients (not dependent on food composition tables)	Very expensive
	Required for metabolic balance studies	Intense supervision required
		May not be usual diet
Weighed inventory	Widely used ∴ able to compare studies	Food composition tables are used
	Precision of portion sizes	
Household measures	No scales needed	Loss of precision compared with weighed inventory

* Reproduced from *Human Nutrition and Dietetics*. Garrow JS, James WPT and Ralph A, table 17.1, p135. With permission from Elsevier.

Table 4.3 Strengths and limitations of retrospective measurements of individual food consumption*

Measurement	Strengths	Limitations
General features	Inexpensive	Biases caused by: • errors in memory, conceptualization of food portion sizes, perception • presence of observer
	Quick	Daily variation not usually assessed
	Lower respondent burden	Dependent on regular eating habits
	Can assess current or past diet	Food composition tables used to estimate nutrients
Diet history	Assesses usual diet	Over-reporting of foods believed to be healthy
24 hour recall	Very quick	Prone to underestimate consumption due to omissions
	Can be repeated to gain measure of daily variation and improve precision	Single observation provides poor measure of individual intake
Food frequency questionnaires	Suitable for large-scale surveys	Requires validation in relation to reference measure
	Can be posted	Literacy and numeracy skills required if self-completed
	Short versions (or screeners) can focus on specific foods, e.g. fruit and vegetables	

* Adapted from Table 17.2, p.137 of Garrow, J.S., James, W.P.T., and Ralph, A. (2000). *Human nutrition and dietetics*, 10th edn. Churchill Livingstone, Edinburg.

Physical assessment

Observation of an individual may offer a gross assessment of nutritional status (see 'Nutritional Screening', Chapter 16).

- *Physical appearance*, e.g. pallor, emaciation, and hair changes may be indicative of long-term energy deficit; loose dentures and loose clothing may indicate recent weight loss; xanthoma or corneal arcus in some types of hyperlipidaemia; nail and teeth changes that occur in bulimia nervosa.
- *Oedema* may be present following protein depletion.
- *Pressure sores or poor wound healing* may be the result of immune response abnormalities or undernutrition.
- *Breathlessness* may be the result of anaemia.
- *Mobility* may be reduced following a ↓ in muscle mass due to immobilization which may present difficulties in food purchasing and preparation.
- *Mood*, e.g. apathy and depression, may be present in patients with eating disorders and other causes of undernutrition.

Biochemical and haematological assessment

Various parameters of nutritional status can be measured by analysis of serum, plasma, whole blood, urine, and faeces. Some measures are dynamic and reflect very recent changes and do not reflect long-term nutritional status. See sections on specific nutrients in Chapter 5 and 'Nutritional Screening' in chapter 16.

- *Vitamin and mineral status* may be assessed by circulating levels although deficiency of some micronutrients must be prolonged before blood levels are affected. For other micronutrients the body is very finely balanced and a dietary deficiency is balanced by ↑ mobilization from tissues, e.g. phosphate, or ↓ excretion.
- *Protein status* may be reflected by serum proteins such as albumin, although levels do not truly reflect changes in protein status; levels are affected by other factors, e.g. infection, CRP levels. Serum transferrin and rapid turnover proteins, e.g. thyroxine, are reasonable markers of protein status but are also affected by metabolic stress and may not be very specific.

Body composition

Body composition is used to establish nutritional status especially when measuring adiposity. A limited number of cadavers have been analysed to establish the true composition of the human body. The cadavers analysed varied in ethnicity, age, gender, and cause of death. While the unsystematic selection of cadavers may be criticized, the enormity of the task coupled with ethical considerations and the difficulty and distastefulness of the procedure makes the analysis remarkable. The data from these analyses have formed the basis for the establishment of modern indirect measures of body composition.

Theoretical models

Theoretical models are used to derive reference data for the development of indirect methods, e.g. anthropometry. The body is divided into compartments; the classic 2 compartment model divides the body into fat mass (FM) and fat–free mass (FFM). Fat mass consists of all extractable lipids and the remainder is FFM. Cadaver analysis was used to derive properties of FM and FFM.
- Density of FM = 0.901 g/ml.
- Density of FFM = 1.10 g/ml.
- Densities of FM and FFM are constant within and between individuals.
- FFM is assumed to be 73.8% water, 19.4% protein, and 6.8% mineral.
  The 3 compartment model estimates FM + total body water (TBW) + 'dry' FFM (protein and mineral).
  The 4 compartment model consists of FM + TBW + protein + mineral. The method used to derive each compartment will vary with more sophisticated methods being needed to differentiate between compartments. Table 4.4 summarizes the methods available.

Direct methods

Until the development of *in vivo* neutron activation analysis (IVNAA) the only direct method of body composition analysis was cadaver analysis. In IVNAA the body is bombarded with fast neutrons of known energy levels. Neutrons are captured by chemicals in the body and the resulting higher energy is emitted as gamma rays. This method can be used to measure many elements including Ca, P, N, O_2, K, and Cl. IVNAA is expensive and the body is irradiated. ∴ there are ethical problems with its use especially in children.

Indirect methods

Densitometry

This method is based on the 2 compartment model but it can also be used for 3 and 4 compartment analysis. By measuring the subject in air and under water it is possible to determine volume and ∴ body density. The densities of FM and FFM are assumed (see above) and it is possible

Table 4.4 Summary of methods for the determination of body composition*

Method	Accuracy	Cost	Radiation	Time	Convenience for subject
Cadaver analysis	+++	–		–	
IVNAA	+++	–	–	++	++
Densitometry	++	+		++	+/–
Dilution	++	+/–	(–)	+	++
TBK	++	–		++	++
DEXA	+++	+/–	–	++	++
CT scanning	++	–	–	++	++
MRI scanning	++	–		++	+
Anthropometry	+	+++		++	+
Infrared interactance	+	++		++	++
BIA	+	+		+++	+++
TOBEC	+	–		++	++
Urinary metabolites	+	+		–	–

+++, Excellent; ++, very good; +, good; +/– reasonable; – bad;
IVNAA, *In vivo* neutron activation analysis; TBK, total body potassium; DEXA, dual energy X–ray absorptiometry; CT, computer assisted tomography; MRI, magnetic resonance imaging; BIA, bioelectrical impedance analysis; TOBEC, total body electrical conductivity.
1 Reproduced from Gibney, MJ, Vorster HH, Kok FJ (2002). *Introduction to Human Nutrition*. 1e. table 2.7, P.27. Permission requested from Blackwell Publishing.

to derive the % body fat by substitution into appropriate equations, e.g. the Siri formula.

Siri formula: % Body fat = (495/body density) − 450.

Traditionally body volume was measured by water displacement. This requires the subject to be totally submerged and requires an estimate of lung volume to be made.

Recently, air displacement plethsymography equipment has become commercially available (BodPod). Subjects sit in an enclosed chamber and air volume displaced by the subject is compared to the volume of air in a reference chamber. This system has the advantage of not requiring under water submersion.

Bioelectrical impedance analysis (BIA)

BIA has become a popular method of measuring hydration and body fat as it is easy to use. A small electric current is passed through the body and the voltage drop is measured by electrodes. The electrodes may be placed on hands and feet or the subject may stand on electrodes. The drop in voltage reflects the body's impedance or resistance. Resistance will be greater in individuals with greater body fat and lower in individuals with more FFM and total body water (TBW). Prediction equations are used to derive TBW and FFM from resistance and subject information, e.g. age, weight, height, and gender. BIA is quick and requires little training and the equipment is becoming relatively cheap. The system can be perturbed by factors such as time since last meal and will be affected by hydration. Segmental and multifrequency models are now available.

Dilution techniques

TBW is assumed to be constant at 73.8% and measurement of the dilution of a tracer in TBW gives an estimate of TBW. Suitable tracers are deuterium, tritium, and ^{18}O-labelled water. A sample of blood, urine or saliva is collected at baseline and after an equilibration period of 3 h.

Total body potassium (TBK)

TBK is constant and is present only in FFM. A known proportion of naturally occurring potassium occurs as the isotope ^{40}K which is radioactive. By measuring this radiation it is possible to estimate TBK and then derive FFM. The subject is required to lie in a whole body counter for 20–30 minutes. Whole body counters are rarely available.

Dual-energy X-ray absorptiometry (DEXA)

The body is scanned with X-rays of 2 energy levels and the chemical composition of tissues will determine the attenuation of the radiation.

Software calculates bone mineral content, bone mineral density, and FM.

Imaging techniques

CT and MRI scanning can be used to determine body composition but are expensive and CT scanning exposes the subject to radiation. They are useful for segmental analysis.

Urinary metabolites

FFM can be estimated from 24 h measurements of nitrogen, creatinine, and N-methyl-histidine. All require 24 h urine collections which are often incomplete and creatinine and N-methyl-histidine. Excretion is variable and requires the subject to be on a meat-free diet. Nitrogen balance is an accurate measure of FFM but requires accurate collection of urine and determination of urinary and faecal nitrogen. This technique is rarely used outside metabolic units.

Other methods

Total body electrical conductivity can also be used to measure body composition although it is rarely used in humans. Infrared interactance has been used but there are questions about its validity.

Anthropometry

Anthropometry simply means the measurement of man and involves the measurement of height, weight, skin fold thicknesses, circumferences and various lengths and breadths of the body. These techniques require relatively cheap equipment and minimal training and are ∴ widely used in clinical practice. The techniques for some anthropometric measurements are shown in Table 4.5.

Children (see the 'Growth reference charts' in 'Infant growth and development', Chapter 10)

For most clinical purposes, the UK90 reference is the only suitable growth chart and it is used from birth for measuring weight, length (<2y)/height(>2y), head circumference (<2y), and BMI (weight relative to height) in the UK. These reference data have been incorporated into the Child Growth Foundation's 9-centile growth charts that have been endorsed by the DH and RCPCH. They are included in the UK Personal Child Health Record (PCHR) issued to each newborn (see Appendix 2). BMI percentile chart should be used to identify obesity and the UK 1990 chart is recommended for routine clinical diagnosis of growth faltering. The cut offs are extrapolated from adult cut offs. Overweight is classified as ≥91st centile and obesity ≥98th centile of the UK 1990 data. Epidemiological studies use an internationally acceptable definition to classify prevalence of child overweight and obesity.[1]

Z-score

Anthropometric measurements can be expressed as Z-scores. A Z-score is the standard deviation (sd) score; the deviation of the value for an individual from the median value of the reference population divided by the sd for the reference population:

Z-score = (observed value − median reference value)/sd reference population

---

[1] Cole, T.J., Bellizzi, M.C., Flegal, K.M., and Dietz, W.H. (2000). Establishing a standard definition for child overweight and obesity worldwide: international survey, *Br. Med. J.* **320**, 1240–3.

Table 4.5 Standardized anthropometric measurements*

Circumferences

Site	Anatomical reference	Measurement
Waist	Narrowest part of torso	Apply tape snugly around waist. Take measure at end of natural expiration
Hip (buttocks)	Maximum posterior extension of buttocks	Apply tape snugly around buttocks
MAC (biceps)	Midpoint between acromion process of scapula and olecranon process of ulna	Arms hanging freely with palms facing thighs

Skinfold measurements

Site	Direction of fold	Anatomical reference	Measurement
Subscapular	Diagonal	Inferior angle of subscapular	Fold is natural cleavage line just inferior to interior angle of scapula with caliper applied 1 cm below
Suprailiac	Oblique	Iliac crest	Fold is grasped behind to midaxillary line and above iliac crest
Triceps	Vertical	As circumference above	Midpoint is measured and fold is 1 cm above line on posterior aspect of arm
Biceps	Vertical	Biceps brachii	Fold is lifted over the belly of biceps at line marked for triceps; caliper is applied 1 cm below fingers

* Adapted from VH Heyward and LM Stolarczyk, *Applied Body Composition Assessment*, table 2.1 (p28–29) and S.1 (p71–74). (Copyright 1996, Human Kinetics) Permission requested from Dr Timothy Lohman.

Adults
Weight
Body weight is a crude measure of body composition; scales require regular calibration and servicing and weight may vary between scales. Monitoring of weight over a period can be a useful indicator of nutritional status.

Height
- A stadiometer is used or the subject is measured against a wall. The floor should be uncarpeted.
- The subject should be barefoot and weight evenly distributed between both feet.
- Arms should be hung loosely.
- Heels are together touching the vertical board or stadiometer. Head, scapula, and buttocks should be touching the vertical board or wall.
- Head erect with eyes focused straight ahead
- Subject should inhale.
- The rod is lowered to the most superior point, compressing hair.

Surrogate measures of height
- Recall height may be used in bed-bound patients. This tends to over estimate height by ~2 cm but this does not effect BMI categorization.
- Ulna length can be measured by bending the left arm across the chest with the palm facing inwards and the fingers pointing to the shoulder. The measurement is taken between the central and post prominent parts of the styloid process and the tip of the olecranon (equations for the predicted height are shown in a box opposite).
- Knee height is measured in sitting subjects. The knee and ankle are bent to 90° and the observers hand is placed flat on the thigh. The tape measure is held between the fingers and the height measured to the floor. On the lateral plane of the leg, in the same plane as the lateral malleolus (prediction equations are given in a box opposite).
- Demispan can be measured in patients sitting in a chair or supine. The right arm is raised until it is horizontal with the wrist in natural flexion and rotation. The tape is placed between the middle and ring finger and runs smoothly along the arm. The measurement is taken from the tip of the finger to the centre of the sternal notch (prediction equations are shown in a box opposite).

Body mass index (Quetelet's index)
BMI reflects body fat stores and is calculated as

$$BMI = weight (kg)/height (m)^2.$$

BMI is correlated to the risk of obesity and underweight-associated morbidity. Overweight subjects have an ↑ risk of associated health problems, this risk ↑ with ↑ BMI. The WHO cut-offs for the definition of overweight and obesity are given in Table 4.6.

BMI is a useful clinical tool and epidemiological tool. Appendix 2 gives BMI calculator. It should be used with caution in the elderly and in muscular subjects. Cut–off values for Asian populations are likely to be lower but this is still being debated by WHO and the International Obesity Task Force (www.iotf.org).

Circumferences

Waist circumference and waist–hip ratio have been proposed as measures of risk of obesity–associated morbidity. The WHO cut–offs for waist circumference are shown in Table 4.7.

Skinfold thickness measurements

Most of the body's fat is stored subcutaneously. The thickness of skinfolds at specific sites are measured (3 measurements are needed at each site) by calipers and can be used to estimate total subcutaneous fat. The most commonly used sites are subscapular, suprailiac, biceps, and triceps. Total skinfolds from these sites can be substituted into prediction equations to give an estimate of % FM. The most commonly used equations are those derived by Durnin and Wormesley (1974).[1] Equations that are appropriate for specific ages and ethnic groups are available. Skinfold measurements are cheap and quick but the technique requires training and skill.

Arm muscle measurement

Midarm circumference (MAC) can be measured as shown in Table 4.5. It is assumed that the arm is a cylinder of muscle covered by adipose tissue and that the double thickness of the fat layer is measured by triceps skin fold thickness (TSF). Midarm muscle circumference (MAMC) can be calculated:

MAMC (cm) = MAC – (3.14) × TSF (cm).

This estimate of FM and FFM is used clinically to monitor nutritional status. Appendix 2 gives reference values.

[1] Durnin, J.V.G.A, and Womersley, J. (1974). Body fat assessed from total body density and its estimation from skinfold thickness: measurements on 481 men and women aged from 16 to 72 years. B. J. *Nutri.* **32**, 77–97.

Equations for the prediction of height from ulna length

- Men (<65 y)   Predicted height (cm) = 79.2 + 3.60 ulna length (cm)
- Men (≥65 y)   Predicted height (cm) = 86.3 + 3.15 ulna length (cm)
- Women (<65 y)   Predicted height (cm) = 95.6 + 2.77 ulna length (cm)
- Women (≥65 y)   Predicted height (cm) = 80.4 + 3.25 ulna length (cm)
- ❶ Equations only validated for ulna length measured on the left side.

Equations for the prediction of height from knee height

- Men (18–60 y)   Predicted height (cm) = 71.85 + (1.88 × knee ht (cm))
- Men (60–90 y)   Predicted height (cm) = 59.01 + (2.08 × knee ht (cm))
- Women (18–60 y)   Predicted height (cm) = 67.85 + (1.87 × knee ht (cm))
- Women (60–90 y)   Predicted height (cm) = 62.25 + (1.91 × knee ht (cm))
- ❶ Equations only validated for knee height measured on the left side.

Equations for the prediction of height from demispan

- Men (16–54 y)   Predicted height (cm) = 68 + (1.3 × demispan (cm))
- Men (>55 y)   Predicted height (cm) = 71 + (1.2 × demispan (cm))
- Women (16–54 y)   Predicted height (cm) = 62 + (1.3 × demispan (cm))
- Women (>55 y)   Predicted height (cm) = 67 + (1.2 × demispan (cm))
- ❶ Equations only validated for demispan measured on the right side.

Table 4.6 WHO cut-offs for BMI

BMI	Weight status	Risk of co-morbidities
Below 18.5	Underweight	Low
18.5–24.9	Normal	Average
25.0–29.9	Overweight	Increased
30.0–39.9	Obese	Moderate–severe
Above 40	Very obese	Severe

Table 4.7 WHO waist circumference cut-offs and risk of associated metabolic complications

	Increased	Substantially increased
Men	≥ 94 cm	≥ 102 cm
Women	≥ 80 cm	≥ 88 cm

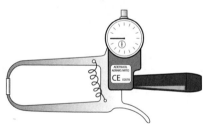

Fig. 4.1 Diagram of calipers.

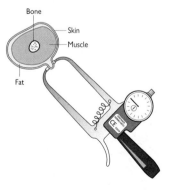

Fig. 4.2 Diagram of skinfold measurement.

Nutrients

Macronutrients: introduction

The macronutrients are protein, fat, and carbohydrate and they are required in gram amounts. They are major sources of energy as well as providing essential nutrients such as amino acids.

Protein

Protein provides approximately 10–15% of the energy in the diet. Protein is essential for numerous structural and functional purposes and is essential for growth and repair of the body. In adults approximately 16% of body weight is protein. 43% of this is muscle, 15% skin, and 16% blood. Protein is in a constant state of flux in the body with protein being synthesized and degraded continuously.

Protein flux (Q) can be described by the following equation:

$$Q = I + D + S + O$$

where I = intake, D = degradation, S = synthesis, and O = oxidation to CO_2 and urinary nitrogen.

Function

Protein has numerous functions in the body. Examples of the different functions of protein are as follows.

- **Structural.** Protein is important for the structure of the body and about half of the body's protein is in structural tissues such as skin and muscle. These structural proteins are collagen (25% of the body's protein), actin, and myosin.
- **Transport.** Proteins act as transport carriers in the blood and body fluids for many molecules and nutrients, e.g. haemoglobin, lipoproteins.
- **Hormonal.** Hormones and peptides are proteins or amino acid chains, e.g. insulin, pancreatic polypeptide.
- **Enzymes.** All enzymes are proteins. Extracellular enzymic proteins include the digestive enzymes, e.g. amylase. Intracellular enzymes are involved in metabolic pathways, e.g. glycogen synthestase.
- **Immune function.** Antibodies are protein molecules. Proteins are also involved in the acute phase response to inflammation.
- **Buffering function.** The protein albumin acts as a buffer in the maintenance of blood pH.

Structure

Proteins are macromolecules consisting of amino acid chains. Amino acids are joined to each by peptide bonds (Fig. 5.1). Amino acids form peptide chains of various lengths from two amino acids (dipeptide), 4–10 peptides (oligopeptides) and more than 10 amino acids (polypeptides). Reactive side groups of the amino acids combine to form links between amino acids in the chain and other peptide chains. The polypeptides form β pleated sheets or α helices. Polypeptides fold and cross-links form between amino acids to stabilize the folds. Proteins are formed by the combination of polypeptides. These cross-links give the peptide a distinctive function and shape (Fig. 5.2). There are approximately 20 amino acids and each has a different side group, size, and different properties, e.g. pH, hydrophilic or hydrophobic. These properties are used in the analysis of amino acids.

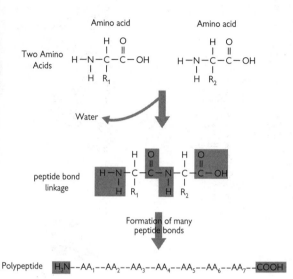

Fig. 5.1 Formation of a polypeptide.

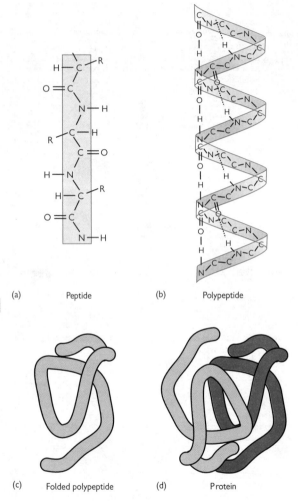

(a)   Peptide   (b)   Polypeptide

(c)   Folded polypeptide   (d)   Protein

Fig. 5.2 Formation of a protein.

Indispensable (essential) amino acids

Some amino acids can be synthesized by the body but others must be supplied by the diet. These are known as indispensable or essential amino acids; there are eight essential amino acids (Table 5.1). Some amino acids are only essential in specific circumstances. In childhood seven other amino acids are essential that are not essential in adults (arginine, histidine, cysteine, glycine, tyrosine, glutamine, proline). These amino acids are essential in children because they are required in amounts larger than can be synthesized because of high demand, immature biological pathways, or a combination. Conditionally indispensable or essential amino acids only become essential in circumstances when the requirement is ↑, e.g. glutamine.

Requirements

The amino acid content of a protein determines its biological value. Proteins that contain all the indspensable amino acids in sufficient quantities have high biological value. High biological value proteins are from animal sources, e.g. meat, eggs, milk, dairy products, and fish. If one or more indispensable amino acids are not present in a protein it will have low biological value. Generally plant proteins are of low biological value. The indispensable amino acid that is in shortest supply is known as the limiting amino acid. By combining foods with low biological value it is possible to provide all indispensable amino acids in the diet; this is important in vegan diets. For example, the limiting amino acid in wheat is lysine and in pulses it is methionine. A diet combining wheat products such as bread with pulses will provide all the indispensable amino acids, e.g. pitta bread and dahl.

As already stated, protein is constantly being turned over; 3–4 g proteins are turned over per kg of body weight per day. Each day 10–15 g of nitrogen are excreted in urine (6.25 g protein is equivalent to 1 g nitrogen). Small amounts are lost in faeces and skin. When nitrogen (protein) intake equals nitrogen excretion the body is said to be in nitrogen balance. Healthy adults will be in positive nitrogen balance. Nitrogen balance studies have been used to derive the recommended requirements that are shown in Table 5.2.

Deficiency

If energy intake is insufficient, protein will be degraded to produce energy; ∴ protein deficiency can occur when the diet does not provide enough protein or energy or a combination of both. Protein energy malnutrition (PEM) is a major cause for concern in developing countries but does occur in the UK amongst at risk groups. These include immuno-compromised individuals (e.g. AIDS), anorexia, and cancer patients with cachexia. Mild PEM is fairly common amongst surgical or elderly hospital patients. Protein deficiency can also occur as the result of ↑ losses in renal disease, ↑ catabolism in trauma, burns or sepsis, or malabsorption. Protein deficiency results in muscle wasting, stunted growth, poor wound healing, susceptibility to infection, oedema, and fatty liver.

Table 5.1 Classification of amino acids

Indispensible/essential amino acids	Indispensible (conditionally essential) amino acids	Dispensible (non-essential) amino acids
Leucine (Leu)	Essential for children:	Glutamic acid (Glu)
Isoleucine (Ile)	Tyrosine (Tyr)	Alanine (Ala)
Valine (Val)	Glycine (Gly)	Aspartic acid (Asp)
Phenylalanine (Phe)	Cysteine (Cys)	
Threonine (Thr)	Arginine (Arg)	
Methionine (Met)	Proline (Pro)	
Tryptophan (Trp)	Histidine (His)	
Lysine (Lys)	Glutamine	
	Other:	
	Serine (Ser)	
	Asparagine (Asn)	

Table 5.2 Recommended nutrient intake of protein for all age groups and average daily intakes of protein of adult men and women in UK*

Age	Weight (kg)	RNI (g/d)
Children (both sexes)		
0–3 months	5.9	12.5
4–6 months	7.7	12.7
7–9 months	8.8	13.7
10–12 months	9.7	14.9
1–3 years	12.5	14.5
4–6 years	17.8	19.7
7–10 years	28.3	28.3
Males		
11–14 years	43.0	42.1
15–18 years	64.5	55.2
19–50 years	74.0	55.5
50+ years	71.0	53.3
Females		
11–14 years	43.8	41.2
15–18 years	55.5	45.4
19–50 years	60.0	45.0
50+ years	62.0	46.5
Additional RNI required for females		
During pregnancy		+6.0
Lactation: 0–6 months		+11.0
Lactation: 6+ months		+8.0
Adults	**Average daily intake UK (g/d)**	
Men	88.2	
Women	63.7	

* Source for RNIs, Department of Health (1991). *Dietary reference values for food and nutrients for the United Kingdom.* HMSO, London; source for average daily intakes for adults, Henderson, L, Gregory , J., and Irving, K. (2003). *The National Diet and Nutrition Survey: adults aged 19 to 64 years.* Vol 2. *Energy, protein, carbohydrate, fat and alcohol intakes.* HMSO, London.

Sources of dietary protein

In the typical UK diet 60% of protein intake has high biological value. High biological protein is supplied by meat and meat products, fish, eggs, and milk and dairy products (Table 5.3). Plants such as cereals and pulses supply proteins of low biological value.

Table 5.3 Contribution of food sources to protein intake[*]

Food group	% Daily intake
Meat and meat products	36
Chicken, turkey and dishes	12
Cereals and cereal products	23
Bread	12
Milk and milk products	16

[*] Source for food sources in adults, Henderson, L., Gregory , J., and Irving, K. (2003). The National Diet and Nutrition Survey: adults aged 19 to 64 years. Vol 2. Energy, protein, carbohydrate, fat and alcohol intakes. HMSO, London.

Fats

Fats are often referred to as lipids. Lipids are described by chemists as substances that are poorly soluble or insoluble in water but are soluble in organic solvents. Fat is the term most often used when discussing foods and lipids metabolism. Over 90% of dietary fats are triglycerides (triacylglycerols); other types of fat include cholesterol, phospholipids, sterols, and carotenoids.

Function

The functions of fat in the diet are:
- Energy source—fat provides 37 kJ (9 kcal) per gram.
- Fat provides essential fatty acids.
- Fat is a carrier for fat soluble vitamins A,D,E, and K.
- ↑ palatability by improving taste perception and appearance of food.
- Some fats are important constituents of cell membranes and can be converted to biologically active compounds such as steroid hormones, interleukins, thromboxanes, and prostaglandins.
- Cholesterol is converted to bile acids, which are important in digestion.

Fatty acids

Fats consist of fatty acids that have carbon chains containing up to 22 carbon molecules in the chain. Triglycerides have glycerol backbone to which are attached three fatty acids. The type of fatty acid attached to the glycerol molecule determines its physical properties, nutritional function, and physiological function. Hydrogen is added to fatty acids to make them more solid when manufacturing some food products such as vegetable spreads; this process is known as hydrogenation.

Fatty acids are carbon molecules with a methyl group at one end and a carboxyl acid at the other (Fig. 5.3). They can have chains of 4–22 carbon molecules although most have 16–18. Hydrogen atoms are attached to the carbon chain; the number of hydrogen atoms determines the degree of saturation (with hydrogen atoms) of the fatty acid. A fatty acid with hydrogen atoms on every arm is said to be 'saturated'. Unsaturated fatty acids contain double carbon bonds where there is no hydrogen (Fig. 5.3). If there is only one double bond the fatty acid is monounsaturated. When more than one double bond is present the fatty acid will be polyunsaturated.

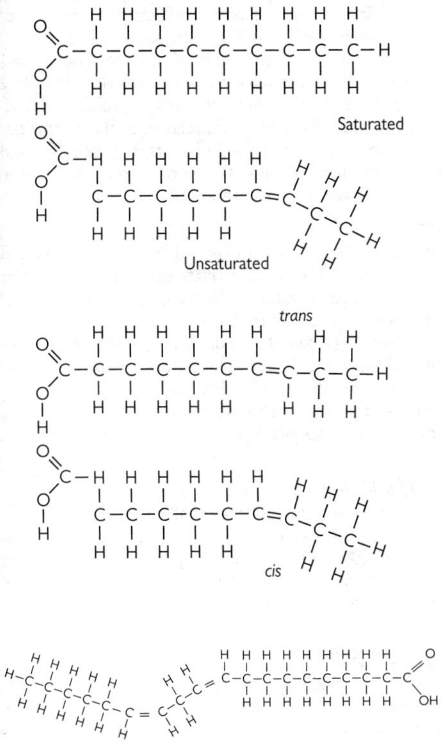

Saturated

Unsaturated

trans

cis

Linoleic acid, a polyunsaturated fatty acid.
Both double bonds are cis

Fig. 5.3 Structure of fatty acids.

Fatty acids have a common name, e.g. linoleic acid, a systematic name, and a notational name. The systematic name reflects the number of carbon atoms, and the number of double bonds, so that linoleic acid becomes octadecadienoic acid. This represents 18 carbons (octadeca-) and two double bonds (di-). The notational name for linoleic acid is 18:2 n6 or 18:2 omega 6; again this represents 18 carbon atoms and two double is now also represented. The position is relative to the methyl (or omega) end of the carbon chain. Linoleic acid has its first double bond between the sixth and seventh carbons. Common names, systematic names, and notational names are shown in Table 5.4.

Saturated fatty acids (SFA)

Saturated fatty acids contain carbon atoms linked by single bonds and hydrogen on all available arms, They have a relatively high melting point and tend to be solid at room temperature. SFA are obtained from animal storage fats and their products, e.g. meat fat, lard, milk, butter, cheese, and cream. Fats from plant origin tend to be unsaturated with the exception of coconut oil and palm oil. Some manufactured margarines and spreads contain significant amounts of SFA. Plasma low-density lipoprotein (LDL) cholesterol, and ∴ plasma cholesterol, tends to be raised by SFA. High intakes of SFA are associated with atherogenesis and cardiovascular disease.

Monounsaturated fatty acids (MUFA)

MUFA contain only one double bond and are usually liquid (oil) at room temperature. Olive oil and rapeseed oil are the most concentrated dietary sources of MUFA. MUFA are present in many foods including meat fat and lard. Dietary MUFA does not raise plasma cholesterol and lowers LDL lipoprotein without a detrimental affect on high density lipoproteins (HDL).

Polyunsaturated fatty acids (PUFA)

PUFA contain two or more double bonds and are liquid at room temperature. They are easily oxidized in foods and in the body. PUFA are involved in the metabolism of cholesterol, are components of phospholipids in cell membranes, and are precursors of biologically active compounds such as prostaglandins, interleukins, and thromboxanes. Therefore they have a vital roles in the immune response, blood clotting, and inflammation. PUFA are derived from the essential fatty acids linoleic acid (n6 or ω6) and α-linoleic acid (n3 or ω3) and are ∴ divided into omega 3 (ω3) or omega 6 (ω6) groups of PUFA. EFA, EPA, and DHA are important in neural development of the fetus and infant. PUFA occur as *cis* or *trans* forms depending on the way the hydrogen atoms are arranged. In *cis* formation the hydrogen atoms are bonded to either end of the double bond on the same side. And in the *trans* form the hydrogen atoms are on opposite side (Fig. 5.3). Most naturally occurring fats are in the *cis* form.

Omega (ω) 3 PUFA

ω3 PUFA (and parent essential fatty acid α -linoleic acid) are found in fish and fish oils and their health benefits are being more fully explored. The health benefits of ↑ consumption of oily fish include improved cardiovascular risk factors. The Western diet contains a high ratio of ω6:ω3 PUFAs; a lower ratio (4:1) is recommended. Research studies have shown benefits in cognitive function but epidemiological studies are required.

Table 5.4 Nomenclature of fatty acids

Common name	Notational name	Systematic name
Saturated fatty acids		
Butyric	4:0	Tetranoic
Caproic	6:0	Hexanoic
Caprylic	8:0	Octanoic
Capric	10:0	Decanoic
Lauric	12:0	Dodecanoic
Myristic	14:0	Tetradecanoic
Palmitic	16:0	Heaxdecanoic
Stearic	18:0	Octadecanoic
Arachidic	20:0	Eicosanoic
Behenic	22:0	Docosanic
Monounsaturated fatty acids		
Palmitoleic	16:1n7	9 cis-hexadecenoic
Oleic	18:1n9	9 cis-octadecenoic
Elaidic	18:1n9	9 trans-octadecenoic
Eicosenoic	20:1n9	11 cis-eicosaenoic
Erucic	22:1n9	13 cis-docosaenoic
Polyunsaturated fatty acids		
Linoleic	19:2n6	9,12 cis, cis-octadecadienoic
Alpha-linolenic	18:3n3	9,12,15 all cis-octadecatrienoic
Gamma-linolenic	18:3n6	5 trans, 9 cis, 12 cis-octadecatrienoic
Arachidonic	20:4n6	5,8,11,14 cis-eicosatetraenoic
EPA	20:5n3	Eicosapentaenoic
DHA	22:6n3	Docosahexaenoic

Trans fatty acids

Trans fatty acids are rare in naturally occurring fats. Some is made in the rumen of cows and sheep and is ∴ found in lamb, beef, milk, and cheese. The most significant source of *trans* fatty acids in the diet is obtained through the hydrogenation of PUFA to produce more solid forms of vegetable oils for spreads, margarines, and some food products. *Trans* fatty acids have been associated with adverse effects on lipoprotein status by elevating LDL and depressing HDL although further research is required.

Essential fatty acids (EFA)

Linoleic and α-linoleic acids are essential fatty acids. Other longer chain fatty acids such as arachidonic, EPA, and DHA are physiologically important but can be synthesized to a limited extent from linoleic and α-linoleic acid. These longer chain fatty acids are not essential fatty acids but their intake may become critical in fatty acid deficiency. EFA are most commonly found in plant and fish oils. Deficiency of linoleic acid has been demonstrated in children although a deficiency of α-linoleic acid has not been seen in healthy people. This has → debate about the essentiality of α-linoleic acid. Deficiency is characterized by a scaly dermatitis. The recommended intake of linoleic acid is at least 11% of total energy and 0.2% for α-linoleic acid.

Sterols

Sterols are relatively simple molecules; the most common sterol is the wax-like cholesterol. Cholesterol and cholesterol ester (cholesterol to which a fatty acid is attached) are only found in animal foods. Phytosterols are found in plant foods. Cholesterol has structural roles in lipoproteins and membranes and is a precursor for bile acids, steroid hormones, and vitamin D. Dietary cholesterol has little influence on plasma levels as most circulating cholesterol is endogenous. Reduction of intake of saturated fat results in lower plasma cholesterol levels.

Lipid transport

Fat digestion and absorption are covered in Chapter 1, 'Digestion'. Lipids are not soluble in water and ∴ complex with apolipoproteins to form water-miscible compounds. Approximately 2% of total plasma lipids are free fatty acids and are transported compounds of albumin. The remainder of lipids is carried in the blood as lipoproteins. Lipoproteins are identified by the apolipoprotein that is present (apo A, apo B, apo C, apo D, and apo E). There are five classes of lipoproteins which vary in density:

- Chylomicrons;
- Very low density lipoproteins (VLDL);
- Low density lipoproteins (LDL);
- High-density lipoproteins (HDL);
- Lipoprotein (a) (LP(a)).

Table 5.5 Average intake for adults compared with DRVs for fat for adults (as a percentage of daily food energy intake) in the UK*

	Average intake (% daily energy)		DRV (% of food energy intake)
	♂	♀	
Total fat	35.8	34.9	35
Saturated fat	13.4	13.2	11
Monosaturated fatty acids	12.1	11.5	13
Polyunsaturated fatty acids	5.5	5.3	6.5
Trans fatty acids	1.2	1.2	<2
Cholesterol†	304	213	<245

* Source: Henderson, L., Gregory, J., and Irving, K. (2003), *The National Diet and Nutrition Survey; adults aged 19 to 64 years.* Vol. 2, *Energy protein, carbohydrate, fat and alcohol intakes.* HMSO, London.
† Cholesterol intake and DRV are expressed in mg/day.

Table 5.6 Sources of total fat and saturated fatty acids in the diet of adults in the UK (NDNS)*.

Food	Total fat (%)	Saturated fatty acids (%)
Meat, meat products, & meat dishes	23	22
Cereal & cereal products	19	18
Milk & milk products	14	24
Fat spreads	12	11

* Source: Henderson, L., Gregory, J., and Irving, K. (2003). *The National Diet and Nutrition Survey: adults aged 19 to 64 years.* Vol. 2, *Energy protein, carbohydrate, fat and alcohol intakes.* HMSO, London.

High and low levels of the lipoproteins have adverse effects on health. High levels of LDL are associated with ↑ health problems and LDL is colloquially known as 'bad cholesterol'. HDL is colloquially known as 'good cholesterol'.

Chylomicrons

Chylomicrons mainly consist of triglycerides as they transport dietary lipids. Plasma levels rise after eating and are negligible in the fasting state. Chylomicrons leave the enterocytes of the small intestine and enter the lymphatic system before transferring to blood vessels. The triglycerides are hydrolysed by lipoprotein lipase so releasing fatty acids that are used for energy or stored in adipose tissue. The life cycle of a chylomicron is 15–20 minutes and the liver clears the remnant from the blood. Fat-soluble vitamins reach the liver as part of the remnant.

Very low-density lipoproteins (VLDL)

VLDL are synthesized in the liver and are large particles that are rich in triglycerides. They deliver fatty acids to adipose tissue, muscles, and heart where lipoprotein lipase facilitates their release from triglycerides. The enzyme in the heart has a high affinity for triglyceride and, when triglyceride concentrations are low, they are preferentially released into heart tissue. Following release of triglycerides the remaining remnants are intermediate density lipoproteins (IDL), which are the precursors of low density lipoproteins.

Low-density lipoproteins (LDL)

LDL contain mainly cholesterol and cholesterol ester as they are the end product of VLDL metabolism. They carry approximately 70% of plasma cholesterol and are taken up by the liver and other tissues by LDL receptors.

High-density lipoproteins (HDL)

The liver and intestine synthesize and secrete HDL. HDL is involved in the reverse transport of cholesterol from tissues to the liver or transfers it to other lipoproteins.

Lipoprotein (a)

This is a complex of LDL with apolipoproteins (a).

Table 5.7 Dietary sources of cholesterol

Cholesterol content	Food
High	Liver, offal
	Eggs, mayonnaise
	Shellfish
	Fish roe
Medium	Meat fat
	Full fat milk and dairy produce, e.g. cream, cheese, butter
	Meat and fish products
	Manufactured meat products, e.g. pies
Low	Skinless poultry
	Skimmed milk and dairy products, e.g. cottage cheese, low fat yoghurt
Cholesterol free	Fruit (including avocados and olives) and vegetables
	Vegetable oils
	Cereals, pasta
	Rice
	Egg white
	Sugar

Table 5.8 Functions of plasma lipoproteins

Lipoprotein	Function
Chylomicrons	Transport dietary lipids to peripheral tissues and liver
VLDL	Transports lipids from liver to peripheral tissues
LDL	Transports cholesterol to peripheral tissues and liver
HDL	Removes cholesterol from peripheral tissues to the liver
Albumin	Transports free fatty acids from adipose tissue to peripheral tissues

Carbohydrate

Carbohydrates are the most significant source of energy in the diet (see 'Energy balance', this chapter). In developing countries up to 85% of energy in the diet is provided by carbohydrate; this figure is as low as 40% in some developed countries. The relationship between dietary carbohydrates and fat is usually reciprocal. Diets rich in fat will have low levels of carbohydrates and vice versa.

Structure and classification

The empirical formula for carbohydrates is $C_x(H_2O)_y$; glucose is the simplest carbohydrate ($C_6H_{12}O_6$ or $C_6(H_2O)_6$) (Fig. 5.4). Simple carbohydrates (monosaccharides) can combine to form disaccharides, e.g. sucrose ($C_{12}H_{22}O_{11}$) from two disaccharides, oligosaccharides, e.g. raffinose which is formed from 3–11 monosaccharides, or polysaccharides, which form from 12 or more saccharides, e.g. starches.

Carbohydrates that can be digested and absorbed in the small intestines and → ↑ in blood glucose levels are referred to as glycaemic carbohydrates (Table 5.9). Plant polysaccharides that cannot be digested (non-glycaemic) are referred to as fibre or non-starch polysaccharides. Sugar alcohols are also classified as carbohydrates although their empirical formula is slightly different.

Sugars (mono-and disaccharides)

Monosaccharides include glucose, fructose, and galactose. The monsaccharide free glucose is found in small amounts in fruit and vegetables but is not abundant in natural foods. It is made from starch and used commercially. Fructose is found in honey, fruit, and vegetables and is manufactured from fructose-rich corn syrup for the food industry. Sucrose is the commonest disaccharide and is extracted from sugar beet or sugar cane. Table sugar is 99% sucrose and the major dietary source of disaccharide. Sucrose is hydrolysed into glucose and fructose. Lactose is found in milk and milk products. It is hydrolysed to glucose and galactose. Maltose is present in malted wheat and barley. Malt extract is used in brewing and in malted products.

Oligosaccharides

Raffinose, stachyose, and verbascose are oligosaccharides that are made of galactose, glucose, and fructose. They are found in legumes and seeds. Humans do not have the enzyme needed to digest them but they may be fermented in the colon. Fructo-oligosaccharides and inulin have been shown to stimulate growth of the potentially beneficial bifidobacteria in the colon.

Table 5.9 Classification of carbohydrates in the diet (FAO/WHO 1998)*

Glycaemic	Non-glycaemic
Monosaccharides	**Oligosaccharides**
Glucose	Raffinose, stachyose, verbascose
Fructose	Human milk oligosaccharides
Galactose	Fructo-oligosaccharides
	Inulin
Disaccharides	
Sucrose	
Lactose	
Maltose	
Trehalose	
Polysaccharides	**Non-starch polysaccharides**
Starch—amylopectin, amylase, modified food starches	Cellulose (insoluble)
	Hemicellulose (soluble and insoluble forms)
	β-glucans (mainly soluble)
	Fructans, e.g. inulin (not assayed by current methods)
	Gums (soluble)
	Mucilages (soluble)
	Algal polysaccharides (soluble)
Sugar alcohols[†]	
Sorbitol	
Xylitol	
Mannitol	

* WHO/FAO (1998). *Carbohydrates in human nutrition,* FAO food and nutrition paper no.66. FAO, Rome.
[†] Sugar alcohols are only partially absorbed.

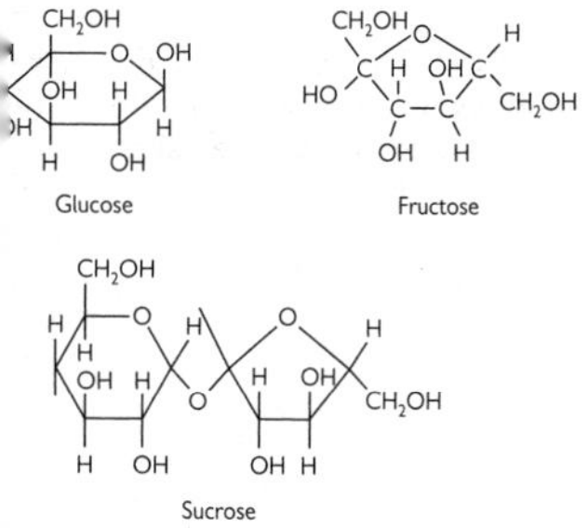

Fig. 5.4 Carbohydrate molecules.

Sugar alcohols

Sorbitol, inositol, and mannitol are sugar alcohols that are only partially absorbed and ∴ provide less energy than the corresponding sugars. Therefore they have been used as sugar substitutes. Small amounts occur naturally but significant amounts in the diet come only from manufactured foods. Large amounts can cause an osmotic diarrhoea.

Starch

Starch is the main storage polysaccharide in plant cells and is found in large quantities in cereal grains, potatoes, and plantains. Starch is the largest source of carbohydrate in the diet. Starch consists of two glucose polysaccharides: amylase and amylopectin. The linkages between the glucose molecules are degraded by the action of α-amylase. Many factors affect the rate at which the linkages are degraded so that some starches are readily digested while others pass undigested into the colon. This has resulted in the classification of starches (Table 5.10) into rapidly digestible starch (RDS), slowly digestible starch (SDS), and resistant starch (RS). Both RDS and SDS are digested in the small intestine while RS passes undigested into the colon where it is available for fermentation.

Non-starch polysaccharide (NSP)—Fibre

In the UK, NSP is the term used in preference to fibre. Dietary fibre is defined as NSP that does not include lignin or resistant starch; the terms are ambiguous. Fibre can be classified as soluble (in water at pH 7.0) or insoluble and it is this classification that categorizes the function of these polysaccharides. Insoluble fibre consists mainly of cellulose and some hemicelluloses. Insoluble fibre binds to water in the colon and swells. This stimulates peristalsis so ↑ transit time in the colon thereby reducing the risk of constipation and possibly reducing the risk of colon cancer. Soluble fibre blunts the response of blood glucose to ingestion. The reabsorption of bile acids is slowed by soluble fibre so ↑ cholesterol losses in faeces and reducing blood cholesterol levels. Table 5.11 lists sources of soluble and insoluble fibre in the diet.

Intrinsic sugars

These are sugars that are present in intact cells, e.g. fructose in whole fruit and sugars in milk, i.e. lactose and galactose.

Non-milk extrinsic sugars (NMES)

Sugars that are in a free or readily absorbable state, e.g. added sugar (usually sucrose), or released from disrupted cells, e.g. fructose in fruit puree or juice. NMES contribute to the development of dental caries.

Table 5.10 Classification of starch

Class	Glycaemic response	Food source
Rapidly digestible starch	Large	Cooked starchy cereals, warm potatoes
Slowly digestible starch	Small	Muesli, oats, pasta, legumes
Resistant starch	None	Unripe bananas, whole grains

Table 5.11 Dietary sources of soluble and in-soluble fibre in the diet

Soluble fibre	Insoluble fibre
Apples	Beans
Barley	Brown rice
Citrus fruits	Fruits with edible seeds
Guar gum	Lentils
Legumes	Maize
Oats	Oats
Pears	Pulses
Strawberries	Wheat bran
	Wholemeal breads
	Wholemeal cereals
	Wholemeal pasta
	Whole wheat flour
	Peas

Table 5.12 Daily carbohydrate and NMES intake of adults (NDNS)*

	Men	Women
Total carbohydrate (g/d)	275	203
% total energy	47.7	48.5
NMES (g/d)	79	51
% total energy	13.6	11.9
DRV (% total energy)	10.0	10.0
NSP (g/d)	15.2	12.6
DRV (g/d)	18.0	18.0

* Henderson, L., Gregory, J., and Irving, K. (2003). *The National Diet and Nutrition Survey: adults aged 19 to 64 years.* Vol. 2, *Energy, protein, carbohydrate, fat and alcohol intakes.* HMSO, London.

Recommended intakes

Sugar and starch   The COMA report recommended that the intake of intrinsic or milk sugars should not be limited in adults. They recommended that infant formulas should contain approximately 40 % energy from sugars; this is similar to the sugar content of breast milk. It is recommended that the average intake of NMES should not exceed 60 g/d or 10% daily energy.

Starches, intrinsic sugars, and milk sugars should provide the balance of dietary energy not provided by alcohol, protein fat, and NMES, which is on average 37% in UK.

NSP   It is recommended that the adult diet contain 18 g NSP/d (12–24 g/d).

Glycaemic index (GI)

The glycaemic index is a method of ranking foods and carbohydrates based on their immediate effect on blood glucose levels. The FAO/WHO (1998)[1] define the GI as 'the incremental area' under the blood glucose response curve of one 50 g carbohydrate portion of a test food expressed as a percentage of response to the same amount of carbohydrate from a standard food taken by the same subject.' The standard carbohydrate is glucose that has a GI of 100. Foods with a high glycaemic index are readily absorbed and raised blood glucose quickly. Low glycaemic index foods are digested and absorbed slowly and raise blood glucose levels slowly. The GI can only be determined by *in vivo* measurement. Foods are categorized into:

- low GI,   55 or less;
- medium GI,   56–69;
- high GI,   70 or more.

[1] WHO/FAO (1998). *Carbohydrates in human nutrition*, FAO food and nutrition paper no.66. FAO, Rome

Table 5.13 Sources of carbohydrate in the diet (NDNS)*

Food group	% Daily intake
Cereals & cereal products	45
Bread	21
Potatoes & savoury snacks	12
Drinks	10

* Henderson, L., Gregory, J., and Irving, K. (2003). *The National Diet and Nutrition Survey: adults aged 19 to 64 years*. Vol. 2, *Energy, protein, carbohydrate, fat and alcohol intakes*. HMSO, London.

Table 5.14 Sources of NMES in the diet (NDNS)*

Food group	% Intake
Drinks	37
Carbonated soft drinks	12
Sugar, preserves, & confectionery	32
Table sugar	19
Cereals & cereal products	19

* Henderson, L., Gregory, J., and Irving, K. (2003). *The National Diet and Nutrition Survey: adults aged 19 to 64 years*. Vol. 2, *Energy, protein, carbohydrate, fat and alcohol intakes*. HMSO, London

Table 5.15 Sources of NSP in the diet (NDNS)*

Food group	Selected food	% intake
Cereals & cereal products		42
	Breakfast cereals	11
Vegetables (excluding potatoes)		20
Potatoes & savoury snacks		16
Fruit & nuts		10

* Henderson, L., Gregory, J., and Irving, K. (2003). *The National Diet and Nutrition Survey: adults aged 19 to 64 years*. Vol. 2, *Energy, protein, carbohydrate, fat and alcohol intakes*. HMSO, London.

Table 5.16 lists examples of GI of these categories. A list of foods that have been tested has been published by Foster-Powell et al. (2002).[2] The way a food is processed, prepared, and cooked will affect the GI of the food. The overall GI of the diet is important rather than aiming to introduce a few low GI foods. The health benefits of a low GI diet include:

- improved diabetic glucose control (see Chapter 18);
- improved risk factors for heart disease (see Chapter 19);
- weight reduction (see Chapter 17);
- there is some evidence to suggest ↓ risk of colon and breast cancers.

Glycaemic load (GL)

GL extends the concept of GI by considering the GI and the amount of carbohydrate have on postprandial blood glucose levels.

$$(GL = \text{Carbohydrate in food portion (g)} \times GI) / 100$$

Blood glucose levels rise more rapidly after a high GL meal than a low GL meal. It is recommended that a healthy diet should have a low GI and a low GL.

[2] Foster-Powell, K. Holt, S.H.A., and Brand-Miller, J.C. (2002). International table of glycaem index and glycaemic load: 2002. *Am. J. Clin. Nutr.* **76**, 5–56.

Table 5.16 Examples of low, medium, and high GI foods

Low GI	Medium GI	High GI
Apples, oranges, pears, peaches	Honey	Glucose
Beans and lentils	Jam	White and wholemeal bread
Pasta (all types made from durum wheat)	Shredded Wheat	Brown rice, cooked
	Weetabix	White rice, cooked
Sweet potato, peeled and boiled	Ice cream	Cornflakes
Sweet corn	New potatoes, peeled and boiled white basmati rice, cooked	Baked potato
Porridge		Mashed potato
Custard	Pitta bread	
Noodles	Couscous	
All Bran, Special K, Sultana Bran		

Energy balance

In order to maintain body weight, energy intake must equal energy expenditure. If energy expenditure exceeds energy intake body weight will be lost. Weight loss is achieved by ↑ energy expenditure or ↓ energy intake. To gain weight the equation is reversed.

The SI unit of energy is the joule (J); the joule is a small amount of energy. Energy in food is usually expressed as kilojoules (kJ) and energy expenditure is expressed as kJ or megajoules (MJ). In practice many people continue to express energy in kilocalories (kcal). A calorie can be defined in several ways although the most frequently used definition is:

- The energy required to raise the temperature of 1 g of water from 14.5°C to 15.5°C.

Energy expenditure can be expressed per unit of time, e.g. kJ per minute or MJ/d or in Watts (W).

Units used in energy balance

- 1000 joules = 1kJ
- 1000 kJ = 1MJ
- 1 kcal = 4.184 kJ*
- 1 kJ = 0.239 kcal
- 1 W = 1 joule per second
- 0.06 W = 1 kJ per min
- 86.4 W = kJ per 24 h

* The Royal Society (London) recommended conversion factor.

Energy expenditure

Total energy expenditure (TEE) has the following components:

- basal metabolic rate (BMR), 50–75%;
- physical activity (PA), 20–40%;
- dietary induced thermogenesis (DIT), 10%.

Growth, pregnancy, lactation, injury, and fever are energy-requiring processes that will ↑ energy expenditure and → ↑ energy intake.

Basal metabolic rate (BMR)

BMR is the amount of energy expended by the body to maintain normal physiological functions. It remains constant throughout the day, under normal conditions, and constitutes 50–75% of total energy expenditure (TEE); it is the largest component of TEE.

BMR is affected by many factors:

- **Body weight**. BMR ↑ or ↓ with ↑ or ↓ body weight;
- **Body composition**. Fat mass is relatively metabolically inactive and expends less energy gram for gram than fat free mass (FFM). Men have a higher FFM to fat ratio than women and ∴ have a higher BMR than women of the same age and weight;
- **Age**. Children have a higher BMR per kilogram than adults due to the energy requirement of growth. As adults age metabolism slows and FFM ↓ ∴ ↓ BMR;

- *Gender*. Men generally have a higher BMR due to differences in body weight and body composition. The BMR of a 65 kg man will be approximately 1MJ/d higher than a weight-and age-matched woman;
- *Genetic factors*. BMR can vary by up to 10% between subjects of the same age, sex, and body weight. Recent research has shown that there are ethnic differences in BMR;
- *Physiological changes*. BMR ↑ during pregnancy and lactation;
- *Disease and trauma*. Fever, sepsis, infection, surgical and physical trauma ↑ BMR;
- *Nutritional status*. The body adapts to changes in energy intake by altering body weight and/or body composition. An individual who is consuming more calories than is required will ↑ weight and ↑ BMR so making further weight impossible unless intake ↑ further;
- *Environment*. The energy cost of maintaining body temperature is influenced by ambient temperature, wind speed, radiant temperature of the surrounding, and clothing;
- *Hormonal status*. Several hormonal factors influence BMR especially thyroid function. BMR is ↑ in hyperthyroidism and ↓ in hypothyroidism. There are small cyclical changes during the menstrual cycle of some women with a rise after ovulation;
- *Pharmacological effects*. Therapeutic drugs and substances such as caffeine and capsaicin can modulate BMR;
- *Psychological effects*. Anxiety will ↑ energy expenditure in the short term. Longer term effects of stress and anxiety have not been established.

Measurement of BMR
- BMR must be measured under standard conditions.
- Post-absorptive state—at least 12 hours after last food or drink. This should also include other stimulants such as caffeine or smoking.
- Thermoneutral environment—20–25°C; comfortably warm.
- Supine—sitting up will ↑ energy expenditure slightly.
- Awake but in a state of complete physical and mental relaxation.
- Heavy physical activity on the day before the measurement may influence the BMR and should be avoided.

In practice BMR is usually measured first thing in the morning before eating and drinking or undertaking physical activity. If any of the conditions are not met the measurement is termed resting metabolic rate (RMR). RMR is slightly higher than BMR while sleeping metabolic rate is 5–10% lower than BMR.

Measurements of energy expenditure
Energy expenditure can be measured directly (the measurement of heat production), indirectly (the measurement of O_2 consumption), or by non-calorimetric methods, e.g. heart rate monitoring. More recently methods have been developed that are indirect measures of gaseous exchange (O_2 consumption), i.e. doubly labelled water technique.

Direct calorimetry
Direct calorimetry is the measurement of heat produced by the body. Subjects are placed in an insulated chamber and heat loss is measured

over a period of at least 24 h. Direct calorimetry is difficult in practice as the chamber must be capable of detecting all heat generated within the chamber and other sources of heat must be eliminated or accounted for. Direct calorimeters are very precise instruments but are expensive and difficult to build and maintain and few are available; ∴ this method is not frequently used.

Indirect calorimetry

Indirect calorimetry is based on the principle that food is oxidized in the body to produce energy and that by measuring oxygen consumption it is possible to calculate energy expenditure. The following equation demonstrates the amount of energy produced by the oxidation of 1 mole of glucose:

$$C_6H_{12}O_6 \quad + \quad 6O_2 \quad \rightarrow \quad 6CO_2 \quad + \quad 6H_2O \quad + \quad heat$$

$$(180 \text{ g}) \qquad (6 \times 22.4 \text{ l}) \quad (6 \times 22.3 \text{ l}) \quad (6 \times 18\text{g}) \quad (2.78 \text{ MJ})$$

The energy produced by the oxidation of 1 g glucose is ∴ 15.4 kJ (2780/180) and 1 litre of oxygen is equivalent to the production of 20.7 kJ (2780/6 × 22.4). Therefore if the amount of oxygen used is known, it is possible to calculate the amount of energy or heat produced. Similar calculations can be made for protein, fat, and alcohol.

Respiratory quotient (RQ) is the ratio of oxygen used to the amount of carbon dioxide produced. From the RQ it is possible to estimate the macronutrient composition of the diet (see Table 5.17). The energy content of a mixed diet is approximately 35% fat, 50% carbohydrate, and ∴ has an RQ of 0.87. To improve the accuracy of the calculations an estimate of nitrogen excretion is used. Substitution into a formula yields energy expenditure (EE). The formulae most frequently used are those of Weir (1949)[1], or Elia and Livesey (1992)[2].

[1] Weir, J.B. De V. (1949). New methods for calculating metabolic rate with special reference to protein metabolism. *J. Physiol. (Lond.)* **109**, 1–9.

[2] Elia, M. and Livesey, G. (1992). Energy expenditure and fuel selections in biological systems: the theory and practice of calculations based on indirect calorimetry and tracer methods. In *Metabolic control of eating, energy expenditure and the bioenergetics of obesity* (ed. A.P. Simonopoulos), pp. 68–131. Karger, Basel.

Weir formula

$$EE (kJ) = 16.489 \, VO_2 \, (l) + 4.828 \, VCO_2 \, (l) - 9.079 \, N \, (g)$$

If nitrogen cannot be measured protein is assumed to be 15% of the energy of the diet and the formula becomes:

$$EE (kJ) = 16.318 \, VO_2 \, (l) + 4.602 \, VCO_2 \, (l)$$

Elia and Livesey formula

$$EE (kcal/24 \, h) = ((15.913 \, VO_2 \, (l) + 5.207 \, VCO_2 \, (l)) \times 1.44 - 4.464 \\ N \, (g)) \times 0.239$$

where $VO_2 = O_2$ consumed, $VCO_2 = CO_2$ produced, and $N =$ urinary nitrogen excretion

Table 5.17 Energy values for oxidation of nutrients*

Nutrient	O_2 consumption (l/g)	CO_2 production (l/g)[†]	RQ	Energy released (kJ/g)	Energy released (kJ/l O_2)
Starch	0.829	0.832	0.994	17.49	21.10
Glucose	0.746	0.742	0.995	15.44	20.70
Fat	1.975	1.402	0.710	39.12	19.81
Protein	0.962	0.775	0.806	18.52	19.25
Alcohol	1.429	0.966	0.663	29.75	20.40

* Reproduced from Human Nutrition and Dietetics, Garrow JS, James WPT and Ralph A, table 17.1, P 135. With permission from Elsevier.
[†]CO_2 is not an ideal gas.6l mole at STP occupies 22.26 l not 22.4 l.

Indirect calorimetry equipment

Various apparatus is available to measure oxygen consumption. The simplest method is the Douglas bag where expired air is collected into a strong non-permeable bag. The volume of expired air over a set period is measured using a dry gas meter and the expired gases are analysed and compared to the ambient air. From this it is possible to calculate O_2 consumption and CO_2 production rates and ∴ calculate energy expenditure. In clinical situations, a ventilated hood, canopy, or tent, e.g. Deltatrac, Gem, Sensormedics, is used which measures gaseous exchange continuously and has a processor to calculate energy expenditure. Other systems are available that can be used during exercise. Respiration chambers are used by some research units; these are small chambers in which a subject stays for several hours or days and gaseous exchange is measured continuously. These chambers are expensive to build and use but give precise measurements.

Non-calorimetric methods

- Heart rate is related to energy expenditure and this relationship has been used to estimate energy expenditure although the results are not very reliable, particularly at low activity levels.
- Accelerometers are often used to measure physical activity; they are small computer motion analysers that measure duration, frequency, and intensity of physical activity. They are used in conjunction with log books that enable the full analysis of activities.

Doubly labelled water

Data is collected on free-living subjects over a period of 10–20 days. It does not require extensive equipment for the collection of gases and ∴ does not restrict the subject. Subjects are given an oral dose of water that has known amounts of the stable isotopes deuterium (^2H) and ^{18}O. These isotopes mix with the body's water and, as energy is used, CO_2 and H_2O are produced. As ^{18}O is in both H_2O and CO_2 it is lost more rapidly than ^2H which is only lost in H_2O. The difference between the rate of loss of ^2H and ^{18}O reflects the rate at which CO_2 is produced. From this it is possible to calculate energy expenditure. This method requires collection of body fluid, either blood, urine, or saliva, before the test period and samples at specified times during the study. It is possible to use this method in babies, hospital patients, field work, and other groups in whom it is difficult to measure energy expenditure by other methods. Specialist equipment is required for the analysis of blood and urine samples and, due to a world shortage of ^{18}O, this method is expensive.

Estimation of energy requirements

Energy requirements are estimated by using prediction equations such as the Schofield equations (1985), see Appendix 14. Table 5.18 shows the Schofield equations with additional data on men aged 60–70 y (DH 1991). Regression analysis of measured BMR against gender, age, and weight was used to generate the equations that estimate BMR. Numerous equations are available; ideally they should be population. specific. They are developed for use in healthy groups; in individuals the accuracy may be ± 10–20%. If equations are extended for use in illness the accuracy may be reduced by 50%.

TEE is calculated by using a physical activity level (PAL) that has been derived from experimental studies, often using doubly labelled water; this is known as the factorial method.

For example, a sedentary male worker, aged 40 y, weight 90 kg, with an inactive lifestyle would have PAL of 1.4 (Table 5.19); ∴ his TEE would be

BMR from prediction equations (7.973 MJ) × 1.4 = 11.16 MJ.

If an activity diary has been kept it is possible to calculate TEE more accurately by partitioning time during the day spent on specific activities and using physical activity ratios (PAR; see Appendix 6) it is possible to calculate a directly related PAL value for the day.

$$TEE = BMR \times [(PAR \times \text{time for activity A}) +$$

$$(PAR \times \text{time for activity B}) + ...]$$

Table 5.18 Formulae for the estimation of BMR*

	Age (y)	BMR prediction equation (MJ/d)[†]
Men	10–17	0.074 (w) + 2.754
	18–29	0.063 (w) + 2.896
	30–59	0.048 (w) + 3.653
	60–74	0.0499 (w) + 2.930
	75 +	0.035 (w) + 3.434
Women	10–17	0.056 (w) + 3.434
	18–29	0.062 (w) + 2.036
	30–59	0.034 (w) + 3.538
	60–74	0.0386 (w) + 2.875
	75 +	0.041 (w) + 2.610

* Equations based on Schofield, W.N. (1985). Predicting basal metabolic rate, new standards and review of previous work. *Hum. Nutr. Clin. Nutr.* **39**C (Suppl. I), 5–41. Additional data on men aged 60–70 y from Department of Health (1991). *Dietary reference values for food and nutrients for the United Kingdom.* HMSO, London.
[†] W, Weight in kg.

Table 5.19 Calculated PAL values for light, moderate, and heavy activity (occupational and non-occupational)*

Non-occupational activity level	Occupational activity level					
	Light		Moderate		Heavy	
	M	F	M	F	M	F
Sedentary	1.4	1.4	1.6	1.5	1.7	1.5
Moderately active	1.5	1.5	1.7	1.6	1.8	1.6
Very active	1.6	1.6	1.8	1.7	1.9	1.7

* Department of Health (1991). *Dietary reference values for food and nutrients for the United Kingdom.* HMSO, London.

Energy intake

Energy is provided by the macronutrients and alcohol.

- Protein, 4 kcal (17 kJ)/g.
- Carbohydrate, 3.75 kcal (16 kJ)/g.
- Fat, 9 kcal (37 kJ)/g.
- Alcohol, 7 kcal (29 kJ)/g.

Polyols (e.g. sorbitol) and volatile fatty acids (produced by gut bacteria by fermentation of some fibre components) contribute small, negligible amounts of energy.

Energy requirements

The DH recommendations are shown in Table 5.20 for babies and children to 10 years. These are given as estimated average requirements (EAR). EARs for men and women are grouped for age, weight, and activity level as shown in Table 5.21.

Energy consumption

The average daily energy intakes for adults in UK are 9.72 MJ (2313 kcal) for men and 6.87 MJ (1632 kcal) for women; this is 93% and 85% of EARs for men and women respectively (NDNS). The sources of energy are shown in Fig. 5.5.

❶ In the UK adults are not energy deficient, as demonstrated by the rising prevalence of obesity. The low percentages of EARs may be due to underreporting and reflect the widely held belief that EARs need revision. The level of physical activity is also important.

Table 5.20 Estimated average requirements (EARs) for energy of children 0–18 years[*]

Age	EAR MJ/d (kcal/d)	
	Boys	**Girls**
0–3 months	2.28 (545)	2.16 (515)
4–6 months	2.89 (690)	2.69 (645)
7–9 months	3.44 (825)	3.20 (765)
10–12 months	3.85 (920)	3.61 (865)
1–3 years	5.15 (1 230)	4.86 (1 165)
4–6 years	7.16 (1 715)	6.46 (1 545)
7–10 years	8.24 (1 970)	7.28 (1 740)
11–14 years	9.27 (2 220)	7.72 (1 845)
15–18 years	11.51 (2 775)	8.83 (2 110)

[*] Source for RNIs, Department of Health (1991). *Dietary reference values for food and nutrients for the United Kingdom.* HMSO, London; source for average daily intakes for adults, Henderson, L, Gregory , J., and Irving, K. (2003). *The National Diet and Nutrition Survey: adults aged 19 to 64 years.* Vol 2. *Energy, protein, carbohydrate, fat and alcohol intakes.* HMSO, London..

Table 5.21 Estimated average requirements (MJ/d) according to body weight and physical activity level (PAL)[†]

Body weight (kg)	BMR* (MJ/d)	PAL 1.4	1.5	1.6	1.8	2.0
Males						
30	4.97	7.0	7.5	8.0	9.0	9.9
35	5.34	7.5	8.0	8.6	9.6	10.7
40	5.71	8.0	8.6	9.1	10.3	11.4
45	6.08	8.5	9.1	9.7	11.0	12.2
50	6.45	9.0	9.7	10.3	11.6	12.9
55	6.82	9.6	10.2	10.9	12.3	13.6
60	7.19	10.1	10.8	11.5	12.9	14.4
65	7.56	10.6	11.3	12.1	13.6	15.1
Females						
30	4.58	6.4	6.9	7.3	8.2	9.2
35	4.86	6.8	7.3	7.8	8.7	9.7
40	5.14	7.2	7.7	8.2	9.2	10.3
45	5.42	7.6	8.1	8.7	9.8	10.8
50	5.70	8.0	8.5	9.1	10.3	11.4
55	5.98	8.4	9.0	9.6	10.8	12.0
60	6.26	8.8	9.4	10.0	11.3	12.5

* BMR, Basal metabolic rate calculated as per Table 5.18.

[†] Henderson, L., Gregory, J., and Irving, K. (2003). *The National Diet and Nutrition Survey: adults aged 19 to 64 years.* Vol. 2, *Energy, protein, carbohydrate, fat and alcohol intakes.* HMSO, London.

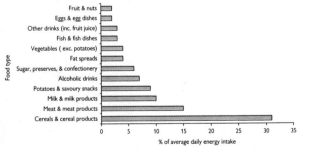

Fig. 5.5 Percentage contribution of food types
to average daily total energy intake of UK adults. Henderson, L., Gregory, J., and Irving, K. (2003). *The National Diet and Nurtrition Survey: adults aged 19 to 64 years.* Vol.2, *Energy protein, and carbohydrate, fat and alcohol intakes.* HMSO. London.

Vitamins: introduction

Vitamins are a group of organic compounds that have a variety of functions in the body and that are chemically different from each other. To show that a compound is a vitamin it is necessary to show a deficiency in experimental subjects and that this can be reversed by restoring the missing compound. The name 'vitamin' is derived from 'vital amine'; as the name suggests these essential compounds were initially thought to be amines. Vitamins can be divided into fat-soluble and water-soluble groups; vitamins A, E, D, and K are fat-soluble and may be stored in the body, the remainder being water-soluble and the body has limited or no stores.

Vitamin A (retinol) and carotenoids

Vitamin A is the term for the biologically active compound retinol and its provitamin (precursor) carotenoids. The most common provitamin A carotenoids are β-carotene, α-carotene, γ-carotene, and β-cryptoxanthin. Only 50 of approximately 600 naturally occurring carotenoids are converted into vitamin A. Carotenoids with no vitamin A activity include zeaxanthin, the pigment in sweet corn, and lycopene, the red pigment in tomatoes. The vitamin A activity of β-carotene is calculated as 6 µg being equivalent to 1 µg of retinol. Other carotenoids are considered to have less activity; 12 µg is considered to be equivalent to 1 µg of retinol.

Function

- Vitamin A is essential for the production of rhodopsin in the rods of the retina. Exposure to light results in a series of changes in the configuration of rhodopsin, which leads to the adaptation of vision in the dark.
- Growth.
- Cell differentiation.
- Embryogenesis.
- Immune response.

Measurement

Biochemical assessment of vitamin A is controversial. The measurement of retinol concentration in serum or plasma is a useful and common measure of vitamin A status. Deficiency is indicated by values below 10 µg/dl (0.3 µmol/l) and values below 20 µg/dl (0.7 µmol/l) are marginal.

Deficiency

- Deficiency of vitamin A is rare in the UK but is common in Latin America, Africa, and Asia especially amongst children.
- Eye changes—night blindness presents when vitamin A status is marginal and, with prolonged or severe deficiency, changes to the cornea and conjunctiva occur. These eye changes are known collectively as xerophthalmia; these changes consist of conjunctival xerosis, Bitot's spots, corneal xerosis, corneal ulceration, and corneal scars
- Epithelial tissues-skin keratinization occurs in vitamin A deficiency. Horny plugs block the sebaceous glands leading to follicular hyperkeratosis.
- Immunity—vitamin A deficiency results in ↑ susceptibility to infectious diseases such as diarrhoea and respiratory infections.
- A deficiency of vitamin A can contribute to nutritional deficiency anaemia.

Requirement and intake (Table 5.22–5.24)

Fat is necessary for the absorption of vitamin A; as retinol is found in foods of animal origin some fat is usually consumed at the same time. Vitamin A absorption is impaired by mineral oils, neomycin, cholestyramine, and commercial fat replacers, e.g. olestra. A low vitamin A intake is associated with lower socio-economic class and low consumption of cereals, milk, eggs, and vegetables.

Toxicity

The early reports of vitamin A toxicity are from polar explorers who ate the polar bears' livers, which are particularly rich in vitamin A. Acute toxicity occurs when more than 200 mg (0.7 mmol) is consumed by adults or more than 100 mg in children. The acute symptoms of vitamin A toxicity include vomiting, abdominal pain, anorexia, blurred vision, headache, and irritability. Chronic toxicity can occur when 10 mg is consumed over periods of a month or more. Symptoms include headache, muscle and bone pain, ataxia, skin disorders, alopecia, liver toxicity, and hyperlipidaemia. Not all the chronic symptoms are reversible. Vitamin A is teratogenic and pregnancy intakes should not exceed 3 mg/d. There is no risk of toxicity from carotenoids in foods although large intakes can → yellow discoloration of the skin.

❶ Vitamin A supplements should not be taken during pregnancy (see Chapter 2).

Liver is not recommended during pregnancy.

Table 5.22 Reference nutrient intakes (RNI) for all ages and average daily intakes for adult men and women for vitamin A provided by food (μg retinol equivalent/d)*

Age (years)	RNI
0–1	350
1–3	400
4–10	500
11–14	600
Males 15+	700
Females 15+	600
Pregnancy	+100
Lactation	+350
	Average daily intake UK
Men	911
Women	671

* Source for RNIs, Department of Health (1991). *Dietary reference values for food and nutrients for the United Kingdom.* HMSO, London; source for average daily intakes for adults, Henderson, L., Irving, K., and Gregory, J. (2003). *The National Diet and Nutrition Survey: adults aged 19 to 64 years.* Vol. 3. *Vitamin and mineral intake and urinary analytes.* HMSO, London.

Table 5.23 Contribution of foods to vitamin A intake*

Food group	% Daily intake
Meat & meat products	28
Liver & liver products	21
Vegetables	27
Cooked carrots	12
Milk & milk products	14
Fat spreads	10

* source for average daily intakes for adults, Henderson, L., Irving, K., and Gregory, J. (2003). *The National Diet and Nutrition Survey: adults aged 19 to 64 years.* Vol. 3. *Vitamin and mineral intake and urinary analytes.* HMSO, London.

Table 5.24 Good food sources of vitamin A

Most concentrated sources of retinol in the diet
Liver and liver products
Kidney and offal
Oily fish and fish liver oils
Eggs
Most concentrated sources of β carotene in the diet
Carrots
Red peppers
Spinach
Broccoli
Tomatoes

Vitamin E

Eight naturally occurring forms of vitamin E are synthesized in plants: four tocopherols (alpha, α-, beta, β-; delta, δ-; and gamma, γ-) and four tocotrienols (α, β, δ, and γ). α tocopherol has the highest biological activity and is used as the standard against which the activity of other forms is measured. Synthetic vitamin E is a mixture of isomers and has biological activities ranging from 20% to 80% .

Function
- Antioxidant. Vitamin E is a powerful antioxidant and protects cell membranes and lipoproteins from damage by free radicals.
- Maintenance of cell membrane integrity.
- Regulation of prostaglandin synthesis.
- DNA synthesis.

Measurement Plasma concentration is the simplest measure and a direct indicator of status. Acceptable levels of intake are indicated by values of 5–20 μg/ml in adults and children aged 12 years and over, and 3–15 μg/ml for younger children.

Deficiency
Experimental, symptomatic vitamin E deficiency has not been induced in humans. Evidence for the essentiality of vitamin E in humans is provided by a genetically inherited disease familial isolated vitamin E (FIVE) deficiency. Sufferers develop reduced tendon reflexes by 3 to 4 years of age. By early adolescence they display symptoms of the nervous system including loss of touch and pain sensation, unsteady gait, loss of coordination, and impaired eye movement. In conditions which → chronic or severe fat malabsorption, cystic fibrosis, cholestatic liver disease, and abetalipoproteinaemia, similar symptoms may develop (especially in children) that can be corrected by vitamin E supplementation (5–25 IU/d).

Requirement and intake (Tables 5.25–5.27) Vitamin E requirements are influenced by the amount of polyunsaturated fatty acids (PUFA); it is estimated 0.4 mg α-tocopherol is required per gram dietary intake of PUFA. The average adult diet in the UK contains 7% energy from PUFA which would mean a vitamin E requirement of 6 mg for women and 8 mg for men. Milk formulas should not be <0.3 mg α-tocopherol equivalents/100 ml reconstituted feed and not <0.4 α-tocopherol equivalents/g PUFA.

Toxicity Vitamin E has low toxicity but at very high doses it acts as an antagonist to vitamins A, D, and K. Symptoms of toxicity include headache, nausea, muscle weakness, double vision, and creatinuria, and gastrointestinal disturbances have been reported at intakes greater than 900 mg per kg of the diet.

Table 5.25 Average daily intakes of vitamin E (mg) for adult men and women provided by food (α-tocopherol equivalents)*

	Average daily intake UK
Men	10.6
Women	8.1

* Henderson, L., Irving, K., and Gregory, J. (2003). The National Diet and Nutrition Survey: adults aged 19 to 64 years. Vol. 3. Vitamin and mineral intake and urinary anallytes. HMSO, London.

Table 5.26 Contribution of foods to vitamin E intake*

Food	% Daily intake
Fat spreads	18
PUFA reduced fat spread	8
Cereals & cereal products	17
Vegetables (excluding potatoes)	13
Potatoes & savoury snacks	13
Meat & meat products	11

* Henderson, L., Irving, K., and Gregory, J. (2003). The National Diet and Nutrition Survey: adults aged 19 to 64 years. Vol. 3. Vitamin and mineral intake and urinary anallytes. HMSO, London.

Table 5.27 Good food sources of vitamin E

Wheat germ oil
Almonds
Sunflower seeds & oil
Safflower oil
Hazelnuts
Peanuts & peanut butter
Corn oil

Vitamin D (calciferols)

The term vitamin D refers to two molecules, ergocalciferol (D_2) and cholecalciferol (D_3). Cholecalciferol is the most effective form of vitamin D and is manufactured in the skin by the action of ultraviolet radiation on 7-dehydrocholesterol. Dietary ergocalciferol and cholecalciferol are biologically inactive and are activated to 25-hydroxyvitamin D in the liver (this has a limited amount of biological activity). Further conversion in the kidney results in the production of the more active form 1,25-dihydroxyvitamin D (calcitrol).

Function

- 1,25-dihydroxyvitamin D maintains plasma Ca by controlling Ca absorption and excretion. Vitamin D and its metabolites are also involved in bone mineralization.
- Children with vitamin D deficiency (rickets) often have impaired immune function that is corrected by the administration of vitamin D.
- It has recently been postulated that vitamin D may inhibit cell proliferation in some forms of cancer.

Measurement

Vitamin D status is assessed by the measurement of plasma 25-hydroxyvitamin D, normal values above 27.5 nmol/l. Plasma vitamin D levels vary with the seasons, being highest in the summer and lowest in winter. Plasma Ca and phosphate fall in severe deficiency and alkaline phosphatase is elevated in mild and severe deficiency states.

Deficiency

Severe deficiency results in rickets in children, which is characterized by reduced calcification of bone epiphyses. It results in skeletal deformities, bone pain, and muscle weakness. In adults deficiency results in osteomalacia which leads to bone pain, and muscle weakness. People who stay indoors and are fully covered are at risk of deficiency due to lack of ultraviolet radiation from sunlight. Supplements are recommended for housebound elderly and some ethnic groups, e.g. Asian and Muslim women due to low sun exposure (see 'DRVs and dietary guidelines during pregnancy' in Chapter 9). Malabsorption ↑ the risk of deficiency.

Requirement and intake   See Tables 5.28–5.30.

Toxicity

Excessive exposure to sunlight does not → vitamin D toxicity as excess D_3 is converted to inert products. Overdose with supplements results in hypercalcaemia, which has symptoms of thirst and anorexia and is accompanied by the risk of soft tissue calcification and urinary Ca stones.

Table 5.28 Reference nutrient intakes (RNI) for all ages and average daily intakes of vitamin D for adult men and women provided by food (µg/d)*

Age (years)	RNI
0–6 months	8.5
7–12 months	7.0
1–3	7.0
4–65	0[†]
65+	10
Pregnancy	+10
Lactation	+10
	Average daily intake UK
Men	4.2
Women	3.7

* Source for RNI's Department of Health (1991). *Dietary reference values for food and nutrients for the United Kingdom*. HMSO, London; source for average daily intakes for adults, Henderson, L., Irving, K., and Gregory, J. (2003). *The National Diet and Nutrition Survey: adults aged 19 to 64 years*. Vol. 3. *Vitamin and mineral intake and urinary anallytes*. HMSO, London.
[†] Certain at risk groups or individuals may require dietary vitamin D.

Table 5.29 Contribution of foods to vitamin D intake*

Food group	% Daily intake
Fish & fish dishes	25
Oily fish	24
Meat & meat products	22
Cereals & cereal products	21
Fat spreads	17
Reduced fat spreads	8

* Source for average daily intakes for adults, Henderson, L., Irving, K., and Gregory, J. (2003). *The National Diet and Nutrition Survey: adults aged 19 to 64 years*. Vol. 3. *Vitamin and mineral intake and urinary anallytes*. HMSO, London.

Table 5.30 Good food sources of vitamin D

Cod liver oil
Oily fish (salmon, mackerel, etc.)
Milk
Margarine
Breakfast cereals
Eggs
Liver

Vitamin K

Naturally occurring vitamin K can be classified into two groups. The major form of vitamin K_1 (phylloquinine) is found in plants while the vitamin K_2 group of compounds (menaquinones) are synthesized by intestinal bacteria.

Function

- Vitamin K promotes the synthesis of γ-carboxyglutamic acid (Gla) in the liver. Gla is an essential part for prothrombin (factor II) and other coagulation factors (VII, IX, and X). Vitamin K is ∴ essential for blood coagulation.
- Other proteins contain Gla and require vitamin K for their synthesis. These include osteocalcin, a bone protein made by osteoblasts.

Measurement

Traditionally, vitamin K deficiency screening was based on coagulation assays of the levels of the active forms of coagulation proteins that require vitamin K. To entirely eliminate a diagnosis of congenital vitamin K deficiency it is necessary to conduct individual factor assays. It is now possible to assay for undercarboxylated vitamin K dependent proteins that are produced when vitamin K is in short supply or blocked by antagonists such as warfarin. A few specialist centres are now able to assay plasma and tissues levels directly by high performance liquid chromatography.

Deficiency

Vitamin K deficiency is characterized by poor blood clotting and results in low prothrombin activity. New born babies are given an injection of vitamin K at birth. Infants are born with very low stores and due to sterility of their intestines do not have bacteria producing vitamin K. Deficiency is rare in adults but does occur in patients with obstructive jaundice as lack of bile can → poor absorption of vitamin K. The anticoagulants warfarin and dicoumarol can → a deficiency as their mode of action is to block some of the enzymes that recycle vitamin K in the liver.

Requirement and intake (Table 5.31)

Studies into vitamin K requirements are not entirely satisfactory as it is difficult to induce deficiency solely by dietary manipulation. It is suggested that the requirements are between 0.5 and 1.0 µg per kg/d. Determination of vitamin K levels in foods and unreliability of estimates of intake in the UK means that a consensus on usual intake is not available. Studies in the USA suggest that intakes vary between 30 and 100 µg/d.

Toxicity

Large intakes of naturally occurring vitamin K do not appear to be toxic. Synthetic preparation of vitamin K_3 (menadione) is used to treat intracranial and pulmonary haemorrhage in premature infants and overdosage can → liver overload and brain toxicity.

❶ Supplements containing vitamin K should not be taken when taking anticoagulant drugs, e.g. warfarin (see 'Drug–nutrient interactions' in Chapter 8).

Table 5.31 Good food sources of vitamin K

Green leafy vegetables (spinach, broccoli, cabbage, & kale)
Vegetable oils especially soya bean oil
Eggs
Meat
Dairy products

Vitamin C (ascorbic acid)

Most animals can synthesize vitamin C from glucose or galactose; humans primates, guinea-pigs, Indian fruit-eating bats, and some birds lack this ability and it is an essential nutrient in these species. L-ascorbic acid and L-dehydroascorbic acid are both biologically active forms of vitamin C.

Function

Vitamin C is a powerful reducing agent (antioxidant) and is essential for many oxidation–reduction reactions.

- Vitamin C is required for the synthesis of collagen, the main protein in connective tissue and ∴ essential for the maintenance of muscles, tendons, arteries, bone, and skin. It is essential for the normal functioning of enzymes involved in collagen synthesis.
- The hydroxylation of dopamine to the neurotransmitter noradrenaline requires vitamin C.
- Vitamin C is required for the production of carnitine. Low levels of carnitine are associated with fatigue and muscle weakness.
- Various peptide hormones and releasing factors require activation by a vitamin C dependent enzyme.
- Numerous other enzymes need vitamin C; these enzymes control many functions including the synthesis of bile and the metabolism of drugs and carcinogens by the liver.
- Vitamin C enhances the absorption of Fe when consumed in the same meal.

Measurement   Vitamin C status is assessed by measurement in plasma and leucocytes; plasma levels are the most practical measure of status. Plasma levels <11 mmol/l show deficiency, >17 mmol/l are adequate. Leucocyte levels of >2.8 pmol/10^6 cells are adequate.

Deficiency   Vitamin C deficiency is uncommon except in populations where there is prolonged lack of fruit and vegetables. Deficiency of vitamin C is characterized by abnormalities of the connective tissue including poor wound healing which are described by the term scurvy. Weakness, fatigue, bleeding gums, and skin haemorrhages are symptoms of scurvy.

Requirement and intake (Tables 5.32–5.34)   Regular smoking ↑ vitamin C turnover and it is estimated that smokers require 80 mg/d.

Toxicity   High doses (1–10 g/day) of vitamin C are sometimes taken in the belief that such doses can prevent the common cold. There is no evidence to support this hypothesis although they may reduce the severity of symptoms to an extent. Sudden cessation of high dose supplements may precipitate rebound scurvy. Intakes at such high levels have been associated with diarrhoea and ↑ risk of kidney oxalate stone formation.

Table 5.32 Reference nutrient intakes (RNI) for all ages and average daily intakes for adult men and women for vitamin C provided by food (mg/d)*

Age (years)	RNI
0–1	25
1–10	30
11–14	35
Males 15+	40
Females 15+	40
Pregnancy	+10[†]
Lactation	+30
Average daily intake UK	
Men	83
Women	81

* Source for RNIs, Department of Health (1991). *Dietary reference values for food and nutrients for the United Kingdom*. HMSO, London; source for average daily intakes for adults, Henderson, L, Irving, K., and Gregory, J. (2003). *The National Diet and Nutrition Survey: adults aged 19 to 64 years*. Vol. 3 *Vitamin and mineral intake and urinary analytes*. HMSO, London.
[†] Last trimester only.

Table 5.33 Contribution of foods to vitamin C intake*

Food group	% Daily intake
Drinks	27
Fruit juice	19
Soft drinks inc. low calorie	8
Vegetables excluding potatoes	22
Fruit & nuts	19
Potatoes & savoury Snacks	15

* Source for average daily intakes for adults, Henderson, L., Irving, K., and Gregory, J. (2003). *The National Diet and Nutrition Survey: adults aged 19 to 64 years*. Vol. 3 *Vitamin and mineral intake and urinary analytes*. HMSO, London.

Table 5.34 Good food sources of vitamin C

Kiwi fruit
Citrus fruit (oranges, lemons, satsumas, clementines, etc.)
Black currants
Guava
Mango
Papaya
Pepper
Brussels sprouts
Broccoli
Sweet potato

Riboflavin (vitamin B$_2$)

Function

Riboflavin is part of two coenzymes that are both oxidizing agents: flavin mononucleotide (FMN) and flavin adenine dinucleotide (FAD). FMN and FAD are contained in flavoproteins, which are involved in many oxidation–reduction reactions in many metabolic pathways. The functions of riboflavin include:

- promotion of normal growth;
- assisting synthesis of steroids, red blood calls, and glycogen;
- maintenance of mucous membranes, skin, eyes, and the nervous system;
- aiding Fe absorption.

Measurement

Riboflavin status can be assessed by the measurement of urinary excretion or by measurement of erythrocyte glutathione reductase activity coefficient (EGRA). FAD is a co-factor for EGR and its activity is directly correlated to riboflavin status. EGRA is the method of choice as it reflects tissue saturation and long-term riboflavin status. Levels <1.3 are acceptable. Recently, doubts about the validity of EGRA in pregnancy and exercise have been expressed.

Deficiency

- Lesions of the mucosal surfaces of the mouth, angular stomatitis, cheilosis, glossitis and magenta tounge, surface lesions of the genitalia, seborrhoeic skin lesions, and vascularization of the cornea.
- Riboflavin deficiency is often accompanied by other nutrient deficiencies, e.g. pellagra.
- In animal studies deficiency is associated with poor growth of the young and it is probable that similar effects occur in human neonates.
- Severe deficiency is unlikely in the UK but the elderly, anorexia nervosa sufferers, and chronic 'dieters' are at risk.

Sources in the diet Riboflavin is unstable when exposed to ultraviolet light and up to 70% will be lost from milk during 4 hours exposure to sunlight.

Requirement and intake See Tables 5.35–5.37.

Toxicity Toxicity is low due to the small amount that can be absorbed by the gastrointestinal tract in a single dose.

Table 5.35 Reference nutrient intakes (RNI) for all ages and average daily intakes for adult men and women for riboflavin (mg/d)*

Age (years)	RNI
0–1	0.4
1–10	0.6–1.0
Males 11–14	1.2
Males 15+	1.3
Females 11+	1.1
Pregnancy	+0.3
Lactation	+0.5
Average daily intake UK	
Men	2.11
Women	1.60

* Source for RNIs, Department of Health (1991). *Dietary reference values for food and nutrients for the United Kingdom*. HMSO, London; source for average daily intakes for adults, Henderson, L., Irving, K., and Gregory, J. (2003). *The National Diet and Nutrition Survey: adults aged 19 to 64 years*. Vol. 3. *Vitamin and mineral intake and urinary analytes*. HMSO, London.

Table 5.36 Contribution of foods to riboflavin intake*

Food group	% Daily intake
Milk & milk products	33
Semi-skimmed milk	16
Cereals & cereal products	24
Meat & meat products	15
Drinks	10

* Source for average daily intakes for adults, Henderson, L., Irving, K., and Gregory, J. (2003). *The National Diet and Nutrition Survey: adults aged 19 to 64 years*. Vol. 3. *Vitamin and mineral intake and urinary analytes*. HMSO, London.

Table 5.37 Good food sources of riboflavin

Eggs
Milk and milk products
Liver & kidney
Yeast extracts
Fortified breakfast cereals

Niacin (nicotinamide, nicotinic acid)

Niacin is the generic term for a group of compounds that prevent pellagra. Nicotinamide and nicotinic acid both occur in food but have different physiological properties. Approximately 50% of niacin in the body is synthesized from the amino acid tryptophan. Sixty milligrams of tryptophan are equivalent to one milligram of niacin or 1 niacin equivalent (NE).

Function

Nicotinamide is incorporated into the pyridine nucleotide coenzymes nicotinamide adenine dinucleotide (NAD) and nicotinamide adenine dinucleotide phosphate (NADP). The coenzymes are involved in numerous oxidoreductase reactions including glycolysis, fatty acid metabolism, tissue respiration, and detoxification.

Measurement

Niacin status is most often assessed by the measurement of its metabolites N'-methylnicotinamide (NMN) and N'-methyl-2-pyridone-5-carboxamide. These metabolites are ↓ in niacin deficiency. A deficiency should be considered when the NMN to creatinine ratio is <1.5 mmol/mol. This assay requires 24 hour urine collection, which may be problematical. Other measures of niacin status include red cell NAD concentration and fasting plasma tryptophan.

Deficiency

Deficiency of niacin is known as pellagra and classically it is characterized by the three Ds.
- Dermatitis—skin that is exposed to the sun becomes inflamed, which progresses to pigmentation, cracking, and peeling. The neck is frequently involved and the distinctive distribution of skin lesions is known as Casal's collar.
- Diarrhoea—this is often accompanied by an inflamed tongue.
- Dementia—symptoms range from mild confusion and disorientation to mania, occasionally psychoses may occur that require hospitalization.

Pellagra is rare in the UK but still occurs in parts of Africa.

Requirement and intake   See Tables 5.38–5.40.

Toxicity   Nicotinic acid intakes of 200 mg/day → flushing due to vasodilatation, higher doses → dilatation of non-cutaneous vessels and can cause hypotension. Doses of 1–2 g/day are used in the treatment of hypertriglyceridaemia and hypercholesterolaemia. Larger doses (3–6 g/d) cause reversible liver toxicity with changes in liver function, carbohydrate tolerance, and uric acid metabolism.

Table 5.38 Reference nutrient intakes (RNI) for all ages and average daily intakes for adult men and women for niacin provided by food (mg niacin equivalent/1000 kcal)*

Age (years)	RNI
All ages	6.6
Lactation[†]	+2.3 mg/d
Average daily intake UK	
Men	911
Women	671

* Source for RNIs, Department of Health (1991). *Dietary reference values for food and nutrients for the United Kingdom.* HMSO, London; source for average daily intakes for adults, Henderson, L., Irving, K., and Gregory, J. (2003). *The National Diet and Nutrition Survey: adults aged 19 to 64 years.* Vol. 3. *Vitamin and mineral intake and urinary analytes.* HMSO, London.
[†] No increment is recommended during pregnancy.

Table 5.39 Contribution of foods to niacin intake*

Food group	% Daily intake
Meat & meat products	34
Chicken, turkey, & dishes inc. coated	15
Cereals & cereal products	27
White bread	7
Cheese	12

* Henderson, L., Irving, K., and Gregory, J. (2003). *The National Diet and Nutrition Survey: adults aged 19 to 64 years.* Vol. 3. *Vitamin and mineral intake and urinary analytes.* HMSO, London.
[†] No increment is recommended during pregnancy.

Table 5.40 Good food sources of niacin

Beef
Pork
Chicken
Wheat flour
Maize flour
Eggs
Milk

Thiamin

Function
Thiamin forms part of the coenzyme thiamine pyrophosphate (TPP), which is involved in major decarboxylation steps in the following pathways.
- Pyruvate → acetyl CoA at the entry to the citric acid cycle.
- α-Ketoglutarate → succinyl CoA, halfway round the citric acid cycle.
- Transketolase reactions in the hexose monophosphate shunt.
- Catabolism of branch chain amino acids, leucine, isoleucine, methionine and valine.
- Thiamin is needed for the metabolism of fat, carbohydrate, and alcohol.

Measurement
Red cell transketolase assay is the most frequently used measure of thiamin status. It is essential to use fresh, heparinized whole blood. Thiamin deficiency is indicated by ↑ in transketolase activity after the addition of TPP. Higher values indicate greater deficiency; in Wernicke's encephalopathy activity can be ↑ by 70–100%.

Deficiency
Thiamin deficiency manifests as beriberi and Wernicke–Korsakoff syndrome. Beriberi is usually classified as either 'wet' (cardiac) or 'dry' (neurological). They rarely occur together.
- Wet beriberi is the acute form of the disease and is characterized by high output cardiac failure, bounding pulse, warm extremities, peripheral oedema, and cardiac dilatation.
- Dry beriberi is the chronic form of the disease and is characterized by progressive, peripheral neuropathy. Foot drop is accompanied by loss of sensation in the feet and absent knee jerk reflexes.
- Wernicke–Korsakoff syndrome is seen in chronic alcoholics who have a poor diet. It is characterized by confusion, low levels of consciouness, and poor coordination (Wernicke's encephalopathy). Paralysis of one or more of the external movements of the eye is a diagnostic criteria. Memory loss (Korsakoff's psychosis) often follows the encephalopathy.

Requirement and intake See Tables 5.41–5.43. Thiamin requirements are related to energy metabolism.

Sources in the diet Thiamin is widely distributed in the diet. In the UK and many other industrialized countries bread flour is fortified with thiamine by law and in practice it is added to many breakfast cereals.

Toxicity Chronic intakes of more than 3 g/d are associated with symptoms of toxicity; these include headache, irritability, insomnia, weakness, tachycardia, and pruritis. Regular large intakes can → an allergic reaction.

Table 5.41 Reference nutrient intakes (RNI) for all ages and average daily intakes for adult men and women for thiamin provided by food (mg/1000 kcal)*

Age (years)	RNI
0–12 months	0.3
1–50 +	0.4[†]
Average daily intake UK	
Men	2.00 mg/d
Women	1.54 mg/d

* Source for RNIs, Department of Health (1991). *Dietary reference values for food and nutrients for the United Kingdom*. HMSO, London; source for average daily intakes for adults, Henderson, L., Irving, K., and Gregory, J. (2003) *The National Diet and Nutrition Survey: adults aged 19 to 64 years*. Vol. 3. *Vitamin and mineral intake and urinary analytes*. HMSO, London.
[†]No increment for pregnancy or lactation.

Table 5.42 Contribution of foods to thiamin intake*

Food group	% Daily intake
Cereals & cereal products	34
White bread	9
Meat & meat products	21
Vegetables excluding potatoes	15
Potatoes & savoury snacks	13

* Source for RNIs, Department of Health (1991). *Dietary reference values for food and nutrients for the United Kingdom*. HMSO, London; source for average daily intakes for adults, Henderson, L., Irving, K., and Gregory, J. (2003) *The National Diet and Nutrition Survey: adults aged 19 to 64 years*. Vol. 3. *Vitamin and mineral intake and urinary analytes*. HMSO, London.

Table 5.43 Good food sources of thiamin

Cereal products (including breakfast cereals and bread)
Yeast and yeast products
Pulses
Nuts
Pork & other meats
Vegetables
Milk

Folate (folic acid)

Folic acid (pteroyl glutamic acid) is the synthetic form of the vitamin and is the parent molecule for a number of derivatives known as folates. Folic acid is a very stable molecule with high biological activity. It is used in the fortification of foods and in supplements. Folates occur naturally as a number of tetrahydrofolates, which have variable biological activities.

Function
- Folates are involved in a number of single carbon transfer reactions particularly in the synthesis of purines, pyrimidines, glycine, and methionine. It is ∴ essential for the synthesis of DNA and RNA.
- The folate derivative 5-methyl tetrahydrofolate requires vitamin B_{12} to enable the use of methionine synthase in the synthesis of methionine and tetrahydrofolate.

Measurement Recent intake is assessed by serum folate; normal levels are 2.0–11.0 µg/l Cellular status is reflected by red cell folate; normal levels are 150–700 µg/l.

Deficiency Dietary deficiency is seen occasionally but secondary deficiency is fairly common. Secondary deficiency can result from malabsorption, the use of certain drugs, and in late pregnancy and some disease states including leukaemia. Deficiency results in megaloblastic anaemia with abnormal neutrophil nuclei and giant platelets. There may also be infertility and diarrhoea.

Benefits of extra folate
Folate supplements in early pregnancy (before the neural tube closes at 24–28 days) have been shown to reduce neural tube defects (see 'Preconceptional and periconceptual nutrition', in Chapter 9).

Large doses (200 µ/day) reduce plasma levels of homocysteine. Raised plasma homocysteine is a risk factor for cardiovascular disease.

Requirement and intake See Tables 5.44–5.46.

Toxicity The toxicity of folates is low. Folate supplements given to patients with developing vitamin B_{12} deficiency may obscure diagnosis.

Drug interactions Chronic use of anticonvulsants has been associated with folate deficiency. Other drugs that interfere with folate metabolism include cytotoxic chemotherapy agents (methotrexate, aminopterin) and antimalarial (pyrimethamine) and antibacterial (co-trimoxazole) agents.

Table 5.44 Reference nutrient intakes (RNI) and average daily intakes for adult men and women for folate provided by food (μg/d)*

Age (years)	RNI
0–1	50
1–3	70
4–6	100
7–10	150
Males 11+	200
Females 11+	200
Pregnancy	+100[†]
Average daily intake UK	
Men	344
Women	251

* Source for RNIs, Department of Health (1991). *Dietary reference values for food and nutrients for the United Kingdom.* HMSO, London; source for average daily intakes for adults,
[†] To prevent first occurrence of NTD: 400 μg during preconception and until the 12th week of pregnancy (on prescription or over the counter). To prevent recurrence of NTD: 5000 μg during preconception and until the 12th week of pregnancy (on prescription only).

Table 5.45 Contribution of foods to folate intake*

Food group	% Daily intake
Cereals & cereal products	33
Whole grain and high fibre breakfast cereals	8
Vegetables excluding potatoes	15
Drinks	14
Potatoes & savoury snacks	12

* Henderson, L., Irving, K., and Gregory, J. (2003) *The National Diet and Nutrition Survey: adults aged 19 to 64 years.* Vol. 3. *Vitamin and mineral intake and urinary analytes* HMSO, London.

Table 5.46 Good food sources of folate

Rich sources >100 μg per serving: Brussels sprouts, kale, spinach

Good sources 50–100 μg per serving: fortified bread and breakfast cereals, broccoli, cabbage, cauliflower, chickpeas, green beans, icebergs, lettice, kidneys, beans, peas, spring greens

Moderate sources 15–15 μg per serving: potatoes, most other vegetables, most fruits, most nuts, brown rice, wholegrain pasta, oats, bran, some breakfast cereals, cheese, yoghurt, milk, eggs, salmon, beef, game

Vitamin B$_6$

There are three naturally occurring forms of vitamin B$_6$: pyridoxine, pyridoxal, and pyridoxamine. These three vitamers are interconvertible in the body.

Function

The three vitamers can be converted to the coenzyme pyridoxal-5-phosphate which is involved in amino acid metabolism. These reactions include:

- transamination of amino acids to produce keto acids and synthesis of non-essential amino acids;
- decarboxylation to yield biologically active amines, e.g., neurotransmitters (adrenaline, noradrenaline, serotonin, and γ–amino butyric acid) and histamine;
- porphyrin synthesis, including haemoglobin.

Vitamin B$_6$ is also involved in the conversion of glycogen to glucose in muscles, the conversion of tryptophan to niacin, and in hormone metabolism.

Measurement   Vitamin B$_6$ status can be assessed by the measurement of plasma concentrations of pyridoxal phosphate (normal values are above 30 nmol/l) or total vitamin B$_6$. Activation of erthyrocyte transaminases can be a useful measure. Metabolism of test doses of methionine can be used but is technically difficult.

Deficiency   Severe deficiency of vitamin B$_6$ is rare. One outbreak was reported in 1954 due to errors in the manufacture of infant's formula feed. The affected infants suffered seizures that responded to treatment with vitamin B$_6$. Patients suffering malabsorption, receiving dialysis, or alcoholics are at risk of deficiency. Clinical signs include lesions of the lips and corners of the mouth and inflammation of the tongue. Peripheral neuropathy may be a sign of vitamin B$_6$ deficiency but as vitamin B$_6$ deficiency is usually associated with other vitamin deficiency the neuropathy may be the result of thiamin deficiency. Sideroblastic (microcytic, hypochromic) anaemia due to poor haem synthesis is associated with vitamin B$_6$ deficiency.

Requirement and intake (Tables 5.47–5.49)   Due to the importance of vitamin B$_6$ in amino acid metabolism requirements are linked to protein intake.

Toxicity   Intakes of 500 mg/d and above have been associated with peripheral neuropathy and loss of sensation in the feet has been reported at higher doses (from supplements). The DH recommends that the daily dose of vitamin B$_6$ should not exceed 10 mg/d.

Drug interactions   Urinary excretion of vitamin B$_6$ is ↑ by isoniazid (used to treat tuberculosis). Penicillamine, L-dopa, and cycloserine are vitamin B$_6$ antagonists.

Table 5.47 Reference nutrient intakes (RNI) for all ages and average daily intakes for adult men and women for vitamin B_6 provided by food (µg/g protein)*

Age (years)	RNI
0–6 months	8
7–9 months	10
10–12 months	13
1–50 +	15†
Average daily intake UK	
Men	33
Women	31

* Source for RNIs, Department of Health (1991). *Dietary reference values for food and nutrients for the United Kingdom*. HMSO, London; source for average daily intakes for adults, Henderson, L., Irving, K., and Gregory, J. (2003) *The National Diet and Nutrition Survey: adults aged 19 to 64 years*. Vol. 3. *Vitamin and mineral intake and urinary analytes*. HMSO, London.
† No increment is recommended for pregnancy or lactation.

Table 5.48 Contribution of foods to vitamin B_6 intake*

Food group	% Daily intake
Cereals & cereal products	21
Meat & meat products	21
Potatoes & savoury snacks	19
Drinks	11
Beer & lager	8

* Source for RNIs, Department of Health (1991). *Dietary reference values for food and nutrients for the United Kingdom*. HMSO, London; source for average daily intakes for adults, Henderson, L., Irving, K., and Gregory, J. (2003) *The National Diet and Nutrition Survey: adults aged 19 to 64 years*. Vol. 3. *Vitamin and mineral intake and urinary analytes*. HMSO, London.

Table 5.49 Good food sources of vitamin B_6

Meat
Wholegrain cereals
Fortified cereals
Bananas
Nuts
Pulses

Cobalamin B$_{12}$

Cobalamin is a complex molecule that contains cobalt; it occurs naturally in usual forms. Cyanocobalamin is the commercially available form, which is converted to the natural forms. It requires salivary haptocorrin and 'intrinsic factor' to be absorbed. 'Intrinsic factor' is secreted by the parietal cells of the stomach.

Function

The functions of vitamin B$_{12}$ include:
- recycling of folate coenzymes;
- normal myelination of nerves;
- synthesis of methionine from homocysteine.

Measurement Serum B$_{12}$ status is assessed by radioligand binding or microbiological assay. Levels >150 pmol/l are considered normal. Absorption of B$_{12}$ is assessed by the Schilling test. Absorption of vitamin B$_{12}$ labelled with radioactive cobalt is measured with and without 'intrinsic factor'.

Deficiency

Vitamin B$_{12}$ does not occur in plant foods and ∴ vegans and strict vegetarians are at risk of deficiency. Few exhibit deficiency symptoms as vitamin B$_{12}$ is also manufactured by intestinal bacteria. Children on macrobiotic diets are at particular risk. The most common cause of deficiency is malabsorption due to atrophy of the gastric mucosa, which leads to inadequate production of 'intrinsic factor' or diseases of the ileum. Deficiency results in pernicious anaemia (megaloblastic) and/or neurological problems. The anaemia is morphologically the same as that seen in folate deficiency and biochemical tests are necessary to establish the cause. The neuropathy is characterized by loss of sensation and motor power in the lower limbs due to degeneration of myelin. Deficiency is easily corrected by monthly injections (100 µg/m).

Sources in the diet Vitamin B$_{12}$ is synthesized by micro-organisms and assimilated into the food chain. It occurs naturally in animal products but it can be found in fortified foods such as breakfast cereals.

Requirement and intake See Tables 5.50–5.52.

Toxicity Toxicity has not been reported in humans.

Table 5.50 Reference nutrient intakes (RNI) for all ages and average daily intakes for adult men and women for B_{12} provided by food ($\mu g/d$)*

Age (years)	RNI
0–1	0.3–0.4
1–3	0.5
4–6	0.8
7–10	1.0
11–14	1.2
Males 15+	1.5
Females 15+	1.5
Lactation	+0.5[†]
Average daily intake UK	
Men	6.5
Women	4.8

* Source for RNIs, Department of Health (1991). Dietary reference values for food and nutrients for the United Kingdom. HMSO, London; source for average daily intakes for adults, Henderson, L., Irving, K., and Gregory, J. (2003). The National Diet and Nutrition Survey: adults aged 19 to 64 years. Vol. 3. Vitamin and mineral intake and urinary analytes. HMSO, London.
† No increment is recommended during pregnancy.

Table 5.51 Contribution of foods to vitamin B_{12} intake*

Food group	% Daily intake
Milk & milk products	36
Semi-skimmed milk	18
Meat & meat products	30
Fish & fish dishes	18
Oily fish	11

* Source for RNIs, Department of Health (1991). *Dietary reference values for food and nutrients for the United Kingdom.* HMSO, London; source for average daily intakes for adults, Henderson, L., Irving, K., and Gregory, J. (2003). *The National Diet and Nutrition Survey: adults aged 19 to 64 years.* Vol. 3. Vitamin and mineral intake and urinary analytes. HMSO, London.

Table 5.52 Good food sources of vitamin B_{12}

Meat and meat products
Eggs
Milk and dairy products
Fish and fish products
Yeast products & fortified vegetable extracts
Breakfast cereals (fortified)

Biotin

Of the eight isomers of biotin only D-biotin is biologically active. Biotin is made by bacteria and yeasts. Biotin is obtained from the diet and synthesized by endogenous bacteria in the colon.

Function Biotin is a coenzyme for several carboxylases involved in fatty acid synthesis and metabolism, gluconeogenesis, and the metabolism of branched chain amino acids.

Measurement Microbiological assays are available to measure biotin in whole blood or urine. The normal range in whole blood is 0.22–0.75 µg/ml.

Deficiency

Biotin deficiency is rare but has been reported in patients receiving total parenteral nutrition and should be added to the infusion solution. Deficiency is associated with a scaly dermatitis, glossitis, hair loss, anorexia, depression, and hypercholesterolaemia. It is possible to induce biotin deficiency by the ingestion of large amounts of raw egg white. Egg whites contain the protein avidin, which binds biotin and prevents absorption. The effect is prevented by heating the egg whites.

Requirement and intake See Tables 5.53 and 5.54. No studies are available on which recommendations on intake can be based. It is believed that intakes of between 10 and 200 µg/day are safe and adequate.

Toxicity There have been no reports of biotin toxicity.

Table 5.53 Average daily intakes for adult men and women for biotin (µg/d) in UK*

| Men | 41 |
| Women | 29 |

* Henderson, L., Irving, K., and Gregory, J. (2003). *The National Diet and Nutrition Survey: adults aged 19 to 64 years*. Vol. 3. *Vitamin and mineral intake and urinary analytes*. HMSO, London.

Table 5.54 Good food sources of biotin

| Liver |
| Kidney |
| Milk |
| Eggs |
| Dairy products |

Pantothenic acid

Function

- Pantothenic acid is part of coenzyme A (CoA) and as such is involved in the tricarboxylic acid cycle.
- The pantothenic acid derivative 4'-phosphopantetheine is part of acyl carrier protein.
- It is essential for reactions involved in carbohydrate and lipid metabolism.

Measurement Pantothenic acid can be measured in blood and urine. Normal urinary excretion is 1–15 mg/day and normal blood values are >100 µg/dl.

Deficiency

Spontaneous deficiency of pantothenic acid has not been described. It is possible to induce a deficiency with experimental diets or by administration of the antagonist ω-methylpantothenic acid. During World War II malnourished prisoners in the Far East developed 'burning feet' parathaesiae which responded to treatment with pantothenic acid.

The symptoms of deficiency include a burning sensation in the feet, depression, fatigue, vomiting, and muscle weakness.

Requirement and intake See Tables 5.55 and 5.56. Information is not available to derive recommended intakes but intake of 3–7 mg/d is considered adequate.

Sources in the diet Pantothenic acid is widely distributed in food but highly processed foods do not contain the vitamin.

Toxicity There are no specific toxic effects although large doses may cause gastrointestinal symptoms such as diarrhoea.

Table 5.55 Average daily intakes of pantothenic acid provided by food (mg/d) in UK*

Men	7.2
Women	5.4

* Henderson, L., Irving, K., and Gregory, J. (2003). *The National Diet and Nutrition Survey: adults aged 19 to 64 years.* Vol. 3. *Vitamin and mineral intake and urinary analytes.* HMSO, London.

Table 5.56 Good food sources of pantothenic acid

Yeast
Offal
Peanuts
Meat
Eggs
Green vegetables

Minerals and trace elements: introduction

Table 5.57 shows the minerals and trace elements known to be essential to humans. Fl is semi-essential in that no physiological requirement is known to exist but there are known beneficial effects. Minerals are required in grams or milligrams while trace elements are required in microgram amounts. Elements that are of biological importance but are not currently considered essential include nickel, vanadium, cobalt, and boron.

Criteria for essentiality of minerals and trace elements

- Present in healthy tissues.
- Concentration must be relatively constant between different organisms.
- Deficiency induces specific biochemical changes.
- Deficiency changes are accompanied by equivalent abnormalities in different species.
- Supplementation corrects the abnormalities.

Table 5.57 Essential minerals and trace minerals

Minerals	Trace elements
Calcium	Copper
Phosphorus	Chromium
Magnesium	Manganese
Sodium	Molybdenum
Potassium	Selenium
Iron	Iodine
Zinc	
Fluorine	

Calcium (Ca)

Ca is the most abundant mineral in the human body (1.4 g/kg) and 99% is deposited, usually as hydroxyapatite, in bones and teeth where it provides structural rigidity. Ca plasma levels are tightly controlled by parathyroid hormone, 1,25 dihydroxycholecalciferol, and calcitonin. Plasma Ca levels are also controlled by the vitamin D metabolite $1,25(OH)_2D_3$ which controls the active absorption of calcium from the intestine and osteoclastic resorption of bone. Causes of abnormal Ca plasma concentrations are shown in Table 5.58.

Function

- Structural rigidity of bones and teeth, as hydroxyapatite.
- Intracellular signalling control of muscles and nerves.
- Blood clotting.
- Co-factor for enzymes, e.g. lipase.

Measurement

The normal plasma range for Ca is 2.15–2.55 mmol/l and 50% of plasma Ca is bound to protein, principally albumin; ∴ plasma value is frequently given as a corrected value. Plasma Ca levels are tightly controlled and are not usually affected by dietary insufficiency in healthy adults. Hypocalcaemia results in symptoms such as tetany and cardiac arrhythmias. Bone mineral concentration can be measured by neutron activation analysis and dual X-ray absorptiometry can be used to directly measure bone mineral density.

Deficiency

In early adulthood Ca deficiency can → stunted growth and failure to achieve peak bone mass. Peak bone mass is achieved in early adulthood and is determined by genetic factors, use of the skeleton, and nutritional factors including Ca intake. Failure to achieve peak bone mass is a risk factor for osteoporosis in later life. Poor Ca absorption due to vitamin D deficiency leads to rickets in children (see 'Vitamin D (calciferols)', this chapter).

Requirement and intake   See Table 5.59.

Sources in the diet   See Tables 5.60 and 5.61. Ca absorption is variable; Ca in milk and dairy foods is more readily absorbed than Ca in plants. The presence of phytates in cereals and oxalates in leafy green vegetables inhibits absorption.

Toxicity   Accumulation in blood and tissues due to dietary excess is virtually unknown due to the tight homeostatic control of Ca. Hypercalcaemia is usually the result of an abnormality in this control as shown in Table 5.58. Milk alkali syndrome (MAS) results from excessive intake of Ca and alkali as antacid tablets, Ca supplements, and milk (which provides vitamin D and → ↑ absorption). MAS has been reported at Ca carbonate intakes of ≥4 g/d or more. A rare cause of MAS is excessive intake of Ca by the ingestion of betel nut paste containing oyster shells. Intakes of up to 2 g of Ca /d have been shown to be safe.

Table 5.58 Causes of abnormal plasma Ca*

Hypercalcaemia	Hypocalcaemia
Malignant disease	Vitamin D deficiency
Primary hyperparathyroidism	Hypoparathyroidism (and pseudohypoparathyroidism)
Sarcoidosis (and other granulomas)	
Vitamin D overdose	
Milk alkali syndrome	
Immobilization	
Thyrotoxicosis	
Hypercalcaemia of infancy	
Familial hypocalciuric hypercalcaemia	

* Reproduced from Human Nutrition and Dietetics. Garrow, JS., James, WPT., and Ralph, A. table 17.1, p.135. With permission from Elsevier.

Table 5.59 Reference nutrient intakes for Ca (mg/d) for all ages and average daily intakes (mg) for adult men and women provided by food*

Age (years) [†]	RNI
0–12 months	525
1–3 years	350
46–years	450
7–10 years	550
Men	
11–18 years	1 000
19 + years	700
Women	
11–18 years	800
19 + years	700
Lactation	+ 550
Average daily intake UK	
Men	1007
Women	777

* Source for RNIs, Department of Health (1991). *Dietary reference values for food and nutrients for the United Kingdom*. HMSO, London; source for average daily intakes for adults, Henderson, L., Irving, K., and Gregory, J. (2003). *The National Diet and Nutrition Survey: adults aged 19 to 64 years*. Vol.3. *Vitamin and mineral intake and urinary analytes*. HMSO, London.
[†] There is no recommendation for an increase in Ca intake during pregnancy, Ca absorption ↓ during pregnancy.

Table 5.60 Contribution of foods to Ca intake (NDNS)*

Food group	% Daily intake
Milk & milk products	43
Semi skimmed milk	17
Cheese	11
Cereals & cereal products	30
White bread	13

* Henderson, L., Irving, K., and Gregory, J. (2003). The National Diet and Nutrition Survey: adults aged 19 to 64 years. Vol.3. Vitamin and mineral intake and urinary analystes. HMSO, London.

Table 5.61 Food and portions that provide approximately 100 mg Ca

85 ml milk
15 g cheddar cheese
50 g yoghurt
100 g cottage cheese
20 g sardines
200 g baked beans
3 large slices white bread
125 g pulses (e.g. chickpeas)
20 g tofu
15 g tahini

Phosphorus (P)

Phosphate is present in every cell in the body although 80–85 % is found with Ca in hydroxyapatite.

Function
- Skeletal rigidity as the Ca compound hydroxyapatite.
- Energy for metabolism is derived from the phosphate bonds in adenosine triphosphate (ADP).
- Constituent of phospholipids and membranes.
- Constituent of nucleic acids.

Measurement   Serum total phosphate levels are measured by colorimetric methods. The normal adult range is 0.7–1.5 mmol/l.

Deficiency   P deficiency is unlikely to occur as it is present in all plant and animal foods. Hypophosphataemia does occur in poorly managed parenteral nutrition and re-feeding syndrome. Some studies have shown that P deficiency at birth is linked to rickets at a later age. Hypophosphataemia can occur in sepsis, liver disease, alcoholism, diabetic ketoacidosis, and excessive use of aluminium-containing antacids.

Requirement and intake   See Tables 5.62 and 5.63 Dietary requirements for P are equal to those for Ca, i.e. 1 mg P:1 mg Ca or l mmol P: 1 mmol Ca.

Sources in the diet   Phosphate is present in all natural foods and is present in many additives. Good sources are shown in Table 5.64. Absorption is approximately 60% of intake; it is ↓ by non-starch polysaccharides (NSP). NSP rich diets are also rich in phosphate so compensating for the reduction in absorption.

Toxicity   Intakes above 70 mg/kg body weight may → high serum levels that are above any likely to be taken in foods. Generally ↑ intakes are balanced by ↑ excretion in urine; this is disrupted in renal patients (see Chapter 24). The P:Ca ratio should not be above 2.2 mg P to 1 mg of Ca.

Table 5.62 Reference nutrient intakes for P (which are equivalent to those for Ca (mg/d) for all ages and average daily intakes (mg) for adult men and women provided by food*

Age	RNI
0–12 months	525
1–3 years	350
4–6 years	450
7–10 years	550
Men	
11–18 years	1000
19 + years	700
Women	
11–18 years	800
19 + years	700
Lactation	+550
Average daily intake UK	
Men	1493
Women	1112

* Source for RNIS, Department of Health (1991). *Dietary reference values for food and nutrients for the United Kingdom*. HMSO, London; source for average daily intakes for adults, Henderson, L., Irving, K., and Gregory, J. (2003). *The National Diet and Nutrition Survey: adults aged 19 to 64 years*. Vol. 3. *Vitamin and mineral intake and urinary analytes*. HMSO, London.

Table 5.63 Contribution of foods to P intake (NDNS)*

Food group	% Daily intake
Milk & milk products	24
Semi-skimmed milk	9
Cereals & cereal products	23
White bread	5
Breakfast cereals	5
Meat & meat products	21

* Henderson, L., Irving, K., and Gregory, J. (2003). *The National Diet and Nutrition Survey: adults aged 19 to 64 years*. Vol. 3. *Vitamin and mineral intake and urinary analytes*. HMSO, London.

Table 5.64 Good food sources of P

Milk & dairy products except butter
Cereals and cereal products
Meat & meat products
Fish
Nuts
Fruits & vegetables

Iron (Fe)

There is approximately 4 g Fe in the body of an adult man of which 2.4
is present as haemoglobin; adult women have approximately 2.1 g of
which 1.6 g is haemoglobin. Haemoglobin consists of 4 units: each unit
contains 1 haem group and 1 protein chain. Fe is also present in the non-
haem form. Fe compounds in the body are shown in Table 5.65.

Transport and absorption

In the free state Fe is toxic; ∴ its transport and storage are closely
controlled. Fe is actively absorbed in the duodenum. When the body
needs Fe it passes directly through the mucosal cells and is transported by
transferrin, with Fe released from old red blood cells, to the bone marrow
(80%) and other tissues. If Fe is not required it is stored in the mucosal
cells as transferrin. It will be lost in faeces when the mucosal cells are
exfoliated. Excess Fe that is absorbed is stored as ferritin or haemosiderin
in the liver, spleen, or bone marrow. Fe can be mobilized from these
stores when demand is ↑. Haem Fe is absorbed directly into the mucosa
cells where Fe is released by haem oxidase and then bound to transferrin.
Haem Fe represents 10–15% of Fe intake but contributes ≥40% total Fe
absorbed (Fig. 5.6). Non-haem Fe is poorly absorbed (1–20% of the total
absorbed) and is influenced by dietary constituents (see Table 5.66).

Table 5.65 Fe compounds in the body (mg)

	Man (75 kg)	Woman (55 kg)
Functional Fe		
Haemoglobin	2400	1600
Myoglobin	350	230
Haem & non-haem enzymes	150	110
Transferrin-bound Fe	3	2
Total functional Fe	~2900	~1940
Storage Fe		
Ferritin & haemosiderin	500–1500	0–300
Total Fe	~4000	~2100

Table 5.66 Factors influencing Fe absorption

		Increased absorption	Decreased absorption
Haem	Physiological factors	Low Fe status	High Fe status
	Dietary factors	Low haem intake Meat	High haem intake Ca Tannins
Non-haem	Physiological factors	Depleted Fe stores Pregnancy Disease states (aplastic anaemia, haemolytic anaemia, haemochromatosis)	Replete Fe stores Achlorhydria
	Dietary factors	Vitamin C Meat, fish, seafood Organic acids: ascorbic, citric, lactic, malic, tartaric	Phytate Fe-binding phenolic compounds Inorganic elements: Ca, Mn, Cu, Cd, Co

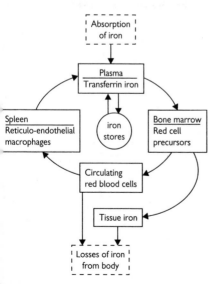

Fig. 5.6 Schematic representation of Fe metabolism.

Function

As haemoglobin:
- transport of oxygen;
- cell respiration.

As myoglobin:
- oxygen storage in muscles.

Other functions:
- component of enzymes, including those involved in immune functions, and cytochromes, which are essential for energy production.

Measurement

Fe deficiency develops in 3 stages and measurements are appropriate to each stage.
- Fe depletion—Fe stores are depleted and serum ferritin levels will fall below 12 µg/l. Other measures of Fe status will be normal.
- Fe deficient erythropoiesis—Fe stores are depleted and supply does not meet needs for haemoglobin production. Serum ferritin levels will be low, serum Fe concentration is low, and transferrin saturation is <16%. Haemoglobin within normal range.
- Fe deficiency anaemia—haemoglobin levels <11.5 mg/l in women and <13 mg/l in men. Red cells are microcytic and hypochromic. Mean corpuscular volume (MCV) <77 fl and mean cell haemoglobin (MCH) <27 pg.

Requirement and intake   See Table 5.67 and 5.68.

Table 5.67 Reference nutrient intakes for Fe (mg/d) for all ages and average daily intakes (mg) for adult men and women provided by food (NDNS)*

Age[†]	RNI
0–3 months	1.7
4–6 months	4.3
7–12 moths	7.8
1–3 years	6.9
4–6 years	6.1
7–10 years	8.7
Men	
11–18 years	11.3
19–50 + years	8.7
Women	
11–50 years	14.8
50 + years	8.7
Average daily intake UK	
Men	13.2
Women	10.0

*Source for RNIs, Department of Health (1991). *Dietary reference values for food and nutrients of the United Kingdom.* HMSO, London; source for average daily intakes for adults, Henderson, L., Irving, K., and Gregory, J. (2003). *The National Diet and Nutrition Survey: adults aged 19 to 64 years.* Vol.3. *Vitamin and mineral intake and urinary analytes.* HMSO, London.
[†] There is no recommendation for pregnancy and lactation as women should have enough Fe stores which will be enhanced by increased absorption and cessation of menstruation. Women with low Hb levels at the start of pregnancy may require supplementation.

Table 5.68 Contribution of foods to Fe intake (NDNS)*

Food group	% Daily intake
Cereals & cereal products	44
Whole grain & high fibre breakfast cereals	13
Meat & meat products	17
Vegetables excluding potatoes	10

* Henderson, L., Irving, K., and Gregory, J. (2003). *The National Diet and Nutrition Survey: adults aged 19 to 64 years.* Vol. 3. *Vitamin and mineral intake and urinary analytes.* HMSO, London.

Deficiency

Fe deficiency anaemia (IDA) is the most common nutritional deficiency i the world. It is estimated that up to 30% of women have IDA, wit prevalence of ~8% in developed countries (see sections on 'Iron def ciency anaemia' in Chapters 10–12 and 'Is a vegetarian diet risky fo health?' in Chapter 13). Up to 15% of pregnant women are Fe deficier (see 'Dietary problems in pregnancy' in Chapter 9).

Physical signs include:

- Pallor of finger nails and mucous membranes in the mouth and under eyelids;
- Tachycardia and in severe cases oedema;
- Fatigue, breathlessness on exertion, insomnia, giddiness, anorexia;
- Paraesthesia of fingers and toes.

Sources in the diet   See Tables 5.69 and 5.70.

Toxicity

Due to the tight metabolic control dietary excess does not occur. F poisoning can occur due to overdose of supplements: the lethal dose i children is 200–300 mg/kg body weight and approximately 100 g in adult High doses of Fe supplements cause gastrointestinal symptoms especiall constipation although nausea, vomiting, and diarrhoea may occur. Th absorption of other micronutrients, e.g. Zn, are reduced by high dose F supplements.

The hereditary disease primary idiopathic haemochromatosis is charac terized by high levels of Fe being absorbed. Fe deposits in the liver an heart and may → cirrhosis, liver cancer, congestive heart failure, an eventually death. Treatment requires regular blood removal.

Table 5.69 Dietary sources of Fe

Very good sources

Meat especially offal*

Fish

Eggs

Meat extracts

Good sources

Bread & flour

Breakfast cereals

Vegetables (dark green) & pulses

Nuts & dried fruit—prunes, figs, apricots

Yeast extract

* Liver is not recommended in pregnancy due to its high vitamin A content.

Table 5.70 Fe content of 50 g portions of foods

Food	Fe (mg)
Liver—cooked*	5
Liver pate	3
Roast or corned beef	1
Boiled egg	1
Sardines in tomato sauce	2
Wholemeal bread—1 slice	1
Bran flakes—30 g	6
Baked beans	1
Frozen peas	1
Lentils—cooked	1.5
Dark green leafy vegetables—cooked	0.5
Dried apricots	2
Tofu	0.5
Dry roasted peanuts	1

*Liver is not recommended in pregnancy due to its high vitamin A content.

Zinc (Zn)

Function

- There are more than 200 Zn enzymes in plant and animal tissues including alcohol dehydrogenase, alkaline phosphatase, aldolase, and RNA polymerase. Zn is ∴ involved in digestion, carbohydrate metabolism, bone metabolism, and oxygen transport and it is a powerful antioxidant.
- Zn is important in the immune response.
- It has other vital functions including structural properties in some proteins. Zn stabilizes the structure of DNA, RNA, and ribosomes; it has a vital role in gene expression.

Measurement

<0.1% of the body's Zn is present in the blood and its measurement in plasma is not a good measure of Zn status. The measurement of thymulin activity is increasingly being used although it is labour-intensive and ∴ not widely available. Thymulin promotes T-lymphocyte maturation and requires Zn for it to be active. Zn supplementation and observation of the subject's response is the most reliable method of diagnosing deficiency.

Deficiency

- Severe deficiency results in growth retardation, failure to thrive, delayed sexual maturation.
- Sore throat and immune defects.
- Circumoral and acral dermatitis.
- Diarrhoea: Zn supplementation has been implemented in areas of the world where children are affected by persistent diarrhoea.
- Alopecia and neuropsychiatric symptoms.

Requirement and intake   See Tables 5.71 and 5.72.

Sources in the diet   See Table 5.73. Zn bioavailability is higher from animal sources than from cereals which contain phytate. Bioavailability estimated to be 50–55% for an omnivorous diet in the UK; vegetarian and vegan diets have an estimated bioavailability of 30–35%.

Toxicity   Zn toxicity can occur following ingestion of water that has been stored in galvanized tanks or if this water is used for renal dialysis. Acute ingestion of 2 grams or more of Zn results in nausea, vomiting, and fever. Intakes of 50 mg of Zn have been shown to interfere with Cu and Fe metabolism. Chronic intakes of 75–300 mg/d have been associated with symptoms of Cu deficiency including microcytic anaemia and neutropenia.

Table 5.71 Reference nutrient Intakes for Zn (mg/d) for all ages and average daily intakes (mg) for adult men and women provided by food (NDNS)*

Age[†]	RNI
0–6 months	4.0
7 months–3 years	5.0
4–6 years	6.5
7–10 years	7.0
11–14 years	9.0
Males	
15+ years	9.5
Females	
15+ years	7.0
Lactation	
0–4 months	+6.0
4+ months	+2.5
Average daily intake UK	
Men	10.2
Women	7.4

*Source for RNIs, Department of Health (1991). *Dietary reference values for food and nutrients for the United Kingdom.* HMSO, London; source for average daily intakes for adults, Henderson, L., Irving, K., and Gregory, J. (2003). *The National Diet and Nutrition Survey: adults aged 19 to 64 years.* Vol. 3. *Vitamin and mineral intake and urinary analytes.* HMSO, London.
[†]No increase is recommended in pregnancy.

Table 5.72 Contribution of foods to Zn intake (NDNS)*

Food group	% Daily intake
Meat & meat products	34
Beef, veal, & dishes	11
Turkey, chicken, & dishes	5
Cereals & cereal products	25.5
White bread	6
Breakfast cereals	5
Milk & milk products	17
Cheese	6
Semi-skimmed milk	6

*Henderson, L., Irving, K., and Gregory, J. (2003). *The National Diet and Nutrition Survey: adults aged 19 to 64 years.* Vol. 3. *Vitamin and mineral intake and urinary analytes.* HMSO, London.

Table 5.73 Food sources of Zn

Source	Food
Very rich	Lamb, leafy & root vegetables, crabs & shellfish, beef, offal
Rich	Whole grains, pork, poultry, milk and milk products, eggs, nuts

Copper (Cu)

An adult has 80 mg of Cu in their body, 40% of which is present in muscle, 15% in the liver, 10% in the brain, and 6% in blood.

Function Cu is incorporated in many metallo-enzymes, which are shown in Table 5.74.

Measurement

A totally reliable, sensitive method of assessing Cu status has yet to be established. Plasma Cu and caeruloplasmin (Cu- containing protein that normally binds 90% of the Cu present in plasma) are frequently used they are both lowered in deficiency but they plateau as levels of Cu and do not reflect high intakes. Neither is very specific. Normal serum Cu levels are 12–26 µg/l but they are ↑ in late pregnancy and in women taking oestrogen-based contraceptives. Other methods include assessment of the activity of Cu enzymes in particular superoxide dismutase.

Deficiency

Cu deficiency is rare although it can occur in premature infants and in patients receiving total parenteral nutrition. Cu is accumulated in the fetus during the late stages of pregnancy and full term babies have large stores in the liver. ↑ Cu losses can occur in diseases such as cystic fibrosis, coeliac disease, and in children with chronic diarrhoea. Cu deficiency occurs in the hereditary condition Menkes disease in which Cu transport is impaired.

The symptoms of Cu deficiency are:
- Failure to thrive in babies;
- Oedema with low serum albumin;
- Fe resistant anaemia;
- Impaired immunity with low neutrophil count;
- Skeletal changes including fractures and osteoporosis;
- Abnormal blood vessels due to defects in collagen and elastin;
- Hair and skin hypopigmentation with steely, uncrimped hair;
- Neurological abnormalities.

Cu deficiency may be a risk factor for coronary heart disease as it has been associated with raised plasma cholesterol levels and heart-related abnormalities.

Table 5.74 Functions of Cu metallo-enzymes

Enzyme	Functions
Blue proteins	Electron transfers
Cytochrome- c oxidase	Electron transport: reduction of O_2 to H_2O
Caeruloplasmin (ferroxidase I)	Fe oxidation and transport
Superoxidase dismutase	Antioxidant
Dopamine-hydroxylase	Hydroxylation of dopa in the brain
Diamine and monamine oxidase	Removal of amines and diamines
Lysyl oxidase	Cross-inking in collagen and elastin, cardiovascular and bone integrity
Tyrosinase	Melanin formation
Chaperone proteins	Intracellular Cu transport
Chromatin scaffold proteins	Structural integrity of nuclear material
Clotting factors V, VIII	Thrombogenesis
Metallothionein	Metal sequestration
Nitrous oxide reductase	Reduction of NO_2^- to NO

From C.Reilly (2004), *The nutritional trace metals*, table 41, p120. Reproduced with permission from Blackwell Publishing.

Requirements and intake See Tables 5.75 and 5.76. No increment for pregnancy is recommended as any ↑ in demand is met by the mother's adaptive responses. The average intake is ↑ to 1.48 mg/d in men and 1.07 mg/d in women by the use of supplements.

Sources in the diet See Table 5.77. Bioavailability ranges from 35 to 70% and ↓ with age. The bioavailability of Cu in milk based formulae is approximately 50%.

Toxicity Cu toxicity occurs either by the deliberate ingestion of Cu salts or by drinking contaminated water. The symptoms of acute toxicity are nausea, vomiting, and diarrhoea and may be fatal in extreme cases. Chronic Cu poisoning, due to contamination by Cu water pipes or cooking utensils can → liver cirrhosis; infants and young children are particularly vulnerable. Wilson's disease is an inherited disease in which there is abnormal Cu transport that results in Cu accumulation in the liver, eyes brain, and kidneys and associated pathology.

Table 5.75 Reference nutrient intakes for Cu (mg/d) for all ages and average daily intakes (mg) for adult men and women provided by food*

Age[†]	RNI
0–12 months	0.3
1–3 years	0.4
4–6 years	0.6
7–10 years	0.7
11–14 years	0.8
15–16 years	1.0
18+ years	1.2
Pregnancy	+ 0.3
Average daily intake UK	
Men	1.43
Women	1.03

* Source for RNIs, Department of Health (1991). *Dietary reference values for food and nutrients for the United Kingdom*. HMSO, London; source for average daily intakes for adults, Henderson, L., Irving, K., and Gregory, J. (2003). *The National Diet and Nutrition Survey: adults aged 19 to 64 years*. Vol. 3. *Vitamin and mineral intake and urinary analytes*. HMSO, London
[†]No increase is recommended in pregnancy.

Table 5.76 Contribution of foods to Cu intake (NDNS)*

Food group	% Daily intake
Cereals & cereal products	31
White bread	8
Meat & meat products	15
Potatoes & savoury snacks	10
Fruits	10

* Henderson, L., Irving, K., and Gregory, J. (2003). The National Diet and Nutrition Survey: adults aged 19 to 64 years. Vol. 3. Vitamin and mineral intake and urinary analytes. HMSO, London.

Table 5.77 Good food sources of Cu

Offal
Nuts
Cereals & cereal products
Meat & meat products

Iodine (I)

Function

- Iodine is a component of the thyroid hormones thyroxine (T4) and triiodothyronine (T3).
- Thyroid hormones maintain the body's metabolic rate by controlling energy production and oxygen consumption in cells.
- They are required for normal growth and development.
- In the fetus and neonate normal protein metabolism in the brain and CNS requires iodine.

Measurement Levels of thyroid-stimulating hormone (TSH) are the most sensitive indicators of iodine status. It is raised in iodine deficiency. In severe deficiency serum T3 and T4 decline.

Deficiency

- Iodine deficiency disorder (IDD) in adults results in hypothyroidism and raised levels of TSH, which cause hyperplasia of thyroid tissues resulting in goitre. Hypothyroidism is characterized by lethargy, poor cold tolerance, bradycardia, and myxoedema.
- In the fetus IDD results in cretinism. This is characterized by mental retardation, hearing, speech defects, squint, disorders of stance and gait, and growth retardation. The degree of cretinism is variable and varying degrees of growth retardation and mental retardation are seen in infants and children with IDD.
- IDD is also linked to ↑ in the rates of still birth, miscarriage, and infertility.
  IDD is now rare in UK although some areas were once associated with IDD, e.g. Derbyshire. It is estimated that 200–300 million people worldwide demonstrate some degree of IDD.

Intake (Tables 5.78–5.80)

The amount of iodine in the diet is affected by the geography of the areas of cultivation. Areas with poor soil content, e.g. mountainous areas such as the Himalayas are often associated with endemic IDD. This is due to iodine being washed from the soil. Supplementation of salt has been introduced in an attempt to reduce IDD. In the UK the iodine content of foods has gradually ↑ due to the supplements of cattle feeds, which are secreted in milk.

Absorption is reduced by the presence of goitrogens in some foods, e.g. brassica vegetables (cabbage, swede, Brussels sprouts, broccoli), cassava, maize, lima beans. Goitrogens are inactivated by heating.

Toxicity High intakes can cause hyperthyroidism and toxic modular goitre; there is a weak relationship between persistently high intakes and thyroid cancer. The safe upper limit is 17 µg/kg/d.

Table 5.78 Reference nutrient intakes for iodine (µg/d) for all ages and average daily intakes (µg) for adult men and women provided by food*

Age	RNI
0–3 months	50
4–12 months	60
1–3 years	70
4–6 years	100
7–10 years	110
11–14 years	130
15+ years	140
Average daily intake UK	
Men	215
Women	159

* Source for RNIs, Department of Health (1991). *Dietary reference values for food and nutrients for the United Kingdom.* HMSO, London; source for average daily intakes for adults, Henderson, L., Irving, K., and Gregory, J. (2003). *The National Diet and Nutrition Survey: adults aged 19 to 64 years.* Vol. 3. *Vitamin and mineral intake and urinary analytes.* HMSO, London.

Table 5.79 Contribution of foods to iodine intake (NDNS)*

Food group	% Daily intake	
	Men	Women
Milk & milk products	35	42
Skimmed milk	18	18
Drinks	19	9
Beer & lager	15	3
Cereals & cereal products	12	12
Fish & fish products	11	11

* Henderson, L., Irving, K., and Gregory, J. (2003). *The National Diet and Nutrition Survey: adults aged 19 to 64 years.* Vol. 3. *Vitamin and mineral intake and ;urinary analytes.* HMSO, London.

Table 5.80 Good food sources of iodine

Milk and dairy products
Sea fish, e.g. haddock, cod
Seaweed
Iodized salt

Selenium (Se)

Function

Se is an integral part of over 30 selenoproteins; the most important of which are:

- glutathione peroxidases, which protect against oxidative damage;
- iodothyronine deiodinases, which are involved in the production of triiodothyronine from thyroxine;
- selenoprotein P, which is involved in antioxidant and transport functions.

Measurement Se levels are measured in whole blood. There is considerable geographical variation in concentration: the range for the UK is 0.091–0.120 μg/ml.

Deficiency Deficiency of Se is associated with two endemic causes: Keshan disease and Kashin–Beck disease.

- Keshan disease—outbreaks in Russia and several parts of Asia; it is characterized by a cardiomyopathy.
- Kashin–Beck disease is an endemic musculoskeletal disorder that has occurred in parts of Siberia and Asia.
- Iatrogenic causes of Se deficiency include patients receiving TPN, phenylketonuric patients receiving a semi-synthetic diet. Patients exhibit symptoms of cardiomyopathy and/or musculoskeletal disorders.

Requirement and intake See Table 5.81 and 5.82. Se intake has ↓ over the last 20 years, due to ↑ consumption of European wheat which is low is Se, and the average intake is below the recommended intake. Epidemiological evidence suggests that this may contribute to ↑ risk of infection and the incidence of some cancers. Interventional studies are being conducted to establish the functional consequences of small supplements. Due to the potential risk of toxicity self-administration of large supplements is not recommended.

Sources in the diet See Table 5.83 Lacto-ova vegetarians and vegans may be at risk of Se deficiency.

Toxicity Acute Se poisoning is characterized by hypersalivation, nausea, vomiting, and garlic-smelling breath. This may be accompanied by diarrhoea, hair loss, restlessness, tachycardia, and fatigue. Chronic poisoning (selenosis) is associated with nail and hair changes, skin lesions, and neurological, effects; numbness, pain, and paralysis may follow. Early nail changes have been observed at intakes of 900 μg/d and the recommended maximum safe intake is 6 μg/kg/day.

Table 5.81 Reference nutrient intakes for Se (µg/d) for all ages and average daily intakes (mg) for adult men and women provided by food*

Age	RNI
0–3 months	10
4–6 months	13
7–12 months	10
1–3 years	15
4–6 years	20
7–10 years	30
11–14 years	45
Men	
15–18 years	70
19+ years	75
Women	
15+ years	60
Lactation	+ 15
Average daily intake UK	29–39 mg

* Source for RNIs, Department of Health (1991). *Dietary reference values for food and nutrients for the United Kingdom*. HMSO, London; source for average daily intakes for adults, Henderson, L., Irving, K., and Gregory, J. (2003). *The National Diet and Nutrition Survey: adults aged 19 to 64 years*. Vol. 3. *Vitamin and mineral intake and urinary analytes*. HMSO, London.

Table 5.82 Contribution of foods to Se intake (MAFF 1995)*

Food	% Daily intake
Meat & meat products	15
Bread	15
Fish	12
Milk & milk products	10

* MAFF (1995). *MAFF UK—analysis of foods for selenium*, MAFF UK Food Surveillance Information Sheet no. 51, February, 1995. MAFF, London.

Table 5.83 Food sources of Se

Offal
Fish
Brazil nuts
Eggs
Poultry
Meat and meat products

Magnesium (Mg)

Function
- Mg is an integral part of bones and teeth; 60% is found in the skeleton.
- Intracellular energy metabolism; a co-factor for enzymes requiring ATP, in the replication of DNA, and synthesis of protein and RNA.
- Essential for phosphate transferring systems.
- Muscle and nerve cell function.

Measurement Serum Mg is the most frequently used index of status. The normal range is 0.7–1.0 mmol/l.

Deficiency

Mg is found in all animal and plant foods and its concentration in the blood is tightly controlled; a dietary deficiency is unlikely to occur. Low serum Mg levels occur when there are ↑ renal losses, malabsorption, or changes in tissue distribution due to disease or use of some drugs, e.g. diuretics, re-feeding syndrome. Hypomagnesaemia has been associated with cardiac arrhythmias and cardiac arrest. Very low levels of Mg are associated with hypocalcaemia.

Requirement and intake See Table 5.84 and 5.85

Sources in the diet See Table 5.86 Hard drinking water may make a significant contribution to Mg intake.

Toxicity If renal function is normal hypermagnesaemia is virtually impossible to achieve by dietary means; it can occur in renal or adrenal disease. Large quantities of some Mg salts (Epsom salts) are used for their cathartic effect.

Table 5.84 Reference nutrient intakes for Mg (mg/d) for all ages and average daily intakes (mg) for adult men and women provided by food*

Age[†]	RNI
0–3 months	55
4– 6 months	60
7– 9 months	75
10–12 months	80
1–3 years	85
4–6 years	120
7–10 years	200
11–14 years	280
15–18 years	300
Men	
19+ years	300
Women	
19+ years	270
Lactation	+ 50
Average daily intake UK	
Men	308
Women	229

* Source for RNIs, Department of Health (1991). *Dietary reference values for food and nutrients for the United Kingdom.* HMSO, London; source for average daily intakes for adults, Henderson, L., Irving, K., and Gregory, J. (2003). *The National Diet and Nutrition Survey: adults aged 19 to 64 years.* Vol. 3. *Vitamin and mineral intake and urinary analytes.* HMSO, London.
[†] No increment is recommended during pregnancy.

Table 5.85 Contribution of foods to Mg intake (NDNS)*

Food	% Daily intake
Cereals & cereal products	27
Breakfast cereals	7
Sugar, preserves, & confectionery	17
Meat & meat products	12
Milk & milk products	11
Potatoes & savoury snacks	10

* Henderson, L., Irving, K., and Gregory, J. (2003). *The National Diet and Nutrition Survey: adults aged 19 to 64 years.* Vol. 3. *Vitamin and mineral intake and urinary analytes.* HMSO, London.

Table 5.86 Good food sources of Mg

Green vegetables
Pulses & whole grain cereals
Meats

Manganese (Mn)

Function
- Mn is a component of several metallo-enzymes including arginase, pyruvate.
- It is needed for enzyme activity including glutamine synthetase and various hydrolases, kinases, decarboxylases, and phosphotransferases.

Measurement There is no accepted measurement of Mn status. Enzyme activity assays have been proposed but none have been accepted into widespread practice.

Deficiency Deficiency has only been observed in experimental studies: fingernail growth slowed, black hair reddened, and a scaly dermatitis developed.

Requirement and intake See Tables 5.87–5.89 No cases of nutritional Mn deficiency have been observed; ∴ no recommended nutrient intakes have been made in the UK. Safe levels are shown in Table 5.87.

Toxicity Mn toxicity is low as absorption is ↓ when intake is high and any that is absorbed is excreted in bile and urine.

Table 5.87 Safe intakes for Mn for all ages and average daily intakes (µg) for adult men and women provided by food*

Age	RNI
Infants & children	>16 µg/kg/d
Adults	>1.4 mg/d
Average daily intake UK (mg/d)	
Men	3.32
Women	2.69

* Source for RNIs, Department of Health (1991). *Dietary reference values for food and nutrients for the United Kingdom.* HMSO, London; source for average daily intakes for adults, Henderson, L., Irving, K., and Gregory, J. (2003). *The National Diet and Nutrition Survey: adults aged 19 to 64 years.* Vol. 3. *Vitamin and mineral intake and urinary analytes.* HMSO, London.

Table 5.88 Contribution of foods to Mn intake (NDNS)*

Food	% Daily intake
Cereals & cereal products	50
Bread	26
Breakfast cereals	11
Biscuits, cakes, etc.	5
Drinks	17
Tea	12
Vegetables excluding potatoes	10

* Henderson, L., Irving, K., and Gregory, J. (2003). *The National Diet and Nutrition Survey: adult aged 19 to 64 years.* Vol. 3. *Vitamin and mineral intake and urinary analytes.* HMSO, London.

Table 5.89 Good food sources of Mn

Cereals & cereal products
Tea
Vegetables

Molybdenum (Mo)

Function Co-factor in xanthine oxidase, sulphite oxidase, and aldehyde oxidase and is ∴ involved in the metabolism of purines, pyrimidines, quinolines, and sulphites.

Measurement Mo can be measured in whole blood and serum. Concentrations in whole blood vary widely although the mean concentration is 0.5 µg/l.

Deficiency Dietary deficiency of Mo has been reported in farm animals but has not been observed in humans, although there is a single case reported following prolonged TPN. The symptoms included defects in sulphur metabolism, mental disturbance, and coma. An inborn error of metabolism results in abnormal production of the coenzyme. It is characterized by abnormal urinary metabolites, neurological and ocular problems, and failure to thrive. The genetic expression and symptoms are varied and in the most severe cases can be fatal at 2–3 years.

Requirement and intake There are no RNIs but safe intakes are believed to be between 50 and 400 µg/d in adults and 0.5 and 1.5 µg/d in children. Mean intakes in adults are reported as 0.12 mg/d.

Sources in the diet Offal, nuts, cereals, and bread are good sources.

Toxicity Little data are available for dietary excess, although intakes >100 mg/kg/d have been reported to cause diarrhoea, anaemia, and high blood uric acid levels; this is associated with gout.

Chromium (Cr)

The essentiality of Cr is widely accepted, although this is still challenged by some scientists. In nutrition the trivalent state appears to have physiological functions but it is interchangeable with hexavalent Cr.

Function

* Cr is believed to be part of an organic complex known as the 'glucose tolerance factor' (GTF), which potentiates the action of insulin. The evidence for essentiality of Cr comes from observations of patients receiving TPN who develop diabetic symptoms. The symptoms respond to Cr treatment but not insulin. Studies on the use of Cr in the management of type 2 diabetes are not conclusive.
* Cr may participate in lipoprotein metabolism.

Measurement There is no totally reliable measure of Cr. Urinary excretion, expressed in terms of creatinine, has been suggested as a measure of chromium status. Hair Cr levels have been used as a measure of long-term exposure although hair analysis is associated with several problems.

Deficiency Deficiency in humans has only been observed in patients receiving long-term TPN. The symptoms included impaired glucose tolerance, weight loss, neuropathy, elevated plasma fatty acids, depressed respiratory quotient, and abnormal nitrogen metabolism.

Requirement and intake There are no RNIs for Cr but the theoretical requirement extrapolated from balance studies is 25–30 µg/d in adults. In children the safe intake is believed to be 0.1–1.0 µg/kg/d. The average daily intake of Cr for adults is estimated as 0.1 mg.[1]

Sources in the diet The richest sources of Cr in the diet are meat, whole grains, legumes, and nuts.

Toxicity The trivalent form is not associated with toxicity, but the hexavalent form is very toxic. Two fatalities have been reported following acute ingestion of very large doses of hexavalent Cr as dichromate (75 mg/kg) and chromic acid (4.1 mg/kg). Symptoms included gastrointestinal haemorrhages, renal and liver abnormalities. Chronic toxicity is associated with renal failure, liver failure, haemolysis, and anaemia.

[1] Ysart, G., Miller, P., et al. (2000). 1997 UK Total Diet Study—dietary exposures to aluminum arsenic, cadmium, chromium, copper, lead, mercury, nickel, selenium, tin and zinc. *Food Addit Contam*. **17**, 775–86.

Fluorine (Fl)

Fl is considered semi-essential as it has biological functions but its essentiality is still debated.

Function Flouride has a role in bone mineralization and protects against dental caries.

Deficiency Low intakes are associated with ↑ incidence of dental caries.

Requirement and intake See Table 5.90–5.92. There are no RNIs for Fl although safe intakes are given in Table 5.90 Total intakes depends on the level of fluoridation in water consumed. 10% of water in the UK is fluoridated or has a natural content above the recommended fluoridation rate of 1 ppm. A recent report (2006) by the FSA reports findings from the 2004 Total Diet Study.

Toxicity Intake 3–5 times the normal intake is mildly toxic. Tooth mottling occurs in mild toxicity and chronic excess (10 mg/d) causes joint and bone abnormalities.

Table 5.90 Safe intakes of Fl (mg/kg/d)

Age	Safe intake
0–6 months	0.22
6–12 months	0.12
>1 year	0.05

Table 5.91 Mean adult intakes of Fl (mg/d).

	Intake
Non-fluoridated water areas	1.82
Fluoridated water areas*	2.90

* Assumes an average daily intake of 1.1 l daily.

Table 5.92 Sources of 1 mg Fl

1 l water (fluoridated at 1 ppm)
1 Fl tablet
1 g Fl toothpaste (accidental consumption)
5 ml Fl mouthwash (accidental consumption)
2–3 cups of tea (depends on strength)
1400 g cooked spinach
250 g tinned sardines

Electrolytes: introduction

The monovalent electrolytes are Na, Cl, and K.

Sodium (Na)

An adult male (70 kg) has total body Na of 4 mol (92 g); 2000 mmol is in extracellular fluid (ECF), 1500 mmol in bone, and 500 mmol in intracellular fluid.

Function
- Cation in extracellular fluid.
- Regulation of blood pressure and transmembrane gradients.
- Acid–base regulation.
- Electrophysiological control of muscles and nerves.

Measurement Na is easily measurable in plasma, with a normal range of 135–150 mmol/l.

Deficiency Na losses requiring repletion can result from excess sweating in extreme conditions of heat and exertion.

Requirement and intake see Table 5.93.

Sources in the diet
Na is present in many food additives, e.g. monosodium glutamate, but most Na in the diet is present as salt (NaCl). Levels are comparatively low in unprocessed foods. Salt is added to food as a preservative and flavour enhancer; it can also be used as a fermentation control agent in bread making, texturizer, binder, and colour developer. 3 g salt ≈ 1.2 g Na.

Toxicity It is a strong emetic but excessive oral loads of Na are potentially fatal. Artificial intravenous load has severe and rapid effects.

Table 5.93 Reference nutrient intakes for Na mg/d (mmol/d) for all ages and average daily intakes of Na(mg/d) and NaCl (g/d) for adult men and women provided by food (NDNS)*

Age	RNI	
0–3 months	210 (9)	
4–6 months	280 (12)	
7–9 months	320 (14)	
10–12 months	350 (15)	
1–3 years	500 (22)	
4–6 years	700 (30)	
7–10 years	1200 (50)	
11–14 years	1600 (70)	
15–50+ years	1600 (70)	
Average daily intakes UK		
	Na	**NaCl**
Men	3313	8.4
Women	2302	5.9

* Source for RNIs, Department of Health (1991). *Dietary reference values for food and nutrients for the United Kingdom.* HMSO, London; source for average daily intakes for adults, Henderson, L., Irving, K., and Gregory, J. (2003). *The National Diet and Nutrition Survey: adults aged 19 to 64 years.* Vol. 3. *Vitamin and mineral intake and urinary analytes.* HMSO, London.

Health implications of excess consumption

Excess Na intake has been linked to hypertension and heart disease
SACN has recommended that salt intake targets should be:

- 0–6 months, < 1 g/d;
- 7–12 months, 1 g/d;
- 1–6 years, 2 g/d;
- 7–14 years, 5 g/d;
- >15 years, 6 g/d.

N.B. Na can roughly be converted to NaCl by multiplying by 2.5.

FSA is working with food manufacturers to reduce the Na content of
processed foods. Table 5.94 shows foods high in salt. A public awareness
campaign 'Sid the slug' was initiated in 2005; more information is available
at the FSA salt information web site (www.salt.gov.uk). The FSA has
recently published voluntary salt reduction targets to encourge food
manufacturers and retailers to reduce the amount of salt in a wide range
of processed foods. Details can be found an the FSA website
(www.food.gov.uk).

Clinical restriction of Na

Some disease states, e.g. renal disease, require the restriction of Na. The
level of restriction can be classified.

- *No added salt*: 80–100 mmol Na/d.
- *Low salt*: 40 mmol Na/d.
- *Low Na*: 22 mmol Na/d.

Table 5.94 Foods high in salt*

Foods where some brands/recipes are high in salt	
Baked beans	Biscuits - sweet and savoury
Breakfast cereals	Cooking sauces
Hot chocolate	Pizza
Ready meals	Soup
Tinned spaghetti	Tinned vegetables and pulses (with added salt)

Foods that are usually high in salt	
Anchovies	Bacon
Cheese	Chips (if salt added)
Crisps	Gravy granules
Olives	Pickles
Pretzels Salted and dry roasted nuts	Salt fish
Sausages	Smoked meat and fish
Soy sauce	Stock cubes
Yeast extract	

* Based on information from the Food Standards Agency, available at: www.salt.gov.uk.

Potassium (K)

Function Intracellular cation that is involved in acid–base regulation, electrophysiology of nerves and muscles, and is essential for the cellular uptake of molecules against concentration and electrochemical gradients.

Measurement Normal plasma concentration is 3.5–5.0 mmol/l. Over 95% of total body K is found in cells; an adult male contains 40–55 mmol/kg (1.6–2.0 g/kg).

Deficiency Lack of K alters the electrophysiology of cell membranes and causes muscle weakness. In cardiac muscle this leads to arrhythmias and cardiac arrest. Motility is lost in the intestine and mental depression and confusion can develop. Dietary deficiency of K is very unlikely as it is found in all foods. Causes of K depletion are shown in table 5.95.

Requirement and intake See Table 5.96–5.98.

Toxicity Toxicity due to dietary excess is unlikely. Acute intake of supplements exceeding 17.6 g (450 mmol) may cause symptoms of hyperkalaemia. Hyperkalaemia causes paraesthesiae around the mouth and muscle weakness although these symptoms may be absent. There is a risk of cardiac arrest.

Table 5.95 Causes of K depletion

Gastrointestinal causes

Diarrhoea

Vomiting

Small bowel or gastric drainage

Ureterocolic anastomosis

Purgatives

Urinary losses

Chronic acidosis or alkalosis

Osmotic diuresis, e.g. uncontrolled diabetes

Renal disease (tubular)

Diuretic drugs

Steroid excess (Cushing's disease, primary and secondary hyperaldosteroidism)

Table 5.96 Reference nutrient intakes for K mg/d (mmol/d) for all ages and average daily intakes (mg) for adult men and women provided by food*

Age	RNI
0–3 months	800 (20)
4–6 months	850 (22)
7–12 months	700 (18)
1–3 years	800 (20)
4–6 years	1100 (28)
7–10 years	2000 (50)
11–14 years	3100 (80)
15–50+ years	3500 (90)
Average daily intakes UK	
Men	3367
Women	2653

* Source for RNIs, Department of Health (1991). *Dietary reference value for food and nutrients for the United Kingdom.* HMSO, London; source for average daily intakes for adults, Henderson, L., Irving, K., and Gregory, J. (2003). *The National Diet and Nutrition Survey: adults aged 19 to 64 years.* Vol. 3. *Vitamin and mineral intake and urinary analytes.* HMSO, London.

Table 5.97 Contribution of foods to K intake (NDNS)*

Food group	% Daily intake
Potatoes and savoury snacks	18
Meat & meat products	15
Drinks	15
Cereals & cereal products	13
Milk and milk products	13
Vegetables (excluding potatoes)	10

* Henderson, L., Irving, K., and Gregory, J. (2003). The National Diet and Nutrition Survey: adults aged 19 to 64 years. Vol. 3. Vitamin and mineral intake and urinary analytes. HMSO,

Table 5.98 Rich food sources of K

Fruit especially bananas, apricots, blackcurrant, rhubarb, fruit juices

Vegetables especially potatoes and potato snacks

Chocolate, cocoa, and chocolate products

Coffee and coffee products

Malted milk drinks

Yeast extracts and spreads, tomato ketchup, stock cubes, bottled sauces

Table salt substitutes

Chlorine (Cl)

Total body Cl is ~33 mmol (1.2 g)/kg. 70% is in ECF.

Function Cl is the anion to the cations Na and K.

Measurement Normal plasma concentration is 97–107 mmol/l.

Requirement and intake There are no specific DRVs for Cl; it is recommended that Cl intake should equal Na intake in molar terms. The average intakes of Cl in foods are 4995 mg/d for men and 3481 mg/d for women.

Sources in the diet Cl is usually consumed with Na as salt (NaCl).

Fluid balance

The human body is mainly water; a 70 kg man is comprised of approximately 45 l water. 72% FFM is water.
- Total body water, 45 l.
- ECF, 15 l.
- ICF, 30 l.

ECF is comprised of plasma and interstitial fluids. The monovalent electrolytes, Na, Cl, and K, determine the body's osmolality and their distribution determines the volume of ECF and ICF. ICF, plasma, and interstitial fluids are separated by semi-permeable membranes and are interdependent. Movement of fluid between the compartments is controlled by plasma osmolality and hydrostatic pressure gradients.

Regulation of fluid balance

Fluid balance is under tight homeostatic control and fluctuates by <1% per day despite large variations in fluid intake. Normally the osmolalities of plasma and interstitial fluids are similar. Plasma osmolality reflects serum Na which reflects total ECF.

Plasma osmolality

↑ in plasma osmolality → thirst and the hypothalamus will be stimulated to ↑ antidiuretic hormone (ADH). This leads to reabsorption by the distal tubules of the kidney which corrects the osmolality. ↓ plasma volume can also → raised osmolality which causes aldosterone to be released. This ↑ Na and water retention.

Hydrostatic pressure

Plasma volume is also controlled by hydrostatic pressure. At the arterial end of the capillaries blood pressure is exerted but less osmotic pressure is exerted by plasma proteins resulting in the movement of fluid out into the interstitial fluid. At the venous end of the capillary the process is reversed and fluid passes back into plasma.

Water balance (Table 5.99)

Thirst

Thirst usually plays only a small role in fluid balance of normal subjects. Fluid is usually consumed for reasons other than thirst, e.g. habit and customs. Local drying of the mouth and throat will also cause thirst, e.g. public speakers often require water to lubricate the mouth and throat.

Table 5.99 Causes of dehydration*

Reason	Cause
Increased fluid losses	Patients with tracheotomies or on ventilators
	Diarrhoea and/or vomiting
	Stomal losses
	Wound or burn exudates
	Pyrexia
	Diabetes insipidus
	Diabetic ketoacidosis
	Prolonged use of diuretics
	Patients receiving high protein high osmolar diets
Lack of awareness or inability to express the need for fluid	Patients who are unable to communicate, e.g. stroke
Low fluid intake	Poor food intake, e.g. anorexia, depression.
	Apathy, chronic illness, physical immobility, etc.
	Eating difficulties
	Swallowing difficulties
	Deliberate fluid restriction to avoid incontinence
	'Nil by mouth' regimens

* Reproduced from B Thomas (2001). *Manual of Dietetic Practice*, table 2.18, p191. Permission requested from Blackwell Publishing.

Fluid losses

Fluid output in urine is controlled by the kidneys but there are also insensible water losses through the skin and lungs and in faeces.

• Sweat glands secrete water in sweat, which evaporates from the skin. This evaporation cools the skin. Water is also lost directly through the skin. 500–750 ml/d of fluid is lost through the skin and ↑ in fever and extreme temperatures or exertion. ↑ in 1°C in body temperature will ↑ fluid requirements by 500 ml/d/

• Healthy adults pass 50–400 g/d of faeces and approx. 75% of this will be fluid.

• Expired air contains 44 mg water /l and this will be ↑ in fever, ↑ respiration rates, and by reduced water content of inspired air, e.g. high altitudes.

Fluid requirements

The amount of fluid consumed is very variable. In normal conditions 30–35 ml/kg body weight is required daily. In some disease states, i.e. cardiac, hepatic, and renal disease, it may be necessary to restrict fluid intake to prevent fluid overload (see Chapters 19, 23, and 24).

Food labelling, functional foods, and food supplements

Food labelling

Food labelling in the UK is controlled by Food Labelling Regulation (1996) and later amendments and more recently by European law Legally these regulations fall under the Food Safety Act of 1990. In th UK foods sold loose are exempt from many labelling regulations.

Information required by law

Product name

This must be clearly stated and products with 'made up' names must give description of the food. If the food has undergone processing, e.g. 'smoke the process must be stated. The name must also distinguish between simila products. For example, 'orange drink' must contain oranges while 'orang flavoured drinks' can be made with artificial flavourings.

Ingredient list and quantity

The net quantity of a food must be present unless it is <5 g. Ingredient are listed in descending order of weight. All ingredients including add tives and water must be listed. A compound ingredient that does no constitute more than 25% of the final product, e.g. pepperoni on a pizz did not have to be listed until recently. New European Union regulation which will affect the UK, came into force in 2004, with a year's transitio period, and ingredient lists must be comprehensive and the presence c the specified allergens must be indicated (see Table 6.1).

Quantitative ingredient declaration (QUID)

An ingredient that is featured in a photograph or drawing on a pack or i the description of the product, e.g. potatoes in cheese and potato pi must state the quantity of the ingredient declared as a percentage. This i required by European Union labelling law and is known as quantitativ ingredient declaration (QUID).

Allergenic ingredients

From November 2005 food and drink labels must state clearly if the contain ingredients to which people may be allergic or intolerant. Th manufacturer will also have to make it clear if, ingredients are made c the allergens, e.g. it is not enough to state 'glaze'; under new regulation the label must state 'glaze made from eggs'.

Shelf life

Labels must give information on how long the product will last once i has been bought or opened. This information is intended to ensure th safety and quality of the food and to prevent food poisoning. The 'use by' label must be used for perishable foods such as cooked meats which deteriorate and can be dangerous to health after a relativel short period. 'Best before' must be expressed as a day, month, an year and is used to indicate that a food's flavour, colour, or textur may not be at its best beyond this period although it is probably sti safe to eat. For products with a shelf life longer than 3 months 'Bes before end' is used. 'Display until' is not required by law but is used b retailers to alert staff to the need to remove products from sale. Win and spirits do not have to be date marked.

Table 6.1 Allergenic ingredients that must be listed

Celery

Cereals containing gluten—wheat, rye, oats, barley

Crustaceans, e.g. lobster, crab

Milk

Eggs

Fish

Mustard

Soybeans

Peanuts

Nuts—almonds, pistachios, brazil nuts, walnuts, hazelnuts, cashews, pecans, macadamia nuts

Sesame seeds

Sulphur dioxide and sulphites at levels above 10 mg per kg or litre.

Storage instructions

Details must be given on the conditions needed to ensure freshness. Following the instructions should ensure that the product's appearance and taste are optimum and prevent spoiling too quickly, so minimizing the risk of food poisoning.

Name and address of manufacturer, packer, or seller These must be stated on the package so that the consumers have a point of contact if they want to make a complaint or need more information.

Country of origin The label must clearly state where the food is from if it would be misleading not to show it, e.g. French onion soup made in Scotland.

Weight or volume

The volume or weight of the product must be shown on the label. This enables consumers to compare the value of different brands. The symbol 'e' shows that the weight complies with EU requirements in that the average pack is at least the declared weight. Some foods, e.g. butter, tea, are sold only in standard amounts. Products that weigh <5 g do not have to have a stated weight.

Instructions for use

Instruction on how to prepare and cook the product must be printed on the packaging when necessary. Oven temperature and cooking time are stated if the product needs heating; instructions on microwave cooking may also be given. The instructions are given so that the food can be consumed at its best and to reduce the risk of food poisoning by usually heating to a core temperature of 75°C.

Genetically modified (GM) ingredients

EU regulations mean that foods that contain genetically modified organisms (GMO) or ingredients made from GMOs must indicate their presence on the label. Foods produced using GM technology and animal products from animals fed GM feed do not have to be labelled. Loose GM food must be displayed next to information that states that it is genetically modified.

Nutrition information labelling

Food manufacturers are not required by law to display nutrition labelling. If a nutrition claim, e.g. high fibre, is made this must be supported by nutrition information on the label. Labels may state recommended daily amounts or guideline daily amounts. EU regulations allow two nutrition labelling systems. The first system requires that the energy content of the food be given in kilojoules (kJ) or kilocalories (kcal) and the amount, in grams (g), of protein, carbohydrate, and fat per 100 g or 100 ml; manufacturers may also show values per item or average serving. The second system supplies these details together with information on sugars, fibre, Na, and saturated fat. Details on starch, monosaturated fat, polyunsaturated fat, cholesterol, and some minerals and vitamins if they are present in significant amounts may also be given.

Nutrition claims

A nutrition claim is any information other than nutrition labelling that implies or states that a food contains, or has a high or low amount of a nutrient. Nutrition labelling must be given if a nutrition claim is made. Nutrient (content), nutrient function, or comparative claims are permissible but in the UK health claims should be substantiated by the Joint Health Claim Initiative (JCHI). Details of substantiated claims can be found on the JHCI web site (www.jhci.co.uk). Nutrient claims refer to the presence of a nutrient, e.g. source of Fe. Nutrient function claims refer to the physiological function of the nutrient, e.g. helps children develop strong bones. Comparative claims use terms such as 'lower' or 'higher' quantities of a nutrient when comparing foods, e.g. contains 25% more Fe.

Terms such as 'low', 'lite', 'light', or 'high' are not defined under the current legislation but new EU legislation will provide definitions and ban statement such as '% fat free' or the term 'diet'. The Food Standards Agency's (FSA) guidelines on nutrition content claims for sugars, fat, saturates, and sodium (salt) are shown in Table 6.2. Table 6.3 shows the FSA guidelines on fibre.

Organic

In the UK the Department for Environment, Food and Rural Affairs (DEFRA) regulates the bodies that can certify organic producers and manufacturers. 75% of certification is administered by the Soil Association. Organic food products can be sold in two categories:

- Category 1: Organic. Must contain at least 95% of organic ingredients by weight and can be labelled 'organic'.
- Category 2: Special emphasis. Product contains 70–95% organic ingredients by weight and can be labelled as 'made from organic ingredients'.

Organic food cannot legally contain GM or irradiated foods.

Table 6.2 FSA guidelines on nutrient content claims

	Low	No added	Free
Sugar (s)	<5 g per 100 g or 100 ml	No sugars or foods composed mainly of sugars added to the food or any of the ingredients	<0.2 g per 100 g or 100 ml
Fat	<3 g per 100 g or 100 ml		<0.15 g per 100 g or 100 ml
Saturates	<1.5 g per 100 g or 100 ml and not more than 10% of the total energy content of the product		<0.1 g per 100 g or 100 ml
Na/salt	<40 mg Na per 100 g or 100 ml	No salt or Na added to the foods or any of its ingredients	<5 mg Na per 100 g or 100 ml

Table 6.3 FSA guidelines on nutrient content claims for fibre

Source	Increased	High
3 g per 100 g or 100 ml or at least 3 g in the reasonable expected daily intake of the food	>25% more than a similar food for which no claim is made and more than 3 g in either the reasonable daily intake of a food which is lower than 100 g or 100 ml or in 100 g or in 100 ml	>6 g per 100 g or 100 ml or at least 6 g in the reasonable daily intake of the food

Guideline daily amounts (GDAs)

Some pre-packaged foods provide information about GDAs. GDAs are derived from the EARs for energy for men and women, aged 19–50 y, normal weight and fitness. The values for fat and saturated fatty acids are derived from DRVs and salt is based on SACN recommendations. They are intended as a guide for the consumer when comparing products. Revised GDAs (Table 6.4) were published by the Institute of Grocery Distribution (IGD) in 2005. GDAs are now available for children. Further details are available from the IGD web site (www.igd.com).

Table 6.4 Guideline daily amounts (GDAs) for adults as used in UK (IGD 2005)*

	GDA	
	Women	Men
Energy (kcal)	2000	2500
Fat (g)	<70	<95
% Total energy	<33	<33
Saturates (g)	20	30
% Total energy	10	10
Total carbohydrate (g)	230	300
% Total energy	>47	>47
‡Total sugars (g)	<90	<120
% Total energy	<19	<19
NMES (g)	<50	<65
% Total energy	<10	<10
NSP/fibre (g)	>18	>18
Salt (g)	6	6

* IGD (2005), GDAs—*Technical working Group report*, IGD, London.

‡ For labelling use.

NMES, Non-milk extrinsic sugars.

Functional foods and nutraceuticals

- Functional foods are foods with health-promoting benefits or disease-preventing properties above their nutrient value.
- Nutraceuticals are foods for which a claim is made for a specific health benefit; they are often sold in the form of a drug, such as a pill or capsule

Many nutrients and foods have nutrient or health claims as functional foods or nutraceuticals but the claims are not always proven. There is currently no law that controls these claims. It is generally accepted that health claims such as 'can help lower cholesterol as part of a low fat diet' can be made if the claim is supported by scientific research and is not misleading (see 'Food labelling', this chapter). Functional or 'novel' foods must go through a safety approval process before they are launched. Products that were on sale before 1997 do not have to undergo this process. In the UK the Joint Health Claims Initiative has established guidance on a voluntary scheme for health claims (www.jhci.co.uk).

Examples of functional foods

Cholesterol-lowering spreads

These spreads contain plant sterols and stanols (saturated sterols) and have been shown to reduce the amount of cholesterol absorbed. They have been shown to lower LDL cholesterol by 10–15% after a few weeks of use. In Australia and New Zealand all plant products with sterols, apart from margarine, have been banned as there was no evidence that high intakes are safe. The Australia and New Zealand Food Authority also require spreads to carry a warning that they are not appropriate for infants, children and pregnant and breastfeeding women as they may interfere with the absorption of beta carotene. At the moment such spreads are expensive compared with normal margarine or butter.

Omega 3 (n 3 or ω 3) enriched eggs and dairy products Fish oils containing omega 3 fatty acids have been shown to have several health benefits (see 'Fats' in Chapter 5). The incorporation of these oils into hen's eggs or dairy produce offers alternative food sources for people who dislike fish.

Isoflavins Soya beans are incorporated into foods and sold as supplements as a source of isoflavins. The health benefits of isoflavins are discussed in 'Food supplements', this chapter.

Food fortification

Some foods are supplemented with nutrients for their benefits above normal health benefits. In the UK flour is fortified with Ca and margarine is fortified with vitamins A and D.

Folate fortification

Folate is frequently added to cereals and there is considerable debate in the UK as to whether or not to fortify all flour and flour products. Flour is fortified with folate in USA, Canada, and Chile. The arguments for and against folate fortification are as follows.

- Arguments for the fortification of flour with folate:
  - prevention of neural tube defects;
  - low folate status is associated with elevated homocysteine which is a risk factor for cardiovascular disease and is linked to some cancers including colon and breast cancer.
- Arguments against the fortification of flour with folate:
  - there is uncertainty about the bioavailability of folate;
  - consumer choice;
  - high consumption of folic acid may mask the diagnosis of vitamin B_{12} deficiency in the elderly.

A recent SACN report has recommended the supplementation of flour in the UK although this has not been ratified by the government. See SACN website for current status (www.sacn.org.uk).

Probiotics

It is estimated that there are 10^{14} bacteria in the human gut and claimed that ingestion of probiotic bacteria improves the balance of bacteria in the gut and thereby reduces the risk of disease. Probiotic bacteria are often described as 'healthy' or 'friendly' and are not potentially pathological bacteria. Probiotics are taken as foods, usually yogurt, and are present as 'live' bacteria which are taken in doses of million colonies. Table 6.5 lists some of the most frequently used probiotic bacteria. Some research has been conducted on the benefits of probiotics although this is limited and conducted mainly in specific disease states. More research is needed, particularly on the use of probiotics by healthy people.

Suggested benefits of taking probiotics for which some evidence is available:

- improving symptoms of lactose intolerance;
- reduction in susceptibility to stomach allergies;
- control of irritable bowel symptoms;
- inhibition of *Helicobacter pylori*, which is responsible for the formation of some peptic ulcers;
- alleviation of some diarrhoea.

Prebiotics

A prebiotic is a food that is not digested by the gut and that stimulates growth of certain bacteria in the colon. Ingredients that have prebiotic properties are inulin and fructo-oligosaccharides (FOS).

Table 6.5 Frequently used probiotic bacteria

Lactobacillus acidophilus
Lactobacillus rhamnosus
Lactobacillus bulgaricus
Lactobacillus salivarius
Lactobacillus casei
Lactobacillus sporogenes
Bifidobacteria bifidum
Bifidobacteria longum
Bifidobacteria infantis
Streptococcus thermophilus
Homeostatic soil organisms

Food supplements

Food supplements are defined by EU law as 'foodstuffs the purpose of which is to supplement the normal diet and which provide concentrated sources of nutrients (vitamins and minerals) or other substances with a nutritional or physiological effect, alone or in combination, marketed in dose form ... designed to be taken in measured small unit quantities'.

The growing interest in diet and health has stimulated ↑ in the market for dietary supplements. In 1991, the market for dietary supplements was £194 million and this had risen to £362 million in 2004. The range of supplements available in health food shops, chemists, and supermarkets is growing with vitamins, minerals, fish liver oils, and evening primrose oil being the most popular. In 2003, 40% of women and 29% of men reported taking supplements in the UK.

Health information

The average diet in UK supplies adequate vitamins and minerals to prevent deficiency and for the majority of people supplements are not necessary. Vulnerable groups, e.g. vegetarians and pregnant women, may benefit from supplements. There is little evidence to support the blanket use of supplements. There are a few well established cases, e.g. additional folate in pregnancy. Most supplements are bought over the counter and are self-prescribed.

The range of nutrition supplements is vast and cannot be adequately covered in this format. Information on the health benefits of specific supplements can be obtained from the National Institute of Health's (USA) Office for Dietary Supplements (www.ods.od.nih.gov/).

Micronutrient supplements

In 2003, the Expert Group on Vitamins and Minerals published its report on the safety of vitamins and minerals in food supplements and fortified foods. Safe upper limits were set for all vitamins and most minerals. The full report can be found at www.food.gov.uk/multimedia/pdfs/vitamin2003.pdf.

Regulation

Food supplements fall between medicines and foods and it is difficult to regulate their marketing. In 2002 the EU issued the Food Supplements Directive and the directive and regulations have applied since August 2005. The directive lists vitamins and minerals that can be used in supplements. It excludes tin, silicon, nickel, boron, cobalt, and vanadium. A second list gives details of the chemical forms that may be used. These forms are considered safe. Manufacturers are required to set maximum doses.

Labelling

Manufacturers must not make claims referring to the prevention, treatment, or curing of diseases or refer to such properties. The label must display:

- Names of the nutrients and substances;
- Portion required for daily use;
- Warning not to exceed stated dose;
- Statement to the effect that supplements should not replace a varied diet;
- Statement that the product should be stored away from children;
- It should not be implied that a balanced and varied diet cannot provide adequate amounts of nutrients;
- Amounts of nutrients available in the recommended dose.

Clinical supplements A range of supplements are available for clinical use, e.g. high energy drinks, which are prescribed or recommended by health-care professionals.

Non-nutrient components of food

Alcohol

The alcohol present in alcoholic drinks is ethanol (ethyl alcohol), C_2H_5OH. Ethanol is produced by the fermentation of glucose in plants. Sugars in grapes and apples are fermented to produce wine and cider; barley starch is hydrolysed to glucose in the production of beer. Other fruits and cereals are used to produce alcoholic drinks, e.g. rice for sake and rye for whisky. The resultant alcohol is diluted to produce the appropriate alcohol content of drinks. By law, drink labels must show the strength of alcohol present; this is expressed as the percentage alcohol by volume (abv). 10% abv is equivalent to 7.9 g of alcohol per 100 ml.

Ciders and beers	4–6% abv
Wines	9–13% abv
Fortified wines	18–25% abv
Liqueurs	20–40% abv
Alcopops	4–13% abv
Spirits, e.g. gin	40% abv

Low alcohol and strong variations of some drinks are now produced. Other substances are added to provide flavour such as juniper berries in gin and hops in beer. Alcoholic drinks may also contain sugars, small amounts of other alcohols, e.g. propyl alcohol, potassium, and small amounts of riboflavin and niacin. In the UK 1 unit of alcohol drink contains 8 grams or 10 ml of pure alcohol (see Table 7.1). Other systems are used by other countries.

Alcohol metabolism

Ethanol is quickly absorbed in the stomach and jejunum and distributed throughout total body water including blood. Alcohol is distributed via the blood to the brain and the liver where it is metabolized by alcohol dehydrogenase (ADH) to acetaldehyde which is converted to acetate by the enzyme aldehyde dehydrogenase (ALDH). ADH is the rate limiting step in the metabolism of alcohol and there is a great deal of variation between individuals in their ability to metabolize alcohol. On average approximately 5–10 g of alcohol (1/2–1 unit of alcoholic drink) is metabolized per hour. The stages of alcohol intoxication are shown in Table 7.2. Alcohol absorption can be slowed by the presence of food in the stomach. Smaller people have smaller livers and ∴ metabolize alcohol more slowly; women have smaller livers than men and ∴ become intoxicated more quickly. Disulfam (Antabuse) antagonizes ALDH and is a drug used to treat alcoholism. The build up of acetaldehyde leads to headache, nausea, and vomiting. Alcoholics have an induced system of alcohol metabolism known as the microsomal ethanol-oxidizing system (MEOS); this system is thermogenic. Some alcohol is excreted in breath, which provides an easy monitor of alcohol intoxication.

Table 7.1 Drink measures equivalent to 1 unit of alcohol

Drink	Bar measure	ml
Spirit, e.g. whisky, gin, vodka	I single optic measure	25
Sherry or fortified wine, e.g. port or vermouth	1 small glass or schooner	50
Wine	1 small glass	125
Strong lager, beer, cider	¼ pint	142
Ordinary strength lager, beer, cider	½ pint	284
Low alcohol lager, beer, cider	2 pints	1136

Table 7.2 Stages of acute alcohol intoxication

Blood alcohol concentration (mg/100 ml)	Stage	Effects
Up to 50	Feeling of well being	Relaxed, talkative
50–80	Risky	Fine movements and judgement affected
80		Legal limit for drink driving prosecution in UK
80–150	Dangerous	Slurred speech, balance affected, blurred vision, drowsiness, nausea and vomiting
200–400	Drunken stupor	Dead drunk, loss of bladder and bowel control, unconscious
450–600	Death	Shock and death

Nutritional value of alcohol Alcohol is an energy source providing 29 kJ (7 kcal) per gram. Alcoholics do not obtain this level of energy from alcohol due to the thermogenic nature of MEOS.

Recommendation on alcohol intake In the UK the Department of Health recommends that men consume no more than 3–4 units of alcohol /d and women no more than 2–3 units. Standard measures of drinks providing 1 unit of alcohol are shown in Table 7.1. It is also recommended that 2 d/wk should be alcohol free.

Alcohol consumption

It is difficult to estimate alcohol consumption due to the social stigma associated with excessive drinking and the effects of alcohol on mental capacity. The National Diet and Nutrition Survey[1] found that on average men consumed approximately 20–21 units per week and women consumed 8–9 units per week; this figure was calculated including non drinkers. Nearly 40% of men and 25% of women exceeded the recommended intakes, with younger people consuming more alcohol than older people.

Acute effects of alcohol

The response to alcohol is variable; this variation is due to the extent of stimulation of the sympathetic nervous system and the rate of production of acetaldehyde and acetate. The most common effects are ↑ in heart rate and peripheral vasodilatation. As a result of the peripheral vasodilatation some people feel excessively warm and some experience facial flushing. The psychological and physiological responses to acute alcohol excess are shown in Table 7.2

Alcohol is a central nervous system depressant and acts as an anaesthetic. Diuresis (increased urine production) results from the action of alcohol on the pituitary gland and leads to dehydration.

Effects of alcohol on health

Light to moderate consumption of alcohol has been shown to have beneficial health effects in reducing the risk of coronary heart disease in men and post-menopausal women. The most established mechanism is that this level of alcohol consumption ↑ plasma high-density lipoprotein. An additional proposed mechanism is that alcohol ↓ platelet aggregation and ∴ ↓ the risk of thrombosis. It has been proposed that polyphenolic compounds in wines have antioxidant properties that reduce the plasma levels of low-density lipoproteins.

Excessive alcohol consumption has been linked to ↑ risk of breast cancer in women and oesophageal and liver cancer in men and women. High intakes of alcohol are strongly associated with ↑ risk of liver disease. Hypertension risk is ↑ by high levels of alcohol intake.

---

1 Henderson, L., Gregory, I., and Irving, K. (2003). *The National Diet and Nutrition Survey: adults aged 19 to 64 years.* Vol. 2. *Energy protein, carbohydrate, fat and alcohol intakes.* HMSO, London.

Table 7.3 Physical health problems associated with excessive alcohol consumption

Body system	Effects
Nervous system	Acute intoxication, dementia, Wernicke—Korsakoff syndrome, cerebellar degeneration
Cerebrovascular system	Strokes, nerve and muscle damage
Liver	Fatty liver, cirrhosis, hepatitis, liver failure, cancer
Gastrointestinal system	Reflux, oesophageal rupture, oesophageal cancer, pancreatitis, gastritis, malabsorption
Nutrition	Reduced food intake and absorption leading to weight loss, obesity in early stages of heavy drinking
Heart and circulatory system	Arrhythmias, hypertension, heart muscle damage leading to heart failure
Respiratory system	Pneumonia from inhalation of vomit
Endocrine system	Overproduction of cortisol, hypoglycaemia, stimulation of the pituitary to cause diuresis
Reproductive system	Loss of libido, atrophy of testicles, reduced sperm count, menstrual abnormalities

The harmful physical effects of alcohol abuse are extensive and some are listed in Table 7.3 Thiamin deficiency can result from chronic, excessive alcohol intake as thiamin is required for ethanol metabolism and dietary intake may be poor. This can → Wernicke's encephalopathy and Korsakoff's psychosis. Other vitamin deficiencies are rare but do occur in alcoholics, e.g. folate and vitamin C. Alcohol is estimated to be a factor in 20–30 % of accidents and has socio-economic consequences including domestic violence.

Alcohol and vulnerable groups

Pregnant women Alcohol may reduce the ability to conceive and excessive consumption is associated with a greater risk of miscarriage. Pregnant women are advised not to drink and to consume no more than 2–4 units per week. Excessive alcohol consumption during pregnancy can → fetal alcohol syndrome which may → facial deformities and growth problems (see 'DRVs and dietary guide lines during pregnancy' in Chapter 9).

Diabetes People with diabetes are advised not to drink excessively as this can → ↑ hypoglycaemic episodes.

Biologically active dietary constituents

Foods contain many chemicals that have no nutrient value but have physiological or pharmacological properties; these are often referred to as 'phytochemicals'. Some of these chemicals have protective properties but some are toxic or may become toxic if taken in excess.

Antioxidants and anticarcinogenic phytochemicals

Epidemiological studies have shown that fruit and vegetables have positive effects on health, particularly the prevention of cancer and heart disease, due to the presence of the antioxidant vitamins, vitamin C, vitamin E, and β-carotene, and probably some as yet to be identified antioxidants or anticarcinogenic compounds. These chemicals prevent damage to body tissues by free radicals. This group of chemicals includes the carotenoids, polyphenols, glucosinolates, phytoestrogens, and sulphides.

Carotenoids

The carotenoids consist of approximately 100 compounds that occur naturally in plants; they often give fruits and vegetables a yellow or orange colour. Some can be converted into retinol (vitamin A; see 'Vitamin A (retionol)' in Chapter 5); the most important of the carotenoids for retinol production is β-carotene. Carotenoids act as antioxidants by reacting with unpaired electrons in free radical and so neutralizing them. Another carotenoid that has received a lot of attention is lycopene; 85% of dietary lycopene is derived from tomatoes. Some studies have shown that lycopene may have anticarcinogenic properties and reduce the risk of heart disease.

Polyphenols

Phenolic compounds are found in many foods and beverages and act as plant's defence system against animals and insects. Polyphenols are either antioxidants or potentiate the effects of other antioxidants. The following chemicals are types of polyphenols.

- Phytosterols are found in seeds and oils and inhibit cholesterol absorption.
- Flavanoids—over 4000 types have been identified. They are found in fruits, vegetables, nuts, and seeds. Onions, apples, and black tea are particular rich sources. Quercetin and catechins are examples of flavanoids.
- Tannins are present in red wines and tea adding colour and flavour. They are antioxidants but bind to Fe and inhibit Fe absorption.
- Phytoestrogens are plant chemicals that are chemically similar to the animal hormone oestradiol. They compete for oestradiol receptors and can either ↑ or ↓ the effects of oestradiol. Isoflavones are phytoestrogens that are found in soya beans and products.

- Soya isoflavones have been shown to have hormonal effects and have been used to alleviate menopausal symptoms.
- Soya isoflavones have been shown to have anticarcinogenic properties in *in vitro* studies but the effects are variable in humans. Some studies have suggested that excessive intakes of isoflavones may in fact be carcinogenic; ∴ concentrated supplements are not recommended.
- Sulphides are present in foods such as onion, leek, and garlic. They have been shown to have anticarcinogenic properties in animal studies. There is some epidemiological evidence to suggest that sulphides reduce the risk of colorectal and gastric cancers.
- Glucosinolates are present in plants of the brassica family such as cabbage, broccoli, kale, Brussels sprouts, and cauliflower. There is some evidence of anticarcinogenic properties of glucosinolates in experimental studies but large intakes may actually be carcinogenic; more studies are required.

Caffeine and methylxanthines

Methylxanthines are a group of chemicals that includes caffeine, theophylline, and theobromine. They occur naturally in foods and drinks such as tea, coffee, cola drinks, and cocoa product (Table 7.5); they are also added to 'energy' drinks. Caffeine is a mild stimulant although there is individual variation in this response. It is mildly addictive and abrupt stoppage of caffeine intake can → mild withdrawal symptoms of headache, fatigue, and irritability. A daily intake of 4–5 cups of coffee is considered moderate; caffeine intake is dependent on the size of cup, the fineness of grinding, brewing method, roasting of beans, and type of coffee beans used. Arabica coffee beans contain less caffeine than Robusta beans. Tea has higher caffeine content than coffee on a dry weight basis but less tea is used to produce a drink.

By law drinks containing caffeine in excess of 150 mg/l must carry a declaration in the same part of the label as the name of the food. Caffeine content, with the amount of caffeine expressed in mg per 100 ml, should be given to identify high levels of caffeine in some drinks. This law does not apply to drinks based on tea or coffee, or coffee or tea extract.

Caffeine is a mild diuretic if taken in quantities above that considered moderate, 4–5 cups per day. The evidence that caffeine reduces fertility is inconclusive. The Food Standards Agency recommends that pregnant women should not have more than 300 mg of caffeine per day (see Chapter 9). Some studies suggest that higher intakes are linked with miscarriage, low birth weight, and premature delivery. This is disputed by some researchers who have suggested that high caffeine intake is an indication of low hormone levels. Many women have a reduced desire for coffee during pregnancy which is believed to be due to high placental hormone levels, ∴ high coffee intake may be a marker of low hormone levels. The National Childbirth Trust recommends that coffee intake during breastfeeding should not be stopped but that intake should not exceed 3–4 cups per day as caffeine passes into breast milk causing the baby to be restless and agitated (see 'Breast versus bottle feeding' in Chapter 10).

Table 7.4 Caffeine content of beverages

300 mg of caffeine is roughly equivalent to
- 4 average cups or 3 average size mugs of instant coffee
- 3 average cups of brewed coffee
- 6 average cups of tea
- 8 cans of regular cola drinks
- 4 cans of so-called 'energy' drinks
- 400 grams (8 standard 50 g bars) of plain chocolate

Household measures of caffeine:
- Average cup of instant coffee—75 mg
- Average mug of coffee—100 mg
- Average cup of brewed coffee—100 mg
- Average cup of tea—50 mg
- Regular cola drink—up to 40 mg
- Regular energy drink—up to 80 mg
- Plain bar of chocolate—up to 50 mg. Caffeine in milk chocolate
  is about half that of plain chocolate

Decaffeinated brands are not totally free of caffeine but usually contain 5 mg caffeine per cup; they contain smaller amounts of the other methylxanthines than normal brands.

Theobromine levels are low in beverages except chocolate products. High cocoa (70% cocoa beans) content brands have higher levels of caffeine and theobromine than average brands.

Vasoactive amines

Tyramine, histamine, tryptamine, and serotonin are all present in foods and are normally deactivated in the body. High intakes and intake in individuals with an impaired ability to deactivate them can → vasoconstrictive effects. Vasoactive amines can trigger migraine in susceptible people. People taking monoamine oxidase inhibitor type A drugs may experience a dangerous hypertensive interaction with vasoactive amine (see 'Drug—nutrient interactions', Chapter 8).

Food additives

Food additives are substances added to food for technological reasons
which may be their organoleptic properties. They are classified into
groups according to their purpose. The numbering system is being
adapted for international use by the Codex Alimentarius Commission.
The International Numbering System (INS) will use the same numbers
used within the European Community but without the E prefix. The use
of food additives is controlled by the Food Standards Agency in the UK
and European Scientific Committee for Food (SCF) in Europe. Food
additives must gain approval before their use in food manufacture is
permitted at specified levels. The approval process is lengthy and detailed
with most of the research being funded by the food manufacturer. Some
additives are naturally occurring substances but they must also undergo
safety testing and approval before they can be used in food manufacture.
Approximately 3500 additives are in use today. Additives are used for the
following reasons:

- the need to keep foods fresh until eaten so widening food choice and
  availability;
- convenience of packaging. storage, preparation, and use;
- attractive presentation;
- economic advantage, e.g. longer shelf life or reduced cost;
- nutritional supplementation.

E numbers

E numbers identify permitted food additives regarded as safe for use
within the European Union. Some additives have a number but no
prefix as they are under consideration by the European Commission.
All food labels must show the additive's name or E number in the list of
ingredients.

Additive groups

Colourings (E100–180) Food is coloured to restore losses that occur in
manufacture and storage, to meet consumer expectations, and to maintain uniformity of products. An example of this is that oranges have green
patches when picked and are coloured orange before sale. Azo, coal tar
based, dyes are frequently linked to food allergy (see Chapter 33). Lists
of natural and synthetic colours are shown in Tables 7.5 and 7.6.

Preservatives (E200–290)[1]
Preservatives are used to prevent food spoilage and enable the consumers to have a wide range of goods that are available out of the usual
season. Traditional preservatives include salt, vinegar, alcohol, and spices.
Acetic acid is the major component of vinegar and may be considered a
a natural additive but it has undergone extensive testing and has an
E number E260. Benzoic acid and benzoates occur widely in fresh foods
e.g. peas, bananas, and berries. Although rare, adverse reactions to benzoates have been seen. Commonly used preservatives are shown in
Table 7.7.

---

1 The preservative lysozyme has the E number, E1105.

Table 7.5 Examples of natural colours*

Name	E number	Food use
Riboflavin (yellow)	E101	Processed cheese
Chlorophyll (green)	E140	Fats, oils, canned & dried vegetables
Carbon (black)	E153	Jams, jellies
α Carotene (yellow/orange)	E160	Margarine & cakes

Reproduced with permission from *Understanding Food and Nutrition*, J Webster–Gandy. Part of the Family Doctor Series Ltd in association with the British Medical Association.

Table 7.6 Examples of synthetic colours*

Name	E number	Food Use
Tartrazine (yellow)	E102	Soft drinks
Sunset (yellow)	E110	Orange drinks
Amaranth (red)	E123	Blackcurrant products
Erythrosine (red)	E127	Glace cherries
Indigo carmine (blue)	E132	Savoury food mixes
Green S	E142	Tinned peas, mint jelly and sauce

Reproduced with permission from *Understanding Food and Nutrition*, J Webster–Gandy. Part of the Family Doctor Series Ltd in association with the British Medical Association.

Sulphur dioxide destroys thiamin and ∴ is not permitted in foods tha are significant sources of thiamies. Sulphur dioxide is used to destro yeasts which can cause fermentation in food products.

Nitrates and nitrites kill the bacteria that cause botulism, a potentia lethal form of food poisoning. They preserve the red colour in meat ar are ∴ used in meat products. A major source of these chemicals in th body is fertilizers that use these chemicals. Nitrites may react with othe chemicals in the gut to form nitrosamines which have been shown t cause cancer in experimental animals. There is no evidence to suppo the suggestion that these preservatives play a role in causing cancer i man.

Antioxidants (E300–322) These additives prevent the unpleasant tast and smell that occur when fats and oils go rancid. The most widely use antioxidants are butylated hydroxyanisole (BHA) and butylated hydrox toluene (BHT). They are used in a wide variety of foods. Table 7.8 show the permitted antioxidants.

Emulsifiers, stabilizers, thickeners, and gelling agents (E400–495)[2] Thes additives are needed to ↑ the shelf life of some foods and are shown Table 7.9. They affect the texture and constituency of products. This the largest group of additives and many are natural substances, e.g. carr geenan, which is derived from seaweed. Polyphosphates have received great deal of attention from consumer groups as they enable products retain water so ↑ the product's weight. They are used in products suc as frozen poultry and cured meats.

Sweeteners

Sweeteners are divided into 2 groups:
- caloric sweeteners: mannitol (E421), sorbitol (E420), isomalt (E953), maltitol (E965), xylitol (E967), and lactitol (E966). These additives add energy to the diet.
- non-caloric sweeteners: acesulfame K (E950), aspartame (951), cyclamic acid and its salts (E952), saccharine and its salts (E954), thaumatin (E957), and neohesperidine (E959).

Sucralose and the salt of aspartame—acesulfame are permitted swee eners in the UK but do not have E numbers as they are not fully autho ized in the European Union. Sucrose, glucose, fructose, and lactose ai all classified as foods rather than sweeteners or additives.

2 Agents with E numbers outside this grouping: lecithins E322, invertase E1103.

Table 7.7 Commonly used preservatives*

Name	E number	Food use
Sorbic acid & derivatives	E200–E203	Cheese, yogurt, soft drinks
Acetic acid	E260	Pickles, sauces
Lactic acid	E270	Margarine, confectionery, sauces
Propionic acid & derivatives	E280–E283	Bread, cakes, flour
Benzoic acid & derivatives	E210–E219	Soft drinks, pickles, fruit products, jams
Sulphur dioxide	E220	Soft drinks, fruit products, beer, cider, wine
Nitrites	E249, E250	Cured meats, cooked meats, meat products
Nitrates	E251, E252	Bacon, ham, cheese (not cheddar or cheshire)

Reproduced with permission from *Understanding Food and Nutrition*, J Webster–Gandy. Part of the Family Doctor Series Ltd in association with the British Medical Association.

Table 7.8 Permitted antioxidants*

Name	E number	Food use
Ascorbic acid (vitamin C) & derivatives	E300–E305	Beer, soft drink, powdered milks, fruit, meat products
Tocopherols (vitamin A) & derivatives	E306–E309	Vegetable oils
Gallates	E310–E320	Vegetable oils & fats, margarine
BHA	E320	Margarine, fat in baked products, e.g. pies
BHT	E321	Crisps, margarine, vegetable oils, convenience foods

Reproduced with permission from *Understanding Food and Nutrition*, J Webster–Gandy. Part of the Family Doctor Series Ltd in association with the British Medical Association.

Table 7.9 Examples of emulsifiers, stabilizers, thickeners, and gelling agents

Name	E Number	Food use
Lecithins (may be used as an antioxidant)	E322	Chocolate, margarine, potato snacks
Citric acid & derivatives	E472c	Pickles, dairy products, baked products
Tartaric acid & derivatives	E472d–f	Baking powder
Alginic acid	E400–E405	Ice cream, instant desserts & puddings
Agar	E406	Tinned ham, ice cream
Carrageenan	E407	Ice cream
Gums	E410–E418	Ice cream, soups, confectionery
Pectin	E440	Preserves, jellies

Other additives

These include:

- flavour enhancers, e.g. monosodium glutamate (E621);
- anti-foaming agents that prevent frothing during processing;
- propellant gases, e.g. in aerosol cream.

A full list of E numbers is available from the Food Standards Agency website http://www.food.gov.uk.

Drug–nutrient interactions and prescription of nutritional products

Drug–nutrient interactions

Both micro- and macronutrients may interact with drug therapy and these interactions may be positive or detrimental (leading to a failure of therapy or drug toxicity). Similarly, drugs may interact with the absorption or metabolism of nutrients. Consequently, nutrition and dietetic therapy should be viewed alongside drug therapy. In the case of disorders such as dyslipidaemia, drug therapy should be used in concert with and not in place of dietary modifications.

❶ The scope for nutrient–drug interactions is large but certain therapies should always cause concern:
- warfarin;
- lithium;
- monoamine oxidase inhibitors (MAOI).

For full information on drug interactions, Stockley's drug interactions should be consulted.[1]

Interactions leading to alterations in drug therapy
- Warfarin and vitamin K containing foods: the anticoagulant warfarin is a vitamin K antagonist and alterations in vitamin K consumption may alter anticoagulant therapy. For example, ↑ consumption of beetroot, green vegetables (e.g. spinach), brussel sprouts, lettuce may ↓ the effects of warfarin. Once patients are stabilized on warfarin they should avoid major variations in the consumption of these foods.
- Potentiation of drug action: inhibition of drug metabolism by nutrients may ↑ drug effects, e.g.
  - Cranberry juice has recently been implicated in deaths through enhancing the effects of warfarin.
  - Grapefruit juice may enhance the actions of Ca channel blockers (especially nifedipine, felodipine, and nicardipine) used in hypertension and angina, the antihistamine, terfenadine, and the immunosuppressant cyclosporin. ↑ plasma concentrations can → toxicity (especially terfenadine and cyclosporin).
- Synergy: fish oils inhibit platelet aggregation and may ↑ bleeding with antiplatelet drugs (aspirin) and warfarin.
- High doses of vitamin E enhance the anticoagulant effects of warfarin.
- Lithium and salt: Na influences the excretion of lithium (used in bipolar affective disorder) such that salt supplements may ↓ plasma lithium and salt-restricted diets may ↑ lithium to toxic levels.

Interactions limiting therapy
- Diuretics and salt: diuretics (such as bendroflumethiazide and furosemide) used for hypertension and chronic heart failure cause salt and water excretion. Their beneficial effects may be undone by consumption of salt in the diet.

[1] Baxter, K. (2005). Stockley's drug interactions, 7th edn. Pharmaceutical Press, London.

- Ca or Fe with tetracycline or 4-quinolones: the antibacterials tetracycline and 4-quinolones (such as ciprofloxacin) should not be taken at the same time as milk, other Ca^{2+} containing substances, or Fe as these antibacterials chelate these ions and are not absorbed.
- Levodopa and pyridoxine (vitamin B_6): the actions of levodopa for the management of Parkinson's disease may be reduced by supplements with pyridoxine. This does not occur when the levodopa is combined with a dopa decarboxylase inhibitor (e.g. carbidopa).

🔴 Interactions with potentially serious events:
- Warfarin and vitamin K containing foods: see above.
- Warfarin and cranberry juice: see above.
- Grapefruit juice and terfenadine or cyclosporin: see above.
- ACE inhibitors/AT_1 receptor antagonists and potassium supplements/salt substitutes: ACE inhibitors (such as ramipril, enalapril) and AT_1 receptor antagonists (e.g. losartan) may cause K^+ retention and this may be exacerbated by K^+ supplements/salt substitutes → to hyperkalaemia.
- Monoamine oxidase inhibitors (MAOI) and tyramine: patients taking MAOI (e.g. phenelzine, moclobemide) for depression (rarely used nowadays) should avoid tyramine-containing foods (e.g. mature cheese, yeast extracts, soya bean products, pickled herring, certain wine) as this may → the 'cheese reaction' with a severe ↑ blood pressure.
- Isotretinoin and vitamin A: isotretetinoin is a retinoid used in acne and should not be used with vitamin A supplements due to the risk of a vitamin A overdose.

Drug therapies requiring nutritional supplements

Certain drug therapies may require nutritional supplements to limit adverse effects.
- Corticosteroids: long term treatment with oral corticosteroids (such as prednisolone) or (potentially high dose inhaled corticosteroids) may → to osteoporosis and Ca supplements may be recommended.
- Methotrexate: this is a folate antagonist used in rheumatoid arthritis, Crohn's disease, anticancer chemotherapy, and psoriasis. Folic acid supplements may be appropriate to prevent megaloblastic anaemia.
- Isoniazid and vitamin B_6: isoniazid (used in tuberculosis) may have anti-vitamin B_6 effects → peripheral neuropathy and so 10 mg pyridoxine is given.
- Antiepileptic drugs in pregnancy: many antiepileptic drugs are associated with birth defects and 5 mg folic acid is prescribed to ↓ the risk of neural tube defects. Carbamazepine, phenytoin, and phenobarbital are associated with ↑ neonatal bleeding (including intracranial bleeds) and vitamin K is given to the mother from the 36th week in pregnancy and to the baby at birth.
- The antimalarial proguanil and pregnancy: 5 mg folic acid supplementation is required.

Drug therapy leading to nutritional deficiencies

Certain drug treatments may reduce the absorption of nutrients.

- Colestyramine and orlistat: colestyramine (for hyperlipidaemia or jaundice) and orlistat may both ↓ the absorption of fat-soluble vitamins (A, D, E, and K). Supplements may be required and taken at a different time to the drug.
- Antiepileptic drugs and Ca: enzyme-inducing antiepileptic drugs (e.g. carbamazepine, phenytoin) may induce the metabolism of vitamin D → Ca deficiencies. This may be overcome by vitamin D supplementation.
- Diuretics such as bendroflumethiazide and furosemide, especially when used at higher doses for chronic heart failure, may → hypokalaemia and K^+ supplements or foods rich in K^+ such as bananas may be recommended.
- The antidiabetic drug metformin may → ↓ absorption of vitamin B_{12}.
- Methotrexate and folic acid: see above.

Diabetes   Insulin and sulphonylureas, e.g. gliclazide and glibenclamide, may → to hypoglycaemia if meals are skipped or insufficient.

Alcohol and drugs

Alcohol may enhance the action of many drugs acting on the brain (e.g. antidepressants, benzodiazepines, and antiepileptic drugs) leading to impaired mental ability and sedation.

It is a misconception that all antibiotics interact with alcohol and, of the commonly used agents, there is only a significant interaction with metronidazole which leads to a severe reaction including nausea and flushing.

Food and drugs

The absorption of many drugs may be retarded by the presence of food or in some cases enhanced. The presence of food may also reduce any gastric damage, for example, with nonsteroidal anti-inflammatory drugs (e.g. ibuprofen and diclofenac). It is for this reason that cautionary labels such as 'with or after food', 'an hour before food or an empty stomach', 'with or after food' should be followed.

Nutritional status and drug therapy

- Dehydration will enhance the actions of diuretics and other anti-hypertensives and may → falls in the elderly.
- Protein restrictions may → hypoalbuminaemia. Many drugs are bound to plasma proteins; this does not necessarily → major changes in therapy although correction may be required in therapeutic drug monitoring.
- Enteral feeding has the scope for drugs to interact with constituents of the feed. When changing from a tablet to a liquid preparation (e.g. digoxin) the bioavailability may be altered and the dose of drug may need to be changed.

Metabolic effects of drugs

Some drugs may alter plasma lipid or glucose levels.
- Drugs that may → dyslipidaemia: β-blockers, corticosteroids, thiazide diuretics, anabolic steroids, certain anti-HIV drugs, retinoids, and oral contraceptives containing levonorgestrel.
- Drugs that may affect glucose tolerance: thiazide diuretics, corticosteroids.

Effects of drug treatment on appetite and feeding

Some drug treatments may affect appetite or eating.
- Anorectic effects: with antiobesity drugs (e.g. sibutramine), digoxin.
- Weight gain: with sulphonylureas, Na valproate, antipsychotic drugs, corticosteroids, tricyclic antidepressants, insulin.
- Taste disturbances may occur with ACE inhibitors, Ca channel blockers, anticancer chemotherapy drugs.
- Dry mouth: antimuscarinic effects (for example with tricyclic antidepressants).
- Oral mucositis: this is a common side-effect of anticancer drugs (especially with alkylating agents, methotrexate, and fluorouracil) where interference with cell division leads to oral ulceration. This may be exacerbated by poor oral hygiene. Saline mouthwashes are often used for relief and in the case of fluorouracil the BNF recommends sucking ice when it is infused.
- Nausea and vomiting: digoxin, anticancer chemotherapy, opioids (such as morphine), certain drugs for Parkinson's disease, SSRIs, erythromycin, theophylline.
- Gastric irritation: nonsteroidal anti-inflammatory drugs in particular are associated with gastric damage.

Common herb–drug interactions

Commonly used herbs are not without adverse events and may interact with conventional medicines. An important example of this is St John's wort which is an important enzyme inducer and may reduce the effects of the following drugs and so concomitant treatment should be avoided.
- Amitriptyline.
- Antiepileptic drugs.
- Certain anti-HIV drugs (protease inhibitors and non-nucleoside reverse transcriptase inhibitors).
- Cyclosporin.
- Digoxin.
- Oral contraceptives.
- Phenytoin.
- Simvastatin.
- Theophylline.
- Warfarin.

St John's wort also has serotonergic effects and so may → ↑ serotonergic side-effects with SSRI antidepressants (e.g. fluoxetine) and triptans (e.g. migraine treatment).

Additional herb–drug interactions include:

- dong quai and warfarin: ↑ actions of warfarin;
- echinacea and immunosuppressants: possible immunostimulation by echinacea may render immunosuppressant less effective and should be avoided;
- garlic and warfarin: ↑ actions of warfarin;
- ginkgo and antiplatelet drugs or warfarin: ↑ bleeding means that gingko should only be used with caution in patients receiving these drugs.

Prescription of nutritional products

All nutritional products within the UK can be bought without a prescription, i.e. none are classified as *prescription-only medication* that can only be obtained if prescribed by a medical practitioner or other specified health-care professional. However, some nutritional products may be prescribed for specific conditions and are then categorized as drugs rather than food. This facility is important for patients with chronic conditions who may need expensive special products over a long period of time, e.g. coeliac disease where gluten-free products are required.

Prescribable nutrition products are listed in the *British National Formulary*, Appendix 7 Borderline Substances, as:
- foods that may be prescribed for clinical conditions, alphabetically by brand name of products;
- conditions for which foods may be prescribed, alphabetically by conditions. If a specific condition is not listed, a broader category should be sought, e.g. Crohn's disease is not included but inflammatory bowel disease and intestinal surgery are present.

Doctors prescribing such products are advised to:
- endorse the prescription with 'ACBS', i.e. prescribed in accordance with the guidelines from the Advisory Committee on Borderline Substances;
- ensure that the patient will be adequately monitored in taking the products and that, where necessary, expert hospital supervision, usually by a dietitian, will be available. Good communication between health-care professionals and patients is required to optimize the products provided and the cost to the prescribing budget.

Diet before and during pregnancy

Pre- and periconceptional nutrition in women

Why is preconceptional nutrition important?

A mother's nutritional status prior to conception, (preconception 3 months before), and immediately afterwards, (periconception 2–3 months after), is critical. The fetus is most vulnerable to nutritional deficiencies in the first trimester of pregnancy, often before a woman realizes that she is pregnant.

There is evidence that poor maternal nutrition has both immediate (e.g. low birth weight) and long-term consequences. The so-called 'fetal origins' or 'Barker' hypothesis proposes that fetal growth plays a major role in determining the risk of some dietary related non-communicable disease, e.g. cardiovascular disease and type 2 diabetes in adulthood.

What dietary changes can the mother make to increase the likelihood of conceiving and giving birth to a healthy infant?

- Take folic acid supplements to protect against neural tube defects (NTDs).[1]
    - To prevent first occurrence of NTD: 400 μg during preconception and until the 12th week of pregnancy (on prescription or over the counter).
    - To prevent recurrence of NTD: 5000 μg during preconception and until the 12th week of pregnancy (on prescription only).
- Foods rich in folic acid should be chosen (see box).

Foods rich in folic acid

- *Rich sources*, >100 μg per serving: Brussels sprouts, kale, spinach
- *Good sources*, 50–100 μg per serving: fortified bread and breakfast cereals, broccoli, cabbage, cauliflower, chickpeas, green beans, iceberg, kidney, lettuce, peas, spring greens
- *Moderate sources*, 15–15 μg per serving: potatoes, most other vegetables, most fruits, most nuts, brown rice, wholegrain pasta, oats, bran, some breakfast cereals, cheese, yoghurt, milk, eggs, salmon, beef, game

---

[1] Expert Advisory Group (1992). *Folic acid and the prevention of neural tube defects.* Department of Health, London.

- Eat a varied diet. Refer to 'Balance of good health' in 'Food-based dietary guidelines' in Chapter 2. The main points are:
  - include 5 portions of fruit and vegetables a day;
  - eat a variety of different foods from all food groups;
  - restrict foods containing too much saturated fat and sugar.
- Achieve and maintain ideal weight at preconception (BMI 18.5–24.9 kg/m^2).
  - Weight needs to be stabilized 3 months before attempting conception.
  - Low body fat content of <22% of body weight can prevent ovulation (average body fat content of post-pubertal women is 28%).
  - Obesity (BMI ≥ 30) can inhibit ovulation due to associated changes in insulin activity and its effect on hormone activity.
  - Obesity at conception can influence the *pregnancy* (high blood pressure, impaired blood sugar metabolism, gestational diabetes; pre-eclampsia), *delivery* (preterm delivery; prolonged labour; unplanned Caesarean), and *infant's health* (stillborn fetus; difficulty initiating and sustaining breastfeeding).
  - Underweight (BMI <18.5) at conception can increase the risk of pre-term delivery and of delivering a low-birth weight infant.
- Reduce alcohol consumption and ideally exclude alcohol.
  - Alcohol intake may be associated with decreased fertility and can affect the growing fetus.
  - Binge drinking in particular is not recommended.
- Avoid excessive intake of retinol/vitamin A (β-carotene is not toxic).
  - Avoid vitamin A supplements, liver, liver pâté, or sausage as retinol is teratogenic at extreme intakes (8000–10000 μg).
  - Avoid drugs that contain vitamin A or its analogues, such as cystic acne medications (isotretinoin; treinoin).
- Women who smoke should seek support for giving up in preparation for pregnancy.
- Women should be encouraged to follow the food safety advice for pregnant women (see 'Food safety in pregnancy and maternal weight gain', this chapter) as a precautionary measure for when conception occurs.

DRVs and dietary guidelines during pregnancy

Dietary recommendations are the same as for a normal healthy diet (see 'Balance of good health' in 'Food-based dietary guidelines' in Chapter 2) except for additional requirements for 6 nutrients (see Table 8.1).

Caffeine

May contribute to low birth weight by increasing fetal heart rate although evidence is inconclusive. Tea, coffee, cocoa, and cola-type drinks are advised in moderation (<4 cups a day of these combined, equivalent to <300 mg/day). Suggest decaffeinated tea and coffee or other alternatives, such as fruit tea, fruit juice, or water. Tea and coffee also reduce iron absorption.

The following contain ~300 mg of caffeine:
- 3 mugs of instant or brewed coffee (100 mg each);
- 4 cups of instant coffee (75 mg each);
- 3 cups of brewed coffee (100 mg each);
- 6 cups of tea (50 mg each);
- 8 cans of cola (up to 40 mg each);
- 4 cans of 'energy drink' (up to 80 mg each);
- 8 (50 g) bars of plain chocolate (up to 50 mg each). Caffeine in milk chocolate is about half that of plain chocolate.

Alcohol

Current optimal advice is abstinence in pregnancy, especially important in the first trimester; however, occasional drinking of small quantities, i.e ≤4 units/week but no more than 2 units at any 'sitting' (see Table 7.1 in 'Alcohol', Chapter 7) is unlikely to harm the fetus.[2]

Excessive binge drinking is most dangerous and can have teratogenic effects leading to fetal alcohol syndrome which affects 1–2/1000 births/year. Risk is elevated in women drinking >8 units/day. Symptoms in the infant are growth retardation, craniofacial and CNS defects, cardiac and genitourinary abnormalities.

Use of vitamin and mineral supplements in pregnancy

Women should try and obtain nutrients from a balanced diet (see 'Balance of good health' in 'Food-based dietary guidelines', Chapter 2) and women need to be advised against taking high dose multivitamin and mineral supplements, some of which can quickly reach toxic levels and may have teratogenic effects (particularly vitamin A). Women should not consume more than 3300 µg/day (UK DH) of vitamin A and supplements are discouraged. However, in areas of the world where vitamin A deficiency is prevalent, supplementation may be beneficial for pregnant women.

[2] Deparment of Health (2005). *The pregnancy book*. Department of Health, London. Available at www.dh.gov.uk.

Table 9.1 RNI for pregnant women

Nutrient	Daily RNI (pre-pregnancy)	↑ in pregnancy
Energy (kcal)	1940–2110	+200 (3rd trimester)
Folic acid (µg)	200	+400 (1st trimester)
		+100 (2nd and 3rd trimesters)
Protein (g)	51	+6
Vitamin C (mg)	40	+10 (3rd trimester)
Vitamin D (µg)	0 (assumed gained from sun exposure)	+10
Vitamin A (µg)	600	+100

NB. No increase recommended for intake of calcium and iron as evidence insufficient that this is needed above RNI. See table x for recommendations for adult women.

Folic acid (400 µg/day) is the only supplement recommended for 'blanket' use by women until the 12th week of pregnancy (see 'Pre-and periconceptional nutrition in women', this chapter).

In the UK, iron supplements are advised only if there is evidence of iron deficiency anaemia (see 'Iron', Chapter 5). Iron stores should be verified preconceptionally and in pregnancy. Iron supplements can cause constipation and other GI changes and may interfere with zinc absorption.

There is inconclusive evidence to recommend vitamin D supplements during pregnancy and currently the D.H recommends that sunlight and dietary sources of vitamin D should be encouraged to meet the increase in requirement of 10 µg/day (see 'Vitamin D (calciferols)', Chapter 5) and that only those on a restricted diet need extra vitamin D. Some Asian women could be at risk of vitamin D deficiency if insufficient skin exposure (see 'Minority ethnic communities', Chapter 13) → neonatal hypocalcaemia and rickets. ∴ may need vitamin D supplements.

However this is controversial and the FSA (www.eatwell.gov.uk) now advises that a supplement of 10 µg of vitamin D should be taken during pregnancy and whilst breastfeeding.

Advise caution about herbal supplements, as these are not generally evaluated for safety in pregnancy.

Food safety in pregnancy and maternal weight gain

Food safety in pregnancy

Besides following normal safe food hygiene practices, pregnant women should be advised to avoid additional practices that have been specifically linked to micro-organisms that can lead to fetal malformations.

- Avoiding salmonellosis. In severe cases can cause premature labour and miscarriage.
  - Avoid raw or undercooked eggs due to salmonella risk. White and yolk should be hard boiled. Raw egg may be found in home-made mayonnaise, ice-cream, mousse,
  - Avoid raw or partially cooked meat, especially poultry.
- Avoiding listeriosis. Caused by *Listeria monocytogenes*. Rare, but even mild infection can lead to miscarriage, still birth, or ill newborn. Women should avoid:
  - all types of pâté (including vegetable);
  - mould ripened soft cheese, e.g. brie, camembert;
  - blue veined cheese, e.g. stilton, roquefort, and other unpasteurized cheese;
  - unpasteurized milk, including cow, goat, and sheep's, and associated milk products;
  - eating uncooked or undercooked ready-prepared meals.
- Avoiding toxoplasmosis (mother has flu symptoms and infant has blindness and mental retardation) caused by *Toxoplasma gondii*.
  - Avoid cats as they can be carriers.
  - Cook poultry and meat thoroughly.
  - Wash salads, fruit, and vegetables to remove all soil.
  - Reheat ready prepared meals and leftovers to avoid listeria.
- Avoiding vitamin toxicity.
  - Avoid liver and its products, as they are rich in vitamin A.
- Reducing likelihood of developing infant allergies. Nut and peanut allergy is increasing in UK. If there is atopic family history, women should avoid:
  - peanuts, nuts, peanut butter, and unrefined groundnut oil;
  - foods containing nuts. Not always easy to follow; patients need to check for 'nut free' label on foods.
- Avoiding mercury poisoning (can affect neural development of fetus).
  - Avoid fish high in mercury: shark, marlin, and swordfish.
  - Limit tuna to ≤4 medium size cans or 2 fresh tuna steaks a week.

Maternal weight gain

How much weight should a woman gain during pregnancy?

It is not always easy to determine women's energy requirements in early pregnancy as BMR falls in some women and rises in others. Weight gained in pregnancy is a combination of maternal and fetal tissues and fluid, as well as maternal fat stores. Rate of weight gain is usually not constant; around 2 kg (5 lbs) are gained in the first trimester and the remainder fairly evenly throughout the second and third trimesters at a rate of around 0.4 kg (1 lb) per week.

An average weight gain of 10–12.5 kg (20–28 lbs) should be anticipated in women of normal BMI in higher income countries. Women who are overweight or obese should not attempt to lose weight during pregnancy but should limit weight gain to 7–11.5 kg (15–25 lbs).

Both too little and too much weight gain can adversely affect the fetus.

Too much maternal weight gain during pregnancy can → postpartum maternal obesity; possibility of caesarean; infant macrosomia; and ↑ risk of gestational diabetes. See 'Balance of good health' in 'Food-based dietary guidelines', Chapter 2 for how to prevent weight gain with healthier eating.

Too little maternal weight gain can → Low birth weight baby with subsequent effects on long-term health ('Pre-and periconceptional nutrition', this chapter).

In the UK, the D.H (see Table 9.1) made a blanket recommendation of an extra 200 kcal per day in the last trimester. However, the best advice is to encourage women to eat to appetite in pregnancy and monitor weight gain within the above ranges.

Weight gain with multiple pregnancy

Multiple births account for 1 in 6 of every births in the UK. Women carrying twins (or more!) will gain even more weight than women carrying one fetus. In the absence of other guidelines, the US Institute of Medicine (IOM) recommendations are used. They advise 16–20.5 kg (25–45 lbs) weight gain for women carrying twins, who begin the pregnancy with a normal weight.[1] Women pregnant with triplets should probably aim for a gain of around a further 4.5 kg (10 lbs). A healthy weight gain is particularly important in multiple pregnancies as they carry a higher risk of premature birth and low birth weight.

Institute of Medicine (1990). *Nutrition during pregnancy, weight gain and nutrient supplements,* report of the Subcommittee on Nutritional Status and weight Gain during Pregnancy, Subcommittee on Dietary Intake and Nutrient Supplements during Pregnancy, and Committee on Nutritional Status during Pregnancy and Lactation, Food and Nutrition Board. National Academic press, Washington DC. (Can be accessed at www.iom.edu/report.asp?id=18257.)

Dietary problems in pregnancy

Food aversions and cravings

Aversions are relatively common especially for tea, coffee, fried food, and eggs. Food cravings can be strong but depend on the individual. There are no nutritional implications as long as not craving and eating a lot of energy-dense foods that result in excessive weight gain.

Pica

Pica is the persistent craving for non-food substances, ranging from coal, clay, candles, matchboxes, to soil. Pica can be harmful if the item craved and eaten is toxic or eaten in large enough quantities to have an impact on nutritional status. Eating soil could carry the risk of toxoplasmosis (see above). Evidence for a physiological basis of need is inconclusive. Pica is often associated with iron deficiency but it is uncertain whether iron deficiency causes pica or conversely whether pica causes iron deficiency via its proposed effect on iron absorption.

Pregnancy (alias morning) sickness

During the first trimester, ~70% of women have pregnancy sickness (nausea and vomiting) as the woman adjusts to higher hormone levels, especially human chorionic gonadotrophin and high oestrogen levels. Although often referred to as 'morning sickness' vomiting can occur at any time of the day: it varies from slight nausea to frequent and severe vomiting. Most cases are mild, but it impacts on the pregnant woman's sense of well-being and daily activities. **Hyperemesis gravidarum** is the most severe form and is defined as persistent nausea and vomiting leading to dehydration, ketonuria, electrolyte imbalance, and weight loss greater than 5% of pre-pregnancy weight.

Advise:[1]

- Frequent small meals and snacks every 2 h, avoiding large meals.
- High CHO foods are best tolerated, e.g. toast, dry biscuits, crackers, low sugar breakfast cereals.
- Avoid smells and foods that exacerbate nausea, e.g. high fat foods. However, these foods will depend on each woman.
- Taking food and drinks separately can help ↓ nausea in some women.
- Encourage plenty of fluid, especially as water and other sugar-free fluids, as dehydration may occur in extreme cases. Recommend at least 35 ml/kg body weight/daily; equivalent to 9 mugs of fluid in a 65 kg woman (1 mug = 250 ml).
- Taking time to rest and relax; take fresh air.
- Reassure women that most cases resolve spontaneously in the first 16–20 weeks of pregnancy.
- When symptoms are persistent, severe, and prevent daily activities, drug treatment should be considered.

---

[1] Further information is available at www.prodigy.nhs.uk/guidance.asp?gt=nausea/vomiting%20in%20pregnancy.

Constipation

5–40% of women suffer during pregnancy, as peristalsis is slower. Encouraging fresh and dried fruit and vegetables for pectins and wholemeal bread and breakfast cereals for cereal fibre will relieve symptoms and plenty of fluid, preferably as water, should be taken. Faecal bulking agents may help.

Women may intentionally restrict their fluid intake to reduce frequency of micturition; this could be a factor in them becoming constipated. See 'Constipation' in 'Disorders of the colon', Chapter 35.

Heartburn

Heartburn is common and 30–50% of pregnant women experience symptoms. This can occur at any stage of pregnancy, but usually in the 3rd trimester.

Suggest
Small, frequent meals.
Eat earlier in the evening and avoid late night meals.
Chew food thoroughly and slowly.
Take fluids between meals, not at mealtimes.
Dairy foods may relieve symptoms.
Avoid spicy and acidic foods that may irritate GI mucosa. Food causing symptoms varies a lot in different women; examples include chilli, vinegar, pepper, acidic fruit juices.
Avoid foods that relax oesophageal muscles before bedtime, e.g. chocolate, fatty foods, alcohol, and mint.
Sleep propped up with cushions.
Avoid bending after eating.

Iron deficiency anaemia

Women with diets poor in iron prior to pregnancy and a history of anaemia will need haemoglobin and ferritin status verifying to assess whether supplements are required. Anaemia is most likely to affect women on a low income (see 'Eating on a low income', Chapter 13), those with low BMI, or vegetarians with an unbalanced diet (see 'Vegetarians', Chapter 13). In the UK, iron supplements are advised only if there is evidence of iron deficiency anaemia (see diagnosis of anaemia in 'Iron', Chapter 5).

However, care should be taken not to 'blanket' prescribe iron supplements (can result in nausea and constipation), as in later pregnancy many women experience haemodilution and ∴ physiological changes may resemble iron deficiency (↓haemoglobin and ↓ferritin). See 'Iron', Chapter 5 for good dietary sources of iron.

Gestational diabetes

Estimated prevalence is 3–5% of pregnancies. Abnormal glucose intolerance occurs in pregnancy and usually disappears after birth, although there evidence that it is a marker for development of type 2 diabetes in later life. Diagnosis is made at fasting blood glucose >7 mmol/l. Women who are obese/overweight, aged ≥30 y, and have a family history of type 2 diabetes are at greater risk of developing gestational diabetes, increased risk of macrosomia at birth, and increased likelihood of Caesarean. See 'Gestational diabetes', Chapter 18.

Vulnerable groups in pregnancy

Adolescents

Pregnancy in adolescence increases risk to:
- *fetus* of low birth weight, perinatal mortality, and premature delivery;
- *mother* of anaemia, difficult labour, and hypertension.

As adolescents are still growing, optimal weight gain is unknown, but is likely to be higher than for adult women (see 'Food safety in pregnancy and maternal weight gain', this chapter). They are less likely to eat healthily and have higher RNIs for calcium and iron than women >18 y ∴ they are less likely to meet requirements for calcium and iron (see Chapter 11). Iron deficiency anaemia can result in low birth weight and preterm delivery. Social problems may have an influence and will compound pregnancy outcome, including:
- reducing energy intake to try and hide pregnancy;
- low income;
- smoking;
- alcohol consumption;
- substance abuse;
- previous dieting leading to low nutrient stores;
- less knowledge of a healthy diet.

The current UK government's *Teenage pregnancy strategy* (2004) has set targets of halving the number of under 18 conceptions by 2010, and getting 60% of teenage parents back into education, training, or employment.

Vegetarians

Being vegetarian should pose no problem in pregnancy, if the woman is well informed and eating a balanced lacto-ovo and lacto-vegetarian diet. Pregnant vegan, fruitarian, and macrobiotic women should be seen by a dietitian to assess overall nutrient adequacy of their diets. They may require supplementation of vitamin B_{12}, iron, vitamin D, or calcium (if <600 mg/day consumed). Some fortified soya milks contain these nutrients. (see 'Vegetarians' in Chapter 13).

Asian vegetarian women could be at risk of vitamin D deficiency if insufficient skin exposure (see 'Minority ethnic communities' in Chapter 13) → neonatal hypocalcaemia and rickets ∴ may need Vitamin D supplements. Pregnant vegetarian adolescents are at particular risk of inadequate diet if they are the only 'veggie' in the house, as they may tend to eat the same as the rest of the family except 'remove' the protein aspect of the meal or replace it with cheese, ready prepared vegetarian sausages and burgers.

Low income and pregnancy

Although it is difficult to generalize, UK women on low incomes may find it harder to achieve an adequate diet (see 'Balance of good health' and 'Food-based dietary guidelines' in Chapter 2 and 'Eating on a low income' in Chapter 13). Key nutrients at risk of low intakes are: zinc and iron, and vitamins A, C, and E and essential fatty acids (EFAs) needed for fetal neural and vascular system development. EFAs are found in green vegetables, oily fish (e.g. tuna, sardines, mackerel, salmon, herring, pilchards, trout, and kippers), and certain vegetable oils (e.g. corn, sunflower, and soya oils). Cheaper blended vegetable oils and margarine are often consumed but they contain less EFAs.

Healthy start scheme

In the UK, the welfare food scheme has been replaced by the healthy start scheme. The healthy start scheme allows beneficiaries to exchange tokens for fresh fruit and vegetables through general retail (see 'Healthy start scheme' in Breast versus bottle feeding' in Chapter 10). Further information on Healthy start see www.healthystart.nhs.uk.

Closely spaced pregnancies

Women having closely spaced pregnancies may have low nutrient stores at conception and in early pregnancy, so taking a dietary history would be useful to assess previous and current diet for nutrient adequacy (including iron status).

Overweight/obese women

Need regular monitoring as there is an increased risk of gestational DM and HT; risk increases with BMI. During pregnancy there is an ↑ risk of pre-eclampsia. At birth there is an ↑ likelihood of caesarean section, post-operative complications, low apgar score, excessive birthweight of newborn (macrosomia), ↑ perinatal mortality (3 fold), and neural tube defects (NTDs). (See 'Food safety and maternal weight gain', this chapter.)

Diabetic women

Regular glucose monitoring and good compliance will result in the same outcome as for non-diabetic mothers. However, poor control can ↑ risk of pre-eclampsia, ↑ fetal problems, and ↑ infant mortality.

Useful websites

DH, *The pregnancy book 2005*; www.dh.gov.uk
NICE 2003 *New guideline for the NHS on the care of pregnant women*
www.nice.org.uk/page.aspx?o=89310
www.eatwell.gov.uk/agesandstages/pregnancy/

Infants and preschool children

Infant growth and development

In the first year of life birth weight increases by 300%, doubling in the fir 4–6 months, and height increases by 50%. Growth then slows down. Th rapid growth involves tissue and organ maturation that mean that energ and nutrient requirements are high relative to body size during the first years of life (see Table 10.1).

Growth reference charts

Monitoring child's growth is essential to identify any faltering growt Length/height, weight, and head circumference should be plotted on growth reference curve. An infant's growth should follow the direction the growth curves. Serial measurements are necessary to determin adequacy of growth as a one-off measurement is only a reflection of siz The chart can be a useful tool for communicating with parents so th they understand the importance of monitoring growth. Parents wit naturally short children will need reassuring that s/he is growing well progressing in parallel with the same centile throughout infancy ar childhood.

Parental height plays a role in determining eventual height (see growt charts in Appendix 2 for how to calculate genetic height potential).

Which growth charts should be used?

The Royal College of Paediatrics and Child Health (www.rcpch.ac.ul commissioned a review of growth reference charts currently in use in th UK.[1] They recommended that, for most clinical purposes, the UK9 reference is the only suitable growth chart and recommend its use in th UK from birth for measuring weight, length (<2 y), height(>2 y), hea circumference (<2 y), and BMI (weight relative to height). These refe ence data have been incorporated into the Child Growth Foundation's ' centile growth charts, that have been endorsed by the DH and RCPCI They are included in the UK Personal Child Health Record (PCHF issued to each newborn (see charts in Appendix 2).

Separate girls' and boys' growth charts have been produced for:
- Birth to 1 year;
- 1–5 years;
- 5–18 years.

The charts have 9 reference centiles of 0.4th, 2nd, 9th, 25th, 50th, 75t 91st, 98th, and 99.9th that mean, for example:
- 98th centile curve, below which 98% of UK children lie (2 in 100 children will be as tall/ heavy as this);
- 50th centile curve, below which 50% of UK children lie (average weight and height for a child of that age).
- 2nd centile curve, below which only 2% of UK children lie (2 in 100 children will be as small/ light as this).

These are available from the Child Growth Foundation (www childgrowthfoundation.org).

[1] Wright, C. M., et al. (2002). Growth reference charts for use in the United Kingdom. Arch, D Child, **86**, 11–14.

Table 10.1 RNI for infants and preschool children*

Nutrient	0–3 mth	4–6 mth	7–9 mth	10–12 mth	1–3 y	4–6 y
Energy (kcal)						
♂	545	690	825	920	1230	1715
♀	515	645	765	865	1165	1545
Energy (kcal/kg/day)	100–115	95	95	95	95	90
Protein (g)	12.5	12.7	13.7	14.9	14.5	19.7
Protein (g/kg/day)	2.1	1.6	1.5	1.5	1.1	1.1
Fluid (ml/kg)	150	130	120	110	95	85
Vitamin C (mg)	25	25	25	25	30	30
Vitamin A (µg)	350	350	350	350	400	400
Folic acid (µg)	50	50	50	50	70	100
Thiamine (mg)	0.2	0.2	0.2	0.3	0.5	0.7
Riboflavin (mg)	0.4	0.4	0.4	0.4	0.6	0.8
Niacin (mg)	3	3	4	5	8	11
Vitamin B_{12} (µg)	0.3	0.3	0.4	0.4	0.5	0.8
Iron (mg)	1.7	4.3	7.8	7.8	6.9	6.1
Calcium (mg)	525	525	525	525	350	450
Phosphorus (mg)	400	400	400	400	270	350
Magnesium (mg)	55	60	75	80	85	120
Zinc (mg)	4.0	4.0	5.0	5.0	5.0	6.5
Selenium (µg)	10	13	10	10	15	20
Copper (mg)	0.2	0.3	0.3	0.3	0.4	0.6

* Department of Health (1991). *Dietary reference values for food and nutrients for the United Kingdom.* HMSO, London.

It is acknowledged that the growth of breastfed babies appears to b slightly slower than that of bottle fed babies, particularly between 3 and months of age. Separate charts have been produced for breastfed babie but they were based on a small population sample, and as such th RCPCH do not recommend their use (www.rcpch.ac.uk). The WHC have produced new growth charts representing growth standards base on the growth of healthy children in optimal conditions, rather tha reference data gained from cross-sectional observations. It is believe that all charts should be based on breastfed infants, as this is the biolog cal norm and all infants should be compared to this. It is not yet know whether the UK will adopt these charts in the future.

How often should infants be measured?

All babies should be weighed at birth, and a weight, length, and hea circumference should also be recorded at the 6–8 week check. Thereafte growth monitoring is no longer required according to Child Health Promotion guidelines until infants are 36–48 months.[2] Babies and your children could however be opportunistically weighed at immunization an surveillance contact, particularly if there is parental or clinical concern Weighing too frequently may cause parental anxiety.

Dietary recommendations for infants and preschool children

Children <5 y need a diet that is higher in fat and lower in fibre than tha presented in the 'Balance of good health' model (see 'Balance of goo health' in 'Food-based dietary guidelines' in Chapter 2) as they need fa for growth and CNS development. However, by the age of 5 they ca follow the dietary guidelines presented. If children are growing normall then >2 y, parents can gradually start introducing low fat/high fibr choices towards 'Balance of good health' recommendations at age 5 Total energy intake should not be restricted.

---

[2] Hall, D.M.B. and Elliman, D. (ed.) (2003). *Health for all children: the report of the Fourth Joir Working Party on Child Health Surveillance*, 4th edn. Oxford University Press, Oxford.

Breast versus bottle feeding

Breastmilk is the best choice for infant feeding for many reasons (see box
Infant formulae have a different composition to breastmilk and do no
provide all the same benefits, particularly the immunological activ
components, nor the same nutritional profile and bioavailability. Th
composition of breastmilk is not homogeneous: colostrum is produce
1–3 days postpartum, eventually becoming mature milk after 3 weeks. Th
immunological factors are not only present in colostrum produced durir
the first few days of lactation, but continue throughout breastfeeding.

Protective factors in breastmilk

- *Immunological active components:* lactoferrin; cytokines; T- and
  B- lymphocytes; neutrophils; macrophages; immunoglobulins;
  lysozymes; growth factors; thyroxin; antiviral lipids; antiprotozoan
  factors; and bifidus factor (promotes growth of protective
  Lactobacillus bifidus in infant's GI tract)
- *Essential long chain fatty acids:* important for cell membrane
  structure, especially CNS development. Most infant formulae only
  contain precursors, i.e. linoleic and alpha linolenic acid
- *Nutrients:* rich in vitamins A, D, E, PUFA, and free amino acids
  compared with infant formula
- *Oligosaccharides:* breastmilk contains >100 different oligosaccharides
  that help normal brain development and to make stools easier to
  pass ∴ reducing constipation (can be a problem in formula fed
  infants)

Benefits of breastfeeding

For the mother

- Encourages bonding between mother and infant.
- Helps women lose excess weight gained during pregnancy.
- Breastfeeding stimulates uterine contractions that help return the
  uterus to normal size.
- Exclusive breastfeeding suppresses ovulation, helping iron stores retur
  to normal.
- Breastmilk is free, except that the mother needs extra nourishment
  (see 'Dietary recommendations for lactating mothers', this chapter).
- Convenience; no preparation required.
- Reduces mother's risk of developing pre-menopausal breast cancer.

For the infant

- Breastmilk offers complete nutrition for the first 6 months and high
  bioavailability of nutrients.
- Infants are less likely to experience gastrointestinal infections, as there
  is no need for access to clean water, which can be a problem in
  developing countries in particular (may also be due to protective
  factors).

Prevention of other infectious diseases, especially respiratory, ear and urinary tract infections (greatest impact is for infants exclusively breastfed for first 6 months).
Breastfed babies are less likely to be obese in later childhood.

Potential obstacles to breastfeeding

Frequent myth of 'not enough milk': usually results from incorrect breastfeeding technique (see 'Promoting and establishing breastfeeding', this chapter). This is a common reason for women stopping breastfeeding.
Freedom of mother: she can feel exhausted as she takes complete responsibility for feeding; ∴will need support of others with housework, especially in the first few weeks.
Mothers may be concerned that they cannot see how much milk the baby is taking.

- Engorged breasts and sore nipples can discourage some mothers; need to make sure that the right position is being used for feeding and latching on.
- High stress levels: mother's mental state will affect the letdown reflex; anxiety→ oxytocin↓. Encourage her to rest more and relax when breastfeeding.
- Glamorous image of infant formula portraying healthy, beautiful babies via advertising.
- Social taboo of breastfeeding in public in some cultures, including the UK.
- Lack of public facilities for breastfeeding, especially needed in colder months.
- Lack of employment legislation supporting breastfeeding mothers in some countries. NB. Mothers are entitled to express breastmilk at work in the UK.
- May be perceived as offensive by some women, their partners, and older children.
- Breastfeeding of boys may be encouraged more in some cultures. Education needs to reinforce that breastfeeding is best for girls and boys.

Contraindications to breastfeeding

- HIV+ women: by vertical transmission from mother to infant, breastfeeding increases risk of transmission by up to 20%. DH advice is that HIV+ women living in the UK should not breastfeed. For further information: www.advisorybodies.doh.gov.uk/eaga/pdfs/hivinfantSep04.pdf. The WHO recommends avoidance of all breastfeeding for HIV-positive mothers when replacement feeding is affordable, feasible, acceptable, sustainable, and safe. These conditions are difficult to achieve in some poor developing countries. In such settings exclusive breastfeeding for 6 months is recommended if HIV+ mothers are unable to provide adequate replacement feed.[1]

[1] Joint WHO–UNICEF statement on HIV and infant feeding (2004). Available at www.who.int/child-adolescent-health/publications/NUTRITION/HIV/IF/WHO/UNICEF.htm.

- Mothers with untreated TB should not breastfeed.
- Mothers with hepatitis C who have cracked or bleeding nipples shoul
  not breastfeed.
- Women who smoke or occasionally drink alcohol *can* still breastfeed,
  however smoking will lower the vitamin C content of breastmilk. Even
  so, it is still preferable to infant formula.
- Certain drugs. Illegal drugs will pass into breastmilk ∴ users should ne
  breastfeed. Other medicines should be checked for suitability in the
  British National Formulary (www.bnf.org/bnf/).
- Some types of breast surgery.
- Infants with galactosaemia (see Chapter 31) as they cannot metabolize
  galactose present in breastmilk. Lactose free infant formulae should b
  used.
- PKU infants should alternate breastmilk with phenylalanine-free
  formula.

Promoting and establishing breastfeeding

Promoting breastfeeding

The DH (2003) recommends exclusive breastfeeding (nothing else but breastmilk, not even water) for the first 6 months (26 weeks) of life following a systematic review conducted by the WHO (2001). An estimated 10% of UK infants meet this recommendation. Although two-thirds of women breastfeed at birth, a third of these stop after the first few weeks and this rapidly declines thereafter. Breastfeeding rates vary greatly and higher social class groups (I and II in the UK) are more likely to breastfeed. More British Asian women (>75%) tend to breast feed at some stage.

Promotion of breastfeeding needs to be part of an effective infant feeding policy. Training needs to target all health professionals to emphasize both the enormous benefits of breastfeeding and appropriate techniques, so that women receive consistent messages throughout their care.

Maternal education needs to begin prenatally by local health-care services providing breastfeeding classes and written support including leaflets. The father, family, and/or friends should be encouraged to participate so that the woman can be offered support.

Focus on changing attitudes and knowledge of the technique and the recommended length of time to continue feeding. Support and education should be targeted at the groups where there is least uptake, i.e. social classes III, V, and VI in UK. Common reasons given by women in the UK (see boxes) for the choice of method and reasons for stopping breast-feeding[1] are useful for targeting public health measures.

Reasons for choice of feeding method

Breast
- Best for baby
- Convenient
- Closer bond
- Cheaper

Bottle
- Others can feed baby
- Dislike idea of breastfeeding

---

[1] Hamlyn, B., et al. (2002). *Infant feeding 2000*. Department of Health. HMSO, London.

Reasons for giving up breastfeeding

Early weeks	*Later weeks (to 4 months)*	*Later months*
Rejecting the breast	Insufficient milk	Returning to work
Painful nipples		

Baby friendly accreditation

Maternity hospitals keen to promote breastfeeding can seek baby friendly accreditation (www.babyfriendly.org.uk/commun.asp#plan), once they have successfully adopted the 'ten steps to successful breastfeeding' (see box).[2]

Ten steps to successful breastfeeding

- Have a written breastfeeding policy that is routinely communicated to all health-care staff
- Train all health-care staff in skills necessary to implement this policy
- Inform all pregnant women about the benefits and management of breastfeeding.
- Help mothers to initiate breastfeeding within an hour after birth
- Show mothers how to breastfeed, and how to maintain lactation even if they are separated from their infants
- Give newborn infants no food and drink other than breastmilk, unless medically indicated
- Practice rooming-in—allow mothers and infants to remain together — 24 hours a day
- Encourage breastfeeding on demand
- Give no artificial teats or dummies to breastfeeding infants
- Foster the establishment of breastfeeding support groups and refer mothers to them on discharge from the hospital or clinic

World Health Organization (1989). *Protecting, promoting and supporting breastfeeding: the special role of maternity services*, a joint WHO/UNICEF statement. World Health Organization, Geneva.

Establishing breastfeeding

Patients' FAQs for establishing breastfeeding

How soon after the birth should I put my baby on the breast?
Start as soon after birth as possible (preferably within 1 h) as suckling stimulates the let down response.

How often should I feed?
Feed as often as the infant wants; not restricting frequency or duration will help fully establish the milk supply initially. Infants usually feed 8–12 times a day including at night. The first 3 weeks are crucial. Dummies should be avoided, as will diminish frequency of baby sucking.

How long should I let the baby feed on each breast?
Always offer both breasts at each feed. Let the baby finish the first breast completely as incomplete emptying of the breasts means the baby may just drink 'foremilk' and not the fat dense 'hind milk'. If this is habitual practice, it may affect infant growth. Babies may seem sleepy but can often coax awake to feed for longer. Start on a different breast from the one last emptied.

Which position is best for feeding the baby?
The most comfortable and convenient position of the baby on the breast will depend on the mother (see Fig. 10.1 and DH breastfeeding leaflets for positions). If baby is restless at the breast and seems unsatisfied, it hurts to breastfeed, or the mother gets cracked nipples, adjust position of baby.

How do I know if my baby is getting enough milk?
Plenty of wet nappies; bright yellow, regular stools (after the first week or two), contented baby after a feed; baby gains weight and looks well.

Does my baby need extra drinks?
No. Foremilk is more watery and thirst quenching and in hot weather, babies tend to take shorter, more frequent feeds.

My breasts are swollen, hard, and painful. Is this normal?
This is known as breast engorgement which occurs when your milk comes in about day 3 and can occur if there has been a delay between feeds. Feeding on demand should prevent it. If there is a lump, it's likely to be a blocked duct. Feed from the breast and massage the lump towards the nipple. If there is a red, hot painful patch it may be a sign of mastitis. Keep feeding from the breast and avoid wearing a bra at night.

I want to carry on breastfeeding but I'm going back to work full-time when the baby is 3 months; what can I do?
If returning to work, exclusive breastfeeding will be challenging, unless the mother is extremely motivated and expresses and freezes breastmilk for use when at work. (NB. Mothers are entitled to express breastmilk at work in the UK.) A high quality breast pump is essential. Mixed bottle/breast may be a more realistic solution in this situation and the woman can continue with pre- and post-work breastfeeds. See 'Combining breast and bottle' in 'Establishing bottle-feeding', this chapter.

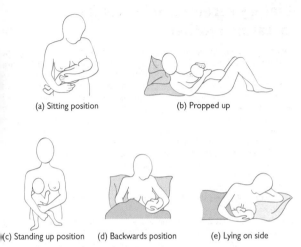

(a) Sitting position   (b) Propped up

(c) Standing up position   (d) Backwards position   (e) Lying on side

Fig. 10.1 Breastfeeding positions. (From Vinther, T. and Helsing, E. *Breastfeeding: how to support success. A practical guide for health workers* (1997). World health Organization. Reproduced with permission (can be accessed at: www.euro.whoint/document/e57592.pdf.)

Further information on breastfeeding

Vinther, T. and Helsing, E. (1997). Breastfeeding: how to support success. A practical guide for health workers. WHO Regional office for Europe, Copenhagen. www.euro.who.int/document/e57592.pdf

Baby friendly initiative: www.babyfriendly.org.uk/commun.asp#plan.

www.breastfeeding.nhs.uk/.

www.dh.gov.uk/Home/fs/en.

Dietary recommendations for lactating mother

Lactating women should follow general healthy eating guidance in the 'Balance of good health' (see 'Food-based dietary guidelines' in Chapter 2), but care should be taken to meet the extra requirements for energy protein, 3 fat-soluble vitamins, 5 water-soluble vitamins and 6 minerals (Table 10.2). In particular, when a woman is breastfeeding exclusively, her nutritional status will be compromised before that of the infant. On a practical level, this can be achieved by women eating larger quantities of the healthy diet suggested earlier.

In addition, women should:

- Limit alcohol to ≤2 units/day as this will pass into breastmilk affecting its smell and potentially the sleep patterns and digestion of the baby;
- Avoid caffeine as this will pass into breastmilk → infant hyperactivity and sleeplessness. Tea, coffee, cocoa, and cola -type drinks are best avoided (<4 cups a day of these combined). Suggest decaffeinated tea and coffee;
- Consume at least 2 litres of fluid a day to avoid dehydration (735 ml/kg body weight). See 'Fluid balance' in Chapter 5.
- Avoid spicy foods that may alter the taste of breastmilk if the infant appears to reject milk as a result;
- Avoid peanuts or foods containing peanuts if there is a family history (siblings, mother, father) of allergy (asthma, eczema, hayfever). See Chapter 32.
- Avoid vitamin and mineral supplements. Exceptions are vegan, macrobiotic, or fruitarian women who may need B12 supplements and women following dietary restrictions, e.g. cow's milk free diet. These and women with poor dietary intakes should see a dietitian.

♦ Controversial advice: the FSA (www.eatwell.gov.uk) now advises that a supplement of 10 µg of vitamin D should be taken whilst breastfeeding.

Table 10.2 RNIs for lactating mothers*

Nutrient	Daily RNI (15–50 y)	↑ in lactation
Energy (kcal)	1940–2110	+450 (month 1)
		+530 (month 2)
		+570 (months 3–6)if exclusively breastfed
Protein (g)†	51	+11 (0–4 months)
		+8 (>4 months)
Vitamin C (mg)	40	+30
Vitamin D (µg)	0 (assumed gained from sun exposure)	+10
Vitamin A (µg)	600	+350
Folic acid (µg)	200	+60
Thiamine (mg)	0.8	+0.2
Riboflavin (mg)	1.4	+0.5
Niacin (mg)	13–14	+2
Vitamin B_{12} (µg)	1.5	+0.5
Calcium (mg)	700–800	+550
Phosphorus (mg)	550–625	+440
Magnesium (mg)	270–300	+50
Zinc (mg)†	7.0	+6.0 (0–4 months)
		+2.5 (>4 months)
Selenium (µg)	60	+15
Copper (mg)	1.0–1.2	+0.3

* Department of Health (1991). *Dietary reference values for Food and nutrients for the United Kingdom.* HMSO, London.
† The RNI for zinc and protein falls after 4 months, which was based on previous DH advice of exclusive breastfeeding up to 4 months. It is likely that the current advice of exclusive breastfeeding up to 6 months will mean these will be revised upwards accordingly.

Establishing bottle-feeding

Women who choose to bottle-feed should not be made to feel guilty or inadequate as a result of their decision. Once this choice is made they need to be advised and supported accordingly. Mother's breasts will return to normal quickly. Modified cows' milk infant formula will meet all nutrient requirements, but all the protective immunological factors will be absent.

Combining breast and bottle

After breastmilk is well established (4–6 weeks), it may be possible to combine breast and bottle where circumstances dictate: e.g. woman returns to work; woman is exhausted (physically or mentally) from feeding continuously; or male partner needs to bond/help with the baby. Introducing 1 or 2 bottle feeds during the day, for example, and regularly continuing with breastmilk before and after returning from work should not affect the woman's ability to breastfeed. NB. This is preferable to stopping breastfeeding entirely, but is not the 'ideal' option as exclusive breastfeeding is recommended for the first 6 months of life.

Choice of infant formula

In the UK, there are three main types of cows' milk formula.
- **Whey dominant**. Ratio of whey to casein of approx 60:40. Whey-based formula is recommended as it most closely resembles the protein structure of breastmilk. Most of these formulae now contain long chain polyunsaturated fatty acids and nucleotides that were previously absent. Some are organic and others contain prebiotics or have been modified to be more 'easily digested' to aid reflux and constipation. The array of choice can be confusing for parents. The advantages of these additional attributes are still to be demonstrated.
- **Casein dominant**. Whey to casein ratio of approx. 20:80; similar to doorstep cows' milk. They are marketed and perceived by parents as milks that can help fill up babies as they get 'hungrier' around 6–10 weeks (but they contain the same kcal as whey dominant milks). They do not usually contain any 'extras'.
- **Follow on and toddler milks**. In the UK, follow-on infant formulae are widely used for infants >6 months. Some parents wish to change their infant's milk at 4–6 months as a symbolic 'developmental milestone'. In these cases, follow-on milk is preferable to the mother introducing solids early or doorstep cows' milk. Such formulae can now come in 4 different stages including for toddlers. There is no evidence of nutritional benefit compared with ordinary infant formula in infants and children who are following an otherwise well balanced diet. However, 'follow on' and 'toddler' milks may be useful in infants who are nutritionally at risk due in particular to their higher iron content.

Soya based formulae

Infant formulae based on soya are not recommended for infants under 6 months of age, due to phytoestrogen content which may have long term effects on the infant's health and sensitization to soya protein. ∴ they should only be used in exceptional circumstances, e.g.

- Vegan mothers who do not breastfeed;
- Infants with cows' milk intolerance/allergy, who consistently refuse elemental formulae.

Goats' milk formulae

Infant formulas based on goats' milk protein are **not** suitable for infants who are intolerant or allergic to cows' milk formulae. Goats milk derived formulae are also unsuitable for babies who are lactose-intolerant.

Infant formulae and energy

Although the energy content of breastmilk is reported to be 70 kcal/ 100 ml, this is based on the energy content of milk obtained by completely expressing the first breast. This is unlikely to be a true representation of suckled human milk, and doubly labelled water studies of suckled human milk have suggested values of 53–58 kcal/100 ml at 6 weeks and 3 months, respectively. The Scientific Committee for Food (SCF 2003) recommends maximum energy content of 60–70 kcal/100 ml for both standard and follow-on infant formulae.

Healthy start scheme

In the UK, the welfare food scheme, established in 1940 as a wartime measure, entitled pregnant women and children <5 y, receiving certain benefits, to tokens for either cows' milk or cows' milk based infant formulae per week and free supplements of vitamins A, C, and D.

This is being replaced by the 'Healthy start scheme'. The NHS Plan 2000 stated that the welfare food scheme needed to be reformed 'to use the resources more effectively to ensure that children in poverty have access to a healthy diet, with increased support for breastfeeding and parenting. The new scheme 'Healthy start' involves a broader range of foods (fresh fruit and vegetables initially, with a plan to increase the range of foods over time) as well as cows' milk and infant formula. Fixed value vouchers are issued so they can be exchanged in a wide range of outlets and are of equal value for both breastfeeding and non-breastfeeding mothers. The age of children eligible will fall from 5 to 4 y. Milk or fruit will be available in nurseries. Free vitamin supplements will continue to be available as part of the scheme, but their formulation is under review.

Healthy start is open to pregnant women and families with children under the age of five who are in receipt of certain income support benefits or are <18 y (see www.healthystart.nhs.uk for further information).

Weaning

When to introduce solids

Six months is the recommended age for the introduction of solid foods for infants (DH 2003) whether they are breastfed, fed solely on infant formula milk, or taking breast and infant formula combined. This choice of milk should continue beyond 6 months, along with solid foods. The DH recommended age for weaning has increased from 4 months and, although waiting until 6 months is recommended, babies should not be weaned earlier than 4 months (17 wks).

Weaning is necessary because at 6 months of age some nutrient requirements increase (see Table 10.1 in 'Infant growth and development', this chapter), especially those for iron, B vitamins, energy, and protein that cannot be met by milk alone. Also, neuromuscular co-ordination is sufficiently developed at 6 months to enable the child to eat solid foods.

Which foods to introduce

The overall aim of weaning is to introduce the infant gradually to a range of foods, textures, and flavours, so that normal family foods are taken at 12 months. The stages of weaning are summarized in Table 10.3. If parents choose to start weaning before 6 months of age, foods should be introduced gradually, starting with fruits, vegetables, rice, and potato. If starting weaning from 6 months of age, babies will need to be exposed to a variety of foods from the outset, especially those containing iron. Foods can be offered 2–3 times a day, of either thick purees or mashed textures and finger foods. Weaning from 6 months of age is simpler as there are few foods that cannot be offered.

As breastfeeding is baby led, baby led weaning is being favoured by some. Emphasis is on the baby self-feeding and discourages the use of spoon feeding. This approach may be extreme and many parents would find it difficult not to feed their baby. A compromise might be to provide a meal containing a combination of finger foods such as vegetables and new potatoes or pasta and some mashed foods, so that the baby can feed him/herself and can also be fed by the parent/ carer.

⚠ Nuts and nut allergy

Peanut allergy appears to be increasing in children (see Chapter 32). Children with a family history (siblings, mother, or father) of allergy (asthma, eczema, hay fever) should not eat peanuts, peanut butter, or groundnut oil, or foods containing these until at least 3 years of age. Other infants can take peanuts and other nuts from 6 months of age. Whole nuts should be avoided until 5 years of age due to the risk of choking.

Weaning preterm infants

Advice on appropriate weaning age should be sought from the specialist paediatric medical and dietetic team caring for the infant. Further information on feeding preterm infants is available from www.bliss.org.uk.

Table 10.3 Summary of guidance for weaning and feeding for under-5s

	6 months*	6–9 months	9–12 months	1–5 years
Milk	Breastmilk or 1 pint of infant formula. Introduce cup or beaker from 6 months			2–3 servings/day from full fat varieties, moving on to lower fat varieties >2 y of: cheese (30 g) , yogurt (pot), 1/3 pint milk.
Dairy foods	Yogurt/custard. No soft unpasteurized cheese <6 months	Cubed/grated hard cheese, cheese spread. Full fat yogurt, fromage frais, custard, fullfat cows' milk in cooking		
	Goat's and sheep's milk should be avoided <12 months			
Fruit & vegetables	Smooth puree of softly cooked	2 servings/day. Mashed with fork/lightly cooked; soft peeled fruit & vegetables as finger foods	3–4 servings/day. No need to peel apple/pear. Raw/lightly cooked	≥4 servings/day. Same form as for adults
Meat, fish & alternatives	After a few weeks: pureed meat, beans & lentils. No eggs, fish, shellfish, nuts, or nut butter <6 months	1 serving/day. Mince/pure meat, beans & lentils; hard boiled egg, fish, tofu	2 servings/day, e.g. mince/chopped red meat, chicken, white fish, eggs, tofu	2 servings/day. As for 9–12 months plus introduce oily fish (sardines, salmon, mackerel) up to twice weekly. No whole nuts <5 y due to choking risk

Table 10.3 (Contd.)

	6 months*	6–9 months	9–12 months	1–5 years
Starchy foods	Baby rice/smooth potatoes. No wheat/gluten based cereal, bread <6 months	2–3 servings/day. Can include gluten-containing foods, e.g. bread, breakfast cereals, toast, pasta	2–3 servings/day, e.g. toast, breadsticks, rice cakes	≥4 servings/day of bread, pasta, potatoes, rice, chapatti
Sugary foods & drinks	No added sugar and no honey <12 months due to infant botulism risks	Drinks should be breast/formula milk or water. Fruit juices should be discouraged but if taken diluted 1 in 10. No sweet biscuits and rusks (including low sugar)		Limit sweet foods & drinks; especially between meals
		Herbal drinks, fizzy drinks, & squashes, including 'diet' drinks with artificial sweetener are not recommended. No tea/coffee		
Salty foods	No salt should not be added; kidneys not mature	Small amounts of gravy/ketchup		Limit crisps & savoury snacks
Vitamin drops	✓If the infant is still breastfed >6 months ✓If a formula-fed infant is taking <1 pint of milk/day			✓ DH recommends for all 1–5yr olds
Texture	Smooth	Mashed, minced, finger foods	Finger foods, lumps, chopped	Family foods

*But no earlier than 4 months (17 weeks) for parents deciding to wean their babies earlier.

Healthier snack suggestions for 1–5 year olds

All fresh fruit
Sticks of carrot, celery
Peppers, cucumber
Cherry tomatoes
Olives without stones
Teacakes/scone
Fruit or malt loaf
Oat cakes
Crackers
Rice cakes, bread sticks
Bagels

Popcorn (unsweetened)
Plain biscuits
Cubes or slices of cheese
Yogurt/fromage frais (lower sugar varieties)
Low sugar cereal and milk
Pitta bread and hummus/cream cheese
Sandwiches, tortilla wraps, toast

Common feeding problems

Prolonged use of feeder bottle and delayed weaning

The DH recommends that infants should be introduced to drinking from a cup from 6 months and actively discouraged from taking drinks in feeder bottles after 12 months. This is part of the natural progression for sipping and swallowing to replace sucking. Delayed weaning (>1 y) is more common in some deprived South Asian communities than for other ethnic groups.

Problems arising from prolonged use of the feeder bottle and delayed weaning include:

Food refusal as the infant may be filling up on milk ∴↓ desire for food;
Iron deficiency anaemia due to increased iron requirements not being met from a mixed diet;
Faltering growth;
Speech development as child's ability to chew and the swallowing reflex may ↓;
Dental caries if sugary/acidic drinks are given in a bottle;
Obesity if sugary drinks are given in a bottle.

Risk of choking

All babies have a sensitive gag reflex and it is normal for them to gag on exposure to increasing textures of food. This should not be a reason for avoiding such textures, and they soon adapt. However, babies should be supervised whilst eating and given softer finger foods at first, such as banana, melon, or avocado. Once the child is able to chew well, s/he can be given non-dissolvable harder finger foods, e.g. apple. Whole nuts or olives containing stones should be avoided until 5 years of age due to risk of choking.

Iron deficiency anaemia

Common causes:
- Mother's diet was inadequate in iron during pregnancy;
- Mother is breastfeeding and is anaemic;
- The baby is weaned late, i.e. >6 months;
- Slow in progressing from weaning foods to family meals;
- Early introduction of cows' milk as the main drink for children <1 y;
- Heavy reliance on sweet baby foods (high in sugar, low in iron and protein), as avoiding savoury products that may have non-*halal* ingredients in some Muslim families.

A varied diet with a regular intake of red meat, fruit, green vegetables, fortified breakfast cereals, and beans and pulses should be encouraged. This is especially important for breastfed babies where, despite good absorption of iron from breastmilk, the iron content is insufficient for infants over 6 months of age. Infant formula is higher in iron, but it should not be relied upon as a sole source of iron in babies over 6 months of age. See 'Iron' in Chapter 5 for foods rich in iron.

Faltering growth

Infants commonly show some weight faltering in the first 12 years, but i may also affect older children. As a guide, population studies show tha 1 in 20 children <2 y shows a sustained fall through 2 centile spaces fo weight. One in 100 children <2 y shows a sustained fall through 3 centile spaces.

Weight faltering is defined as weight falling through centile spaces, low weight for height, or no catch-up from a low birth weight. Growth faltering is defined as crossing down through length/ height centile(s) as well a weight, a low height centile, or a height less than expected from parenta heights.

Consensus statement by a multidisciplinary group of experts in the field of faltering weight and growth in young children is available.[1]

Only 5% of young children whose weight/growth falters will have an organic root to the problem. It is estimated that a further 5% will need the support of Child Protection Agencies. As a result, it is recommended that management for the majority of faltering growth should occur in primary care, rather than in hospitals.

Triggers for primary care assessment
- A weight or height below the 0.4th centile, noted for the first time, should always trigger an evaluation.
- A sustained fall through 2 centile spaces should usually trigger an evaluation.
- Evaluation should be considered if weight or height is below the 2nd centile.

---

[1] Children's Society (2002). *Recommendations for best practice for growth faltering in young children.* Children's Society, London. Also PIER guideline: www.pier.shef.ac.uk/home.htm.

Possible dietary and social causes of faltering growth

- Insufficient calorie intake is major cause
- Formula milk too weak/too concentrated
- Late weaning >6 months
- Prolonged use of feeder bottle
- Fussy eating/behavioural problems at mealtimes
- Physical feeding problems, e.g. gastro-oesophageal reflux, oral motor dysfunction
- Over health conscious parent/carer → diet low in fat and high in fibre
- Inadequacy of the nutritional content or frequency of meals
- Poor inherent feeding drive
- Developmental difficulties
- Illness—although it is rare for serious organic disease to present with weight and/or growth faltering alone
- Abuse and/or neglect (minority of cases)
- Unhealthy parent/carer–child relationship

Managing faltering growth in primary care

In the UK, health visitors are best placed to identify and support infants because of their key responsibility for the health and well-being of children under 5 years of age. It will depend on suspected cause as to whether the dietitian or paediatrician gets involved first; see Fig. 10.2

In those children where weight gain is a concern, the family's health visitor should negotiate home visits at meal/feed times to allow observations. A range of data should be collected including:

- Feeding and symptom history since birth;
- Growth history since birth;
- Any relevant medical or domestic details;
- Food diary outlining food/drinks offered and taken and when;
- Details of mealtime routines, including observation of food preparation and mealtime interactions;
- Family's concerns/anxieties;
- Interaction between parents/carers and child, with description of any behavioural problems.

Having identified areas where there is potential for change, the health visitor should offer appropriate advice and ongoing support. This is likely to include strategies that address:

- Insufficient nutrient intake, e.g. faddy eating, excess drinking, poor parent–child interaction, strict adherence to a low fat-high fibre diet or
- Insufficient nutrient offered, e.g. lack of parent/carer knowledge or skills on good nutrition, stressful social situations, including neglect or abuse.

When a health visitor becomes concerned, h/she should be able to discuss or refer to the most relevant member of the multidisciplinary team (see Fig. 10.2).

The dietitian's role is to use motivational interviewing and counselling techniques to address the following:

- Establishing food attitudes, value systems, and beliefs;
- Ensuring appropriate parent/child interactions, particularly related to food and drink;
- Exploring drinking habits and discouraging prolonged use of a bottle;
- Advising on age-appropriate structured mealtimes, snacks, and drinks;
- Increasing nutrient density of meals using foods where possible;
- Identifying any micronutrient deficiencies and correcting for them where possible;
- Considering use of nutritional supplements if there is no improvement in growth as a result of the above interventions.

Also see 'Fussy eaters', this chapter.

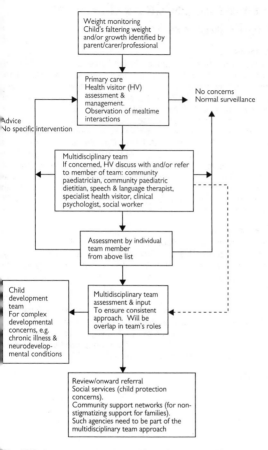

Fig. 10.2 Care pathway for young children's faltering growth/weight. Reproduced from the *Recommendations for best practice for growth faltering in young children* (Copyright 2002). With permission from the Children's Society.

Constipation, toddler's diarrhoea, and milk intolerance

Constipation

Constipation is much more common in fed babies infant formula compared with breastfed babies. Potential contributing factors include fatty acid position on the triglyceride molecule (sn-2 position fatty acids being absorbed more readily), LCPs, and prebiotics that are lower in most formula milk. The energy content of breastmilk may also be lower than originally thought, and hence fluid intake may differ.

Constipation due to low fibre intake and sometimes low fluid intake is relatively common in UK infants. A higher fibre diet should be encouraged, containing foods that are acceptable to the child. Encouraging fresh and dried fruit and vegetables for pectins, bread and breakfast cereals for cereal fibre, will relieve symptoms along with plenty of fluid, preferably as water. Fluid requirements vary with age (see Table 10.1); for example, an average 4 year old boy will need at least 85 ml/kg body weight/daily; equivalent to 5 mugs of fluid for a 15 kg boy (1 mug = 250 ml).

Toddler's diarrhoea

Symptoms: frequent, loose stools, containing undigested foodstuffs.

Usually a self-limiting problem, occurring in otherwise well infants <3 y, who are gaining weight and growing satisfactorily; commonly due to immaturity of the gastrointestinal tract. As well as reassuring parents that the condition will cease spontaneously, dietary treatment is to:
- avoid large quantities of sucrose, fruit and fruit juice;
- reduce dietary fibre intake (choose white bread and avoid high fibre cereals, fibre-dense fruit and vegetables, such as peas, sweetcorn and temporarily reduce consumption of fruit and vegetables in general);
- ensure sufficient fat in the diet. Where this is not possible, a fat-based nutritional supplement can be a useful addition.

Milk intolerance   See Chapter 32

Nutritionally vulnerable groups

South Asian families

There is evidence that certain infant feeding practices in some South Asian families increase the risk of iron deficiency anaemia, faltering growth, and constipation. These include:

- Late weaning, slow to move on to family foods;
- Late progression from a bottle on to a feeder cup;
- Adding honey/sugar to sweeten milk;
- Adding solids to formula milk;
- Choosing sweet commercially prepared baby foods so as to avoid running the risk of using non-*halal* meat products; ∴ lack of iron and protein in weaning foods;
- Use of cows' milk as the main drink with infants <1 y.

The vegetarian baby

Infants consuming a well balanced vegetarian diet should meet all requirements for growth. See 'Vegetarians' in Chapter 13.

❶ Diets that are unbalanced or more restrictive than this, e.g. strict macrobiotic or fruitarian, are likely to result in nutrient deficiencies and need particular attention in infants. Referral to a dietitian for assessment is essential.

Low income families

Children from families living on a low income are at a greater risk of having an unvaried, unbalanced diet, developing micronutrient deficiency and faltering growth. See 'Eating on a low income' in Chapter 13.

Sure Start[1] is a Government programme that aims to help service development in disadvantaged areas alongside financial help for parents to afford childcare by:

- Increasing the availability of childcare for all children;
- Improving health and emotional development for young children;
- Supporting parents, both as parents and in their search for employment.

[1] Further information: www.surestart.gov.uk

Fussy eaters

Patients' FAQs for fussy eaters/behavioural tips for mealtimes

Every meal time is like a battle of wills; how can I break the cycle?
Encourage parents to avoid arguments and try to keep calm. Mealtimes should actually be fun! The child is probably trying to either gain attention or show that s/he has control over parents. It is important not to give in and to ignore the behaviour. The child should not detect that his/her behaviour causes anxiety. Reassure parents that as long as a child is gaining weight overall there isn't too much cause for concern. Never force feed children.

Should I let him have his dessert if he doesn't finish his main course?
Advise parents to put the food on the table and; if it is not eaten after 20–30 minutes, simply remove with no comment. Suggest not giving sweet foods if savoury meal is rejected completely. Trying the savoury meal may be acceptable and deserve a dessert. This will help change behaviour long term. Cooking an alternative meal should be avoided, as this is just as likely to be refused.

I am worried about my 2 year old daughter going hungry if she doesn't eat her meal, is it okay to let her have in between snacks?
Children can go for days without eating, and if they are hungry their behaviour deteriorates. If they refuse their meal, having a small snack (see box with healthy snack suggestions in 'Weaning', this chapter) a couple of hours later will not impact on mealtimes, and it is far enough off for them not to associate snacks with not eating meals. This helps relieve parental anxiety too, as their child is getting something to eat. Mealtimes are approximately 4 hours apart, and snacks (mid am, mid pm, and supper) fall between these, but should not be given any closer than 1½ hours before a meal. This applies to drinks too.

Is it okay to reward my child with sweets for eating his dinner?
Parents should avoid using sweet foods as a bribe to encourage children to eat their meals. Other non-food rewards could be used, like a cuddle, playing a game, or reading a story.

Could it help if he eats on his own, so that we can eat in peace later?
A young child should never be left alone whilst eating as there is a risk that s/he might choke. It is preferable if the whole family tries to sit down and eat together, ideally the same food, so that they are acting as role models and can share food. Inviting friends to eat can help as children often copy each other (as long as the guest is not a fussy eater too!). Parents need to try and create an enjoyable environment.

Is it okay to feed him myself whilst he watches TV, because at least that way he eats his dinner?

Parents should not feed the child (when s/he is capable of doing so) as the attention will be enjoyed and there will be little incentive to self-feed. It is normal for children to make a mess when they feed, and they like to eat with their fingers. This should be encouraged and avoid wiping their hands and mouth until the end of the meal, as it can upset the child. The TV should be switched off during eating as this is distracting and the meal is a good opportunity for parent-child interaction.

Promoting Healthy infant feeding

See 'model of a local infant feeding policy for under 5s' (in examples of nutrition policy in different settings) on p336.

Websites and literature for parents

More information
www.babyfriendly.org.uk
www.publications.doh.gov.uk/pregnancybook/
www.nctpregnancyandbabycare.com/
www.surestart.gov.uk
www.laleche.org.uk
www.dh.gov.uk

Literature for parents
Department of Health publications (www.publications.dh.gov.uk):
- *The pregnancy book* (2005);
- *Birth to five book* (2005);
- Breastfeeding and bottle feeding leaflets.

FSA leaflet: *Eating for breastfeeding* (www.food.gov.uk).
BDA Paediatric Group fact sheets (www.bda.uk.com/pubs_resource.html).

School-aged children and adolescents

Why diet is important in childhood and adolescence

- Children need a balanced diet to meet requirements for growth and development.
- Health-related behaviour and attitudes towards food are formed in childhood.
- The processes for some adult diseases may start early in life.

Growth and development

Each year of life from 1 year to adolescence, a child grows taller by 5–8 cm. Girls' growth spurt begins at 10–11 years. Boys' growth spurt begins at 12–13 years. About 25% of height is gained in adolescence. This requires increases of energy, protein, and several vitamins and minerals (see Table 11.1 in 'Dietary recommendations for children and adolescents', this chapter). If energy needs are not met this can result in stunting or delayed growth. Once the growth spurt is over, nutrient requirements become those of adults. During this period there is ↑ muscle growth in boys and adipose fat in girls. Genes have the strongest influence on onset of menarche.

See girls' and boys' growth charts (5–18 years chart) in Appendix 2. These have been endorsed by the Royal College of Paediatrics and Child Health and the DH. These are available from the Child Growth Foundation (www.childgrowthfoundation.org). See discussion in 'Infant growth and development' in chapter 10.

The charts have 9 reference centiles of 0.4th, 2nd, 9th, 25th, 50th, 75th, 91st, 98th, and 99.9th, e.g.
- 98th centile curve, below which 98% of UK children lie;
- 50th centile curve, below which 50% of UK children lie;
- 2nd centile curve, below which only 2% of UK children lie.

What children and adolescents are eating

The UK National Diet and Nutrition Survey of 4 to 18 year old (DH, 2000)[1] found the following.

- Children are not eating enough fruit and vegetables (~2 portions/day).
- One in five children does not eat any fruit in a week.
- Children in the lowest income groups are about 50% less likely to eat fruit and vegetables.
- Diets are high in total fat and saturated fat, non-milk extrinsic sugars, and salt; low in NSP.
- Boys are less likely to consume a healthy diet.
- Girls are most at risk from inadequate calcium and iron intakes.

Other features of children's habits

Missing breakfast   In the UK ~8% of younger children and up to 20% of adolescents miss breakfast every day. This has been linked to poor concentration and ↓ cognitive performance late morning.

Drinking alcohol   Especially binge drinking in adolescence. Weekly alcohol consumption amongst Welsh adolescents is higher than for any other European country, with England and Northern Ireland not far behind. The WHO[2] estimated that 47% of boys and 36% girls aged 15 drink alcohol ≥once/week. In the UK, alcohol consumption and smoking are increasing, particularly in girls. Alcohol provides extra calories (could lead to weight gain) and could displace nutrient rich foods in the diet.

Sedentary behaviour   The Chief Medical Officer recommends that all young people aged 5–18 years should participate in physical activity of at least moderate intensity *for one hour a day*. This can be accumulated throughout the day, e.g. 4 times 15 minutes, and can be through structured exercise, sport, or everyday physical activity as part of habits.

- Only about 70% of boys and 61% of girls (2–15 years old) are meeting this recommendation[3].
- Physical activity levels tend to fall with age and by age 15, only 50% of girls achieve the recommended levels of activity. Boys' activity levels are fairly constant up to 15 years, when they start to decline.
- Children can practise sport or exercise but still have an otherwise sedentary way of life, e.g. television and computer viewing. High number of hours of television viewing is associated with ↑ risk of obesity.

Snacking   Adolescents eat at least 3 snacks/day, contributing ~25% of daily dietary energy. Snacking can have a negative effect on the nutritional value of the diet as snacks are often low in calcium, iron and high in saturated fat and sugar. Most popular are crisps, sweets, biscuits, sandwiches, fruit, and milk chocolate. The box lists some healthy alternatives.

[1] Gregory, J. and Lowe, S. (2000). National Diet and Nutrition Survey: young people aged 4–18 years. HMSO, London.
[2] Jernigan, DH. (2001). Global status report: alcohol and young people. WHO, Geneva.
[3] Department of Health (2003). Health Survey for England 2002. HMSO, London.

Healthy snack suggestions

- Fruit
- Vegetables: sticks of carrot, celery, cucumber; cherry tomatoes
- Toast, teacakes, scone
- Fruit or malt loaf
- Oat cakes
- Crackers
- Rice cakes
- Bread sticks
- Bagels
- Mixed nuts and raisins
- Popcorn (unsweetened)
- Plain biscuits
- Glass of milk
- Cubes or slices of cheese
- Yogurt/fromage frais (lower sugar varieties)
- Low sugar cereal and milk

Dietary recommendations for children and adolescents

The 'Balance of good health' eating model (in 'Food-based dietary guide lines' in chapter 2) applies to older children (≥5 years) and adolescent as there is evidence that early atherosclerotic plaques can develop fro adolescence → CVD in later life.

In addition to a balanced diet, advise:

- Extra calcium requirements gained from drinking the equivalent of 1 pint of milk a day (see 'Calcium' in chapter 5 for equivalents);
- Regular meals if possible, healthy snack meals if not (see box on previous page);
- Offering praise when a healthy food is offered as this leads to ↑ consumption of the food in younger children;
- Parents to make healthy foods easily available and serve these foods i positive mealtime situations;
- As children prefer familiar foods, repeated exposure to new foods can alter the response from rejection to acceptance;
- Interventions promoting familiarity with foods, e.g. fruit and vegetable tasting, can increase consumption;
- Eating with peers can have a positive effect on eating behaviour.

RNIs vary for age and gender and are related to growth needs; ∴ the reflect differences in growth rates and body composition (Table 11.1).

Table 11.1 RNI for school-aged children and adolescents*

Nutrient†	7–10y		11–14y		15–18y	
	Male	Female	Male	Female	Male	Female
Energy (kcal)	1970	1740	2220	1845	2755	2110
Protein (g)	28.3	28.3	42.1	41.2	55.2	45.0
Fluid (ml/kg)	75	75	55	55	50	50
Vitamin C (mg)	30	30	35	35	40	40
Vitamin A (µg)	500	500	600	600	700	600
Folic acid (µg)	150	150	200	200	200	200
Thiamine (mg)	0.7	0.7	0.9	0.7	1.1	0.8
Riboflavin (mg)	1.0	1.0	1.2	1.1	1.3	1.1
Niacin (mg)	12	12	15	12	19	14
Vitamin B12 (µg)	1.0	1.0	1.2	1.2	1.5	1.5
Iron (mg)	8.7	8.7	11.3	14.8	11.3	14.8
Calcium (mg)	550	550	1000	800	1000	800
Phosphorus (mg)	450	450	775	625	775	625
Magnesium (mg)	200	200	280	280	300	300
Zinc (mg)	7.0	7.0	9.0	9.0	9.5	9.5
Selenium (µg)	30	30	45	45	70	60
Copper (mg)	0.7	0.7	0.8	0.8	1.0	1.0

Department of Health (1991) Dietary reference values for food and nutrients for the United Kingdom. HMSO, London.
† In the UK there is not much evidence of difference in requirements for different ethnic groups except for vitamin D supplements for those Asian schoolchildren who have a lack of sunlight exposure.

Nutritional problems of children and adolescents

Obesity/overweight

↑ in childhood obesity worldwide as widespread transition to energy dense diet and ↓ in physical activity. This is also the case in the UK where an estimated sixth (16%) of boys and girls aged 2–15 y are obese and almost a third (30%) are either overweight or obese[1]. Prevalence of obesity increases with age.

Classification of childhood obesity

Assigning cut-off points for childhood obesity is more complex than for adults. BMI percentile chart should be used to identify obesity and the UK 1990 chart is recommended for routine clinical diagnosis. Overweight is classified as ≥91st centile; and obesity ≥98th centile of the UK 1990 data. For epidemiological studies, an internationally acceptable definition to classify prevalence of child overweight (≥85th centile) and obesity (≥95th centile) of the 1990 data is recommended.[3]

Immediate effects on health In extreme cases of childhood obesity children can develop cardiomyopathy, pancreatitis, orthopaedic disorders, upper airway obstruction, or chest wall restriction.

Effects on well-being

Besides physical aspects, children also suffer from ↓ self-esteem, ↓ social interaction, and poorer academic achievement. Earlier puberty may also → emotional problems as a mismatch between physical and emotional development can → higher expectations from adults. However obesity limited to childhood has little impact on social, psychological, economic and educational outcomes in adult life. Persistent child to adult obesity associated with poorer employment and relationship outcomes in females only.

Long-term effect on health

The ↑ prevalence of obesity and overweight combined with a diet low in fruit and vegetables, high in saturated fat, and low in calcium and low physical activity means that it is likely that there will also be an ↑ risk of type II diabetes, CVD, suboptimal peak bone mass, osteoporosis, gall stones, and diet-related cancers in later life, especially if the increase in obesity is sustained in adult life. Older obese children are at a higher risk of becoming obese adults, but not all obese children become obese adults.

---

[1] Department of Health (2003). *Health survey for England 2002*. HMSO, London.
[2] Cole, T.J., *et al.* (2000). Establishing a standard definition for child overweight and obesity worldwide: international survey. *Br. Med. J.* **320**,1240–3.
[3] For further information: Management of obesity in children and young people report. A clinical national guidelines available at www.sign ac.uk.

Not achieving peak bone mass

Adolescence is a critical period with ~25–40% of peak bone mass laid down at this time in ♀, whilst ~90–95% of peak bone mass is attained by 30 years of age. Adequate calcium and phosphate intake is necessary combined with weight-bearing physical activity to maximize peak bone mass.

In the UK, more girls than boys do not achieve the lower RNI for calcium, as 24% of 11–14 y old girls and 19% of 15–18 y old girls do not meet requirements (~half of this for boys).

Chronic dieting to lose weight in girls is also likely to contribute to suboptimal peak bone mass and osteoporosis in later life.

Iron deficiency anaemia

Iron is the most prevalent nutrient deficiency in UK girls: 45–50% of 11–18 y olds do not meet the lower recommended intake (LRNI).

27% of 15–18 y old girls have low iron stores and 9% are anaemic.

Low intakes in UK girls are often due to lower meat consumption and restricted energy intakes as iron requirement ↑ with onset of menstruation.

Low iron intakes are associated with ↓ physical activity → ↓ peak bone mass.[4]

Adolescent girls living in the UK who are non-Caucasians or vegetarian have poorer iron status than Caucasians or meat eaters.

Foods rich in iron (see 'Iron' in Chapter 5 for full list)

- Peanut butter sandwiches
- Fortified breakfast cereals
- Dried apricots and raisins
- Red meat, e.g. beef, pork, lamb, lean mincemeat, ham
- Egg yolk
- Leafy green vegetables
- Peas, beans, and lentils
- Tinned tuna and salmon

Constipation

Constipation due to low fibre intake and sometimes low fluid intake is relatively common in UK children. Encouraging fresh and dried fruit and vegetables for pectins, bread and breakfast cereals for cereal fibre, will relieve symptoms along with plenty of fluid, preferably as water. Children's access to fluid may be restricted during the school day; if so, they should be encouraged to carry bottled water/sugar-free fluids with them. They may intentionally restrict their fluid intake to reduce frequency of micturition.

Data from Gregory, J. and Lowe, S. (2000). *National Diet and Nutrition Survey: young people aged 4–18 years.* HMSO, London.

Unnecessary dieting
Around a fifth of UK female adolescents are dieting to lose weight at any time with little evidence of a structured weight-reducing plan. Inappropriate approaches are common, such as crash diets, binge eating, chaotic eating plans, missing meals, eating slimming products (alongside energy dense foods), replacing meals with high sugar and fat snacks. This can lead to low intakes of several nutrients, especially iron, calcium, vitamin B_6, and riboflavin, as well as ↑ risk of developing eating disorders. See 'Eating disorders' in Chapter 27.

Underweight
Undernutrition in childhood and adolescence can result in stunting, i.e. inability to achieve inherited potential. Undernutrition may also impact on school achievement.
Diagnosis of stunting in adolescents: height for age <3rd centile of WHO reference data or <−2 Z-scores.
Diagnosis of thinness in adolescence: BMI < 5th centile of WHO reference data. See 'Malnutrition universal screening tool' and 'Undernutrition' in Chapter 16.

Vegetarianism
Vegetarian adolescents are at particular risk of inadequate diet if they are the only vegetarian in the house, as they may tend to eat the same as the rest of the family except 'remove' the animal protein part of the meal and replace it with too much cheese or vegetarian ready meals such as burgers, sausages, or pizza. They should replace it with suitable alternatives (See 'Vegetarians' in Chapter 13). They may have less knowledge of balanced vegetarian diet than adults resulting in low intakes of iron, zinc, protein, and vitamin B_{12}. Vegan children should be referred to see a dietitian as careful planning is needed to supply nutrient requirements.

Acne
Young people often link acne with a diet high in fat and sugar, but there is no evidence that diet is a factor in causing acne. Reassure them their eating pattern is not responsible for their acne; genes are an important determinant and this is one thing they can blame on their parents!

Dental health
In the UK, dental health in young people is improving, due to the introduction of fluoride toothpaste in the 1970s. However, it's still a public health concern, particularly in socially deprived groups, possibly because less preventive dentistry is practised; frequent consumption of sugary foods and ↓ regular brushing → ↓ fluoride intake.

Targeting for dental caries prevention is recommended as decay is unevenly distributed in the UK population: 9% of 5 y olds and 6% of 14 y olds have 50% of the disease (www.sign.ac.uk/pdf/sign47.pdf).[5]

There is ongoing debate in the UK concerning introduction of fluoride in non-water-fluoridated areas.

Causes of dental caries

• Frequent consumption of non-milk extrinsic sugars (glucose, sucrose, fructose) plays an unequivocal role in dental caries development as NMES act as a substrate for oral bacteria.

• Both quantity and stickiness of sugar affect length of time it takes for surface pH to ↑ to normal. Sticky foods may become stuck in-between teeth and are in contact with teeth for longer.

Guidelines for good dental health

Advise children to:

• Decrease both quantity and frequency of sugar intake
• Avoid sugary foods in-between meals and just before bedtime
• Avoid drinks that are carbonated, acidic, or high in sugar in-between meals (→ dental erosion); water and milk are better choices
• Eat sweet foods (including dried fruit) with meals rather than in-between (↑saliva at end of meal → buffer of low pH)
• Avoid eating sticky and chewy foods
• Choose sugar-free medicines
• Regular flossing and brushing with fluoride toothpaste, but not immediately after consuming sweet foods/acidic drinks as ↓ mineralization.
• Regular dental visits

Promoting healthy eating in children

See 'model of a local school food policy' (in examples of nutrition policy in different settings) on p337 and see targeting children in national food and nutrition policy for information on school meals and national programmes.

[5] Further information is available from SIGN guideline 'Preventing dental caries in children at high caries risk' 2000. www.sign.ac.uk. Also See 'Eating on a low income' in Chapter 13, 'Eating disorders' in Chapter 28, and Chapter 33.

Influences on children's food choices

The key factors influencing the eating habits of children and adolescent are shown in figure 11.1

Media and advertising
Children spend on average 2 h/day watching TV
Food adverts during children's programmes are mainly for high fat and sugar food and drink.
Unrealistic ideals of body image portrayed of ♀ and subsequent desire for thinness.

Environmental issues
~10% of teenage girls are vegetarian/vegan, often due to concern over animal welfare

Food choice in children and adolescents

School
Influences food availability, e.g. school meals, vending machines, tuck shops, classroom rewards.
School meals/whole school approach encouraged

Family–parents
Parents influence the availability of food and act as role models for their children. They determine whether the family eats together: children eating dinner with their families ↓with age and has ↓ over time. This ↑ likelihood for 'convenience' foods and erratic eating patterns → diets higher in saturatedfat/sugar and poorer in micronutrients

Peer group
Influence of peer pressure increases with age and adolescent girls are more likely to see friend's support as key to maintaining dietary change.
Eating with peers can have a positive effect on eating behaviour

Available income
1 in 3 children in the UK live in poverty, which is associated with poor nutrition. Convincing evidence that parents make sacrifices so that children have similar foods/snacks as other children to avoid feeling excluded

Implications for nutrition education/health promotion A holistic approach needs to be used to tackle the multitude of influences on food choice See 'Influences on food choice' in Chapter 14.

Older people

Older people: introduction

The United Kingdom has an ageing population. The number of older people (>65 y) is increasing and has doubled over the last 70 years. Between 1971 and 2003 the number of people aged 65 and over rose by 28% while the number of under-16s fell by 18%. Life expectancy is increasing steadily: men who are aged 65 can expect to live to the age of 81, while women can expect to live to the age of 84 (2003) and this is projected to increase further. The vast majority of older people live in the community, either with family or in their own homes, but around 5% live in nursing and residential care homes, although this increases to over 26% of those aged >85 y.

The ageing process

The ageing process involves a range of physiological and biological changes that vary between individuals. These influence digestive capacity, ↓ taste and nasal sensitivity and ↓ LBM, ↑ the relative proportion of adipose tissue and subsequently ↓ BMR.

What older people are eating

Older people are not a homogeneous group and the majority are adequately nourished and meet the RNI for most vitamins and minerals. However, those living in institutions and in lower socio-economic groups tend to have lower intakes of energy, protein, fibre, some vitamins and minerals. Housebound and 'institutionalized' older people have poorer vitamin D status, which is needed for the absorption of calcium and for bone health. In some older people (>85 y), B vitamin status is poor, particularly for folic acid. (See 'Folate (folic acid)' in Chapter 5 for good sources.)

A traditional diet is common, especially amongst older people in institutions, and the most commonly consumed foods are potatoes, white bread, biscuits, and tea.

There are categories of older people who are 'at risk' of malnutrition (see 'Undernutrition', this chapter) and some of these depend on whether the individual is 'fit' or 'frail'.

1 Department of Health (1998). *National diet and nutrition survey: people aged 65 years and over.* HMSO, London.

Dietary recommendations for older people

Some of the RNIs vary with age; ∴ they reflect differences in body composition and needs. In adulthood, requirements fall for calcium, phosphorus, niacin, thiamin (♂ only) and iron (but not before 50 y in ♀). Requirements for copper and selenium increase in adult males. See Appendix 6 for full dietary reference values for adults and older adults aged >50 y. Vitamin D is the only nutrient where dietary requirement increases (from zero to 10 µg from age 50 y) because some older people will have less exposure to the sun and therefore their vitamin D requirement will not necessarily be met by sunlight alone.

General healthy eating guidance (see 'Balance of good health' in 'Food based dietary guidelines', Chapter 2) applies to well older people (≥65 years), as it a balanced, nutrient rich diet to meet requirements. In addition to a balanced diet based on the 'Balance of good health', older people who are housebound will need to eat foods rich in vitamin D, e.g. milk (doorstep deliveries if available), eggs, fortified margarines, oily fish. The DH recommends regular sunlight exposure during May–September and vitamin D supplements during winter months, if housebound.[1] If fresh fruit and vegetable consumption is difficult due to preparation or eating difficulties, juices and frozen and canned produce should be encouraged as the nutrient value is just as rich.

Older people who are 'frail' are at higher risk of malnutrition, so the aspects of healthy eating guidelines related to reducing consumption of energy dense foods (from fat and sugar) are inappropriate. In practical terms this means that full-fat milk and margarines will be preferable, and sugar in the diet may provide useful calories and may help where taste sensitivity is ↓. However, sweet foods need to be part of a nutrient-rich diet and ideally eaten with meals (see dental health section).

[1] Department of Health (1998). *National diet and nutrition survey. People aged 65 years and over*, HMSO, London.

Undernutrition in older people

There are categories of older people who are 'at risk' of malnutrition.

- *People with difficulty eating*, e.g. poor dentition or sore mouth, masticating or swallowing disorders (see section on 'Dysphagia' in 'Cerebrovascular accident/stroke' in Chapter 19), sensory loss, disorders of the upper limb, difficulty manipulating cutlery (could be from arthritis).
- *People who depend on others*, e.g. living in institutions (hospitals, nursing, or residential care homes); depending on others to shop for food (around half of older people rely on someone else to do some of their food shopping).
- *Older age groups* (> 75 y).
- *Lower socio-economic groups*: there is evidence that intakes of a range of nutrients are less in older lower socio-economic groups, especially magnesium and potassium in women. Access to shops may be worse.
- *People with illness-related malnutrition*, e.g. malignancy, Parkinson's disease, pressure sores (↑requirements).
- *People in a vulnerable psychosocial situation*, e.g. loneliness, depression, dementia, bereavement → ↓ appetite.
- *People with physical difficulty in preparing food*, e.g. painful/frail hands from arthritis or reduced muscle strength, could → ↓ intake of fresh fruit and vegetables.
- *People on certain medication* affecting appetite, taste, GI tract (see 'Drug–nutrient interactions' in Chapter 8).

However, in most cases, the causes of undernutrition are multifactoria but an awareness of some specific contributory factors is a valuable firs step in prevention. (see 'Undernutrition' in Chapter 16).

Nutrition screening for malnutrition risk factors in older people

Classifying undernutrition in older people is concerned with establishin risk. The consequences of failing to identify and treat undernutrition ar potentially serious and therefore caution should be used when interpre ing results. Vulnerable older people living in the community need regula nutritional assessments by a member of the PHCT using a routine nutr tional screening tool (see 'Malnutrition universal screening tool' in Chap ter 16). Older people in residential homes should be assessed on entr (dietary intake and weight) and then weighed monthly.

Consequences of malnutrition in older people

The effects of undernutrition vary from subclinical, with no apparent clinical impairment to death, and are dependent on the type, length, and degree of nutritional inadequacy and the nutritional and health status of the individual.

In addition to a significant increased risk of mortality, undernutrition is associated with greater morbidity:

- Weight loss (predominantly fat and muscle), e.g. poorer mobility, ↑ risk of falls, ↑ risk of chest infection;
- Reduced immune function, e.g. ↑ rates of infection;
- Impaired synthesis of new protein, e.g. poor wound healing;
- Prolonged recovery from illness and hospital stays;
- Psychological, e.g. depression, anorexia, ↓ motivation.

See 'Undernutrition' in Chapter 16.

Treatment of malnutrition

There is good evidence that nutritional support in older people can ↑ energy and protein intake, ↓ weight loss, ↑ functional outcomes (muscle strength, walking distances, activity levels, mental health) and clinical outcomes (mortality, complications) in hospital and community settings.

Treatment options could include:

- *Improving food access*, e.g. arranging support through appropriate carers, e.g. shopping, cooking, company whilst eating;
- *Supplementation of food and/or drink using ordinary food items*, e.g. increasing energy /protein density of meals by fortifying, e.g. adding butter and grated cheese to mash potato;
- *Supplementation using proprietary products*; some are available on prescription or over the counter, e.g. milk or juice-based drinks, soups, desserts.

Also see 'Enteral feeding in Chapter 16.

Tips for overcoming institutional factors contributing to malnutrition in care homes and hospitals

✓ A named individual needs to be responsible for nutritional care
✓ Staff breaks do not coincide with mealtimes
✓ Adequate staff to assist patients/residents with eating
✓ Avoid medical rounds or investigations at mealtimes
✓ Food served needs to meet nutritional recommendations (catering staff may need extra training), i.e. average day's food intake, estimated over a 1 week period should meet EAR for energy and RNI for other nutrients (Appendix 6)
✓ Food needs to be at the right temperature for eating
✓ Offer patients adequate choice with a varied meal cycle
✓ Provide facilities for patients/residents (who are able) to make drinks and snacks
✓ Provide storage facilities for patients'/residents' own food
✓ Evening meal should not be so early that patients/residents are not yet hungry
✓ A bedtime snack should be available for those who are hungry later in the evening
✓ Residents/patients should be consulted when devising new menus
✓ Portion size should be flexible to allow for smaller and larger appetites and needs
✓ Environment should be conducive to eating, i.e. clean, light, relaxing, as the social aspects of eating are important for well-being

Other nutritional problems in older people

Constipation
Constipation is relatively common in older people. Fibre and fluid intake need to be assessed and increased consumption encouraged. (see 'Disorders of the colon' in Chapter 21).

Iron deficiency anaemia
Around 10% of older people were found to be anaemic in a population survey.[1] May be due to poor intake or ↓ absorption from GI disorders, GI blood loss. Encourage iron-rich foods and vitamin C consumption (see Iron' in Chapter 5).

Arthritis   See 'Osteoarthritis' and 'Rheumatoid arthritis', Chapter 33.

Osteoporosis
Osteoporosis and the subsequent fractures (hip, wrist, spine) are an important cause of morbidity and mortality in older people. Calcium and vitamin D intake, along with sunlight exposure, are important means of maintaining bone health in older people. The DH recommends regular sunlight exposure during May to September and vitamin D supplements during winter months if housebound.[1] Being under and overweight can influence risk of osteoporosis. See 'Osteoporosis' in Chapter 33.

Dehydration
The risk of dehydration is more common in older people, especially those dependent on others or where there is mental impairment. A daily intake of 1500–2000 ml is recommended, around 6–8 mugs (1 mug = 250 ml).

Dementia   See 'Dementia' in Chapter 27.

---

[1] Department of Health (1998). National diet and nutrition survey' people aged 65 years and over. HMSO, London.

Community support strategies for promoting a healthy diet for older people

Possible strategies include:

- Community shopping facilities/home delivery: serving isolated shoppers, usually grocery produce.
- Community cafés: where older people can eat a cheap meal in a sociable setting, e.g. at pensioners clubs, community centre.
- Community transport: to help bring older people that are isolated from shops nearer to them. Could be run by a local supermarket or local authority funded.
- Cooking club: practical group cooking sessions to improve food skills working with a health professional. Members of the group will cook and taste different recipes.
- Box schemes: customers receive a weekly box of fresh fruit and vegetables from a farmer that is distributed to a central place in the community. A group of people have to buy food regularly. Prices are more affordable as bought directly from the farmer.
- Lunch clubs and meals on wheels: provide hot meals for older and disabled people; may be run by the local authority or a voluntary organization such as Age Concern or the WRVS (largest provider). The average meal over a 1–2 week period should provide ≥33% of RNI, except that energy, folate, vitamin C, calcium, and iron should be higher.
- Grow your own, e.g. growing food in allotments and back gardens.
- Developing a food policy for older people including guidelines for care homes (see Fig. 12.2 and box in 'Undernutrition', this Chapter).

Model of a food policy for older people

The composition of working party could be as follows.

- Dietitians working with older people.
- GPs, hospital doctors.
- Social services; social worker.
- Community dental health service.
- Community nurses.
- Older people's hospital nurses.
- Age Concern representative.
- Representative of residents/patients.
- Residential care home representative.
- Occupational therapist.

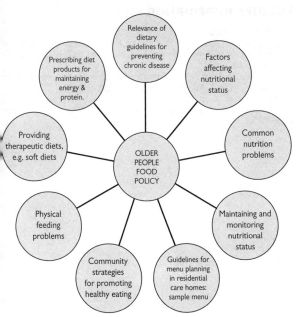

Fig. 12.1 A suggested format for a joint community–hospital-based food policy for older people.

Further information

www.ageconcern.org.uk
Caroline Walker Trust (1995). *Catering for older people in residential Accommodation. CORA menu planner.* Available from CWT, Abbots Langley Herts. WD5 ODQ.
Caroline Walker Trust (1998). *Eating well for older people with dementia.* Available from CWT, Abbots Langleys Herts. WD5 ODQ.
Caroline Walker Trust (2004). *Eating well for older people—nutritional and Practical guidelines.* Available from CWT, Abbots Langley, Herts. WD5 ODQ.

Nutrition in special groups

Minority ethnic communities

Traditional dietary habits and food restrictions

Traditional food restrictions for ethnic minority communities that are predominant in the UK are shown in Tables 13.1–13.3. There is a great deal of variety in dietary habits within all communities, including those of minority ethnic and religious groups; it is essential to find out the nature of the individual's restrictions; ∴ one cannot assume anything. However it is important to be aware of these orthodox food restrictions, even though there is great diversity in following them within UK minority ethnic communities. Younger generations of some ethnic groups are more likely to adopt a mixed diet incorporating that of the majority culture.

Implications for nutrition education

- Promote positive aspects of traditional diets and eating patterns
- Encourage use of readily available fruit and vegetables to incorporate into traditional eating patterns
- Encourage cooking and food preparation methods that reduce fat and sugar consumption of some traditional practices, e.g. oil/ ghee/ butter in curry or spread on chapattis
- Respect and take into account religious and cultural food restrictions (see Tables 13.1–13.3)
- Take account of the diverse patterns of responsibility for food shopping and cooking, e.g. men in some communities may be responsible for buying food
- Promote healthy eating within the whole family, not just centred on individuals
- Cannot assume anything: each individual is different. Need to acknowledge this heterogeneity in nutrition education campaigns/interventions
- Identify target groups that may be nutritionally at risk: low income groups, pregnant and lactating women, young children, older people
- Need to have good knowledge of health issues for each community to conduct evidence-based interventions
- Members of local minority ethnic community should be employed as community or health workers where possible
- Information as leaflets, video, and audio should be available in the mother tongue and recognize the diversity of food consumption in a given community
- For interventions using one-to-one communication, use interpreters where possible and necessary

Table 13.1 Traditional food restrictions of Asians living in Great Britain (4% of population in 2003)*

	Indian	Indian	Pakistani	Bangladeshi
Religion	Hindu	Sikh	Muslim	Muslim
Origin	Gujarat	Punjab	Pakistan	Bangladesh
Language (besides English)	Hindi/Kutchi	Punjabi; Hindi	Urdu, Punjabi	Bengali/ Sylheti
Fasting	✓ Certain holy days, especially month of Shravan	No religious obligation to fast	Especially month of Ramadan: no food during daylight. Pregnant, lactating & menstruating women, prepubescent children, diabetics and those needing regular medication are exempt	
Staple cereals	Chapatti, rice	Chapatti, rice	Chapatti, rice	Rice
Eggs	✗ If strict	✓ Probably; no if strict.	✓	✓
Dairy	✓ Milk, yogurt (may be home-made) but no cheese with rennet.			
Fish & shellfish	✗ If strict	✓ Possibly	✓ Possibly	✓ Often eaten
Poultry	✗	✓ But no if strict.	✓ halal†	✓ halal†
Red meat	✗ Most often lacto-vegetarian. Beef is prohibited.	✗ Except no beef. May be lacto-vegetarian. No if strict.	✓ halal† only, but pork and pork products prohibited.	

Table 13.1 (contd.)

	Indian(Hindu)	Indian(Sikh)	Pakistani	Bangladeshi
Alcohol	✗ If strict	✗ If strict	✗	✗
Caffeine	✗ If strict	✓	✓	✓
Nutritional implications	If unbalanced vegetarian diet, possible deficiencies in protein & energy (faltering growth in infants), B_{12} & iron (anaemia), Calcium & vitamin D (rickets/osteomalacia). See 'vegetarians', this chapter and 'Nutritionally vulnerable groups', Chapter 10		Attention for infant feeding: commercially prepared baby foods with non-halal meat may be replaced with sweet baby foods, low in iron and protein. See 'Nutritionally vulnerable groups', Chapter 10	

If curry cooked for a long time → ↓ folic acid, vitamins B_{12} and C.

↑ Risk of developing obesity, type 2 diabetes and CHD in later life; ∴ advise ↓ in fried foods (e.g. samosa, sev, bhaji, ganthia, puri, chevda, chips, crisps) and sweets (e.g. Indian sweets, including jelabi, burfi, gulab jamen, kulfi and laddo, and gur, jaggery, honey, chocolate, cakes and biscuits)

* There is great diversity in following food restrictions; they should be used as a guide and not a substitute for discussing individual dietary patterns.
† halal, slaughtered in a prescribed way.

Table 13.2 Traditional food restrictions of African Caribbeans and Black Africans living in Great Britain (2% of population in 2003)*

	African Caribbean	African Caribbean	African Caribbean	Black African
Religion	Christian	Rastafarian	Seventh Day Adventist	Muslim, Christian
Origin	West Indian Islands, especially Jamaica (60%), Dominica, Barbados, Trinidad.			Mainly Nigeria, Ghana, Somalia
Language (besides English)	Patois			Nigeria: Hausa, Yoruba, Ibo. Ghana: Twi. Somalia: Somali
Fasting	–	–	✗	✓ Especially month of Ramadan: no food during daylight. Pregnant, lactating & menstruating women, prepubescent children, diabetics and those needing regular medication are exempt
Staple cereals	Rice, plantain, yam, potato, pasta			Cassava, yam, plantain
Eggs	✓	✗	✓	✓
Dairy	✓ But condensed and evaporated milk may be used instead of fresh milk	✓ Unless vegan	✓	✓ Milk, yogurt but possibly no cheese with rennet.
Fish & shellfish	✓ Including salt fish	✓ If fins & scales. No shellfish	✓ If fins & scales. No shellfish	✓ possibly
Poultry	✓	✗	✓	✓ halal† if Muslim
Red meat	✓	✗ Mostly vegetarian; some are vegans.	✓ Mostly vegetarian, but some may eat meat but no pork	✓ If Muslim, possibly halal† only, but pork and pork products prohibited

Table 13.2 (contd.)

	African Caribbean	African Caribbean	African Caribbean	Black African
Religion	Christian	Rastafarian	Seventh Day Adventist	Muslim, Christian
Alcohol	✓	✗ If strict	✗	✗ If strict Muslim
Caffeine	✓	✗ If strict	✗	✓
Nutritional implications	Can be high in fat, sugar and salt. ↑ Risk of developing hypertension, CVD, and type 2 diabetes later	B₁₂ deficiency seen in strict adherent to Ital diet		Attention for Infant feeding; commercially prepared baby foods with non-halal meat may be replaced with sweet baby foods, low in iron and protein. See 'Nutritionally vulnerable groups', Chapter 10

Possibly higher prevalence of primary lactase deficiency (see Chapter 32)

* There is great diversity in following food restrictions; they should be used as a guide and not a substitute for discussing individual dietary patterns.
† halal, slaughtered in a prescribed way.

Table 13.3 Traditional food restrictions of Chinese and Jewish communities living in Great Britain (0.4% of population in 2003)*

	Chinese	Jewish
Religion	Include Taoism, Confucianism, Buddhism, Christianity, Islam	Judaism
Origin	Hong Kong, Malaysia, Singapore, China, Taiwan, Vietnam	Europe, Middle East
Language (besides English)	Written Chinese is common to all. Cantonese or Hakka are often spoken	Hebrew, Yiddish
Fasting	✗	✓ 1 day for Yom Kippur and Tish'ah B'av
Staple cereals	Rice	–
Eggs	✓	✓
Dairy	✓ But not frequently. Warm milk may be taken	✓ Some, but no cheese with rennet. Dairy foods not consumed at a meal with meat. Separate dishes & pans may be used for meat and dairy foods
Fish & shellfish	✓ Also salted fish.	✓ If fins & scales. No shellfish
Poultry	✓	✓ Chicken, turkey, goose, & duck. No birds of prey. Don't eat fish and meat at the same meal.
Red meat	✓ Mostly; except some religions	✓ kosher† only meat, but pork and its products prohibited
Alcohol	✓ Mainly for celebrations	✓ Wine (ideally approved by the rabbi)
Caffeine	✓ But coffee not commonly drunk	✓
Nutritional implications	Low calcium intake could result from low consumption of dairy foods. High sodium intake could be a problem (from monosodium glutamate in soy sauce), NB. food is seen as contributing to the body's balance, i.e. yin (foods that have a hot effect on body) & yang (cold affect). Cold food is often avoided	Traditional diet is high in total fat, saturated fat, and salt. ↑ Risk of obesity, type 2 diabetes and cardiovascular disease

* There is great diversity in following food restrictions as they should be used as a guide and not; a substitute for discussing individual dietary patterns.
† kosher, slaughtered in a prescribed way.

Vegetarians

Trends in vegetarianism

In the UK, the number of vegetarians has increased over the last few years and is now estimated at about 7% of the population, most prevalent in ♀, young people and adolescents, black and minority ethnic groups, and higher socio-economic groups. It is important to respect the individual's choice when giving dietary advice.

Common reasons for choosing a vegetarian diet include:

- Religion (e.g. strict Hindus, Buddhists, and 7th Day Adventists);
- Cultural;
- Ethical, moral, or political beliefs;
- Environmental concerns for use of world resources;
- Animal welfare;
- Perceived health benefits;
- Food safety scares;
- Limited availability of halal or kosher meat;
- Financial constraints.

Types of vegetarian diets

One cannot always categorize individuals along these lines, as there is a large variation, so health professionals should avoid making assumptions about which foods are acceptable, but generally vegetarians fall into the groups shown in Table 13.4.

Table 13.4 Types of Vegetarian diet

Type of vegetarian	Eggs*	Dairy	Fish and shellfish	Poultry	Red meat†
Vegan	✗	✗	✗	✗	✗
Lacto-vegetarian	✗	✓	✗	✗	✗
Lacto-ovo-vegetarian	✓	✓	✗	✗	✗
Demi-vegetarian	✓	✓	✓	✓	✗
Piscatarian	✓	✓	✓	✗	✗
Macrobiotic	✗	✗	✓‡	✗	✗
Fruitarian	✗	✗	✗	✗	✗

* Possibly free-range only.
† Beef, lamb, pork; also sometimes their derivatives, e.g. gelatine, rennet.
‡ Eaten at certain lower 'levels' of macrobiotic diet. Highest level eliminates everything except brown rice and water.

Is a vegetarian diet a risk for health?

A well balanced vegetarian diet can be nutritionally adequate for all age groups **BUT** times of extra nutritional requirements need specific attention: pregnancy, lactation, infancy, childhood, and adolescence. Children consuming a well balanced vegetarian diet should meet all requirements for growth. A well-planned vegetarian diet is more likely to comply with food-based dietary guidelines for reducing long-term risk of certain nutrition-related chronic diseases (NCD). There is evidence that vegetarians suffer less NCD than non-vegetarians, but this may be due to vegetarians adopting other health-promoting behaviours, e.g. being physically active, avoiding smoking, or drinking less alcohol. However, those who rely heavily on full-fat cheese and dairy foods could have a high saturated fat diet.

Diets that are unbalanced or more restrictive, e.g. strict macrobiotic, fruitarian, are likely to result in nutrient deficiencies and need particular attention, especially in infants, children, and pregnant and lactating women. Referral to a dietitian for assessment is essential.

Vegetarian groups at risk of an unbalanced diet

- Vegans
- Macrobiotics
- Fruitarians
- Strict Asian vegetarians
- Pregnant and lactating vegans
- Vegan infants and children
- Adolescent vegetarians
- 'New' vegetarians
- Vegetarians with an erratic eating pattern

Possible nutrients needing special attention for vegetarians

The main nutrients to keep an eye on are: protein, energy, vitamin B_{12}, vitamin D, calcium, and iron. Iodine (vegans) and zinc intakes should also be verified.

Energy

Energy intake is only usually of concern for vegans and those with more restrictive macrobiotic and fruitarian diets. They need to avoid a low energy diet that is too bulky and rich in fibre for infants and children as this could restrict growth; vegan children tend to be leaner than omnivores. See 'Nutritionally vulnerable groups' in Chapter 10.

Protein

Protein intakes usually meet recommendations in well-balanced vegetaria diets. Protein is usually adequate if the diet contains a variety of th following (2–3 serving/day):

- Nuts and seeds, peanut butter;
- Beans and pulses, e.g. baked beans, red kidney beans, soya beans, chick peas, lentils, hummus;
- Soya products, e.g. bean curd (tofu), textured vegetable protein (TVP);
- Eggs;
- Dairy products: milk, cheese, yogurt, fromage frais.

For vegans, high quality protein (see 'Protein' in Chapter 5) can b achieved by 'protein complementing' but energy intakes need to b adequate; otherwise protein is used for energy. Protein complementing foods must be consumed on the same day, but not necessarily at th same meal.

High quality protein = grain (insufficient lysine) + pulse (insufficient
methionine)

e.g. rice and dhal, beans on toast or rice and peas.

Vitamin B_{12}

Animal foods are the main source of vitamin B_{12}. (see 'Cobalamin B_{12} Chapter 5). Deficiency is rare but vegans and those following stricte macrobiotic and fruitarian diets need to be advised to consume suitabl fortified foods:

- Yeast extracts/fortified vegetable stocks;
- Fortified rice and soya milks;
- Breakfast cereal fortified with B_{12};
- Fortified blackcurrant cordial;
- Fortified tinned spaghetti;
- Almonds.

If vitamin B_{12} supplements are recommended these should not excee the RNI. See DRV tables (Appendix 6).

NB. Vitamin B_{12} analogues in seaweed and algae are not well absorbed.

Vitamin D

Vegetarians are no exception to the UK RNI for vitamin D that adult <65y and children >3y should meet their vitamin D requirement by sola UV radiation if living a normal lifestyle.

At risk groups that should take a daily supplement of Vitamin D are:

- Asian vegetarian children, adolescents, and women (see 'DRVs and dietary guidelines during pregnancy', Chapter 9);
- Children on strict vegan diets, especially African-Caribbean infants;
- Older vegetarians who are housebound or live in residential care.

Calcium

Vegetarians who consume dairy products regularly are not at risk of calcium deficiency. Vegans, fruitarians, and macrobiotics may be at risk of deficiency. Three servings should be eaten daily from a variety of sources:

- Dairy products: milk, cheese, yogurt (if lacto-vegetarian);
- Tofu;
- Nuts: almonds, brazil, hazelnuts;
- Fortified soya or rice milks;
- Fortified bread;
- Green leafy vegetables, e.g. broccoli, spinach, rocket, watercress;
- Peas, beans and pulses, e.g. baked beans, red kidney beans, soya beans, chickpeas, broad beans;
- Sesame seeds, tahini;
- Dried fruit, e.g. apricots, figs;
- White bread and white flour products.

As vitamin D enhances calcium absorption, vegetarians at risk of poor vitamin D status in particular need to be encouraged to eat a variety of the above foods regularly. Vegan children and pregnant women should be referred to a dietitian who may recommend calcium supplements if dietary sources are insufficient.

Iron

UK vegetarians generally consume similar intakes of dietary iron to UK non-vegetarians. However, non-haem iron (plant sources) is absorbed less readily than haem iron (animal sources). Vegetarians should be encouraged to consume a good source of vitamin C to help absorption, e.g. citrus fruits and juices, and avoid drinking tea at the same meal ($\downarrow$ absorption). See 'Iron' and 'Vitamin C (ascorbic acid)', Chapter 5.

Good vegetarian sources of iron:

- Eggs;
- Wholemeal flour and bread;
- Breakfast cereals fortified with iron;
- Dark green leafy vegetables;
- Beans and pulses;
- Dried prunes, figs, and apricots;
- Yeast extract;

Iodine

As milk is an important source of iodine in the UK, vegans, fruitarians, and macrobiotics are at risk of low intakes $\rightarrow$ $\uparrow$ levels of thyroid-stimulating hormone. Encourage vegans to use iodized salt or take iodine supplements.

Zinc

Intakes of zinc by vegetarians and vegans are not lower than for omnivores. However, there is low bioavailability from plant sources due to phytates inhibiting zinc absorption; ∴ intakes of at least the RNI should be encouraged (7–9.5 mg/day in adults, depending on age and gender; see DRV tables, Appendix 6).

Dietary guidelines for a balanced vegetarian diet see 'Balance of good health' in 'Food-based dietary guidelines', Chapter 2.

Vegetarians and pregnancy

Being vegetarian should pose no problem in pregnancy if the woman is well informed and eating a balanced lacto-ovo and lacto-vegetarian diet (see above). Pregnant vegan, fruitarian, and macrobiotic women should be seen by a dietitian to assess the overall nutrient adequacy of their diets. They may require supplementation of vitamin B_{12}, iron, vitamin D, or calcium (if <600 mg/day consumed). Some fortified soya milks contain these nutrients.

Asian vegetarian women could be at risk of vitamin D deficiency if there is insufficient skin exposure → neonatal hypocalcaemia and rickets, ∴ may need vitamin D supplements (see 'Minority ethnic communities', this chapter).

Vegetarianism in childhood and adolescence See 'Vegetarianism' in 'Nutritional problems of children and adolescents', Chapter 11.

The vegetarian baby See 'Nutritionally vulnerable groups' in Chapter 10.

Eating on a low income

Scale of the problem

Some UK families and children are at much higher risk of poverty than others, particularly larger families, families of Pakistani and Bangladeshi origin, and families with one or more disabled adults and/or one or more disabled children. An estimated 20% of children in the UK live in poverty[1] and >2 million older people receiving a pension are still living below the poverty line. However, the poor are not a homogeneous group and people can move in and out of poverty with changing employment, relationships, or other circumstances. This impacts on financial resources and therefore reduces opportunities for eating a healthy diet.

Causes of food poverty

Causes of food poverty are multifactorial, but poverty is strongly related to income, social exclusion, and physical access to food (proximity of shops selling healthy foods of good quality at affordable prices). Studies have shown that the poorest 10% of UK households spend almost a third of their income on food compared with a fifth in the richest. A typical basket of food purchased in local shops can cost around 25% more than from a large supermarket; this difference can rise up to 60% if supermarket economy lines are compared.

Nutritional problems that are associated with food poverty do not arise because money is spent poorly on food, but because there is not enough money to spend. Several studies have shown that spending is often based on maximizing value for money in terms of energy intake and ∴ compromising micronutrient intake. Several key influences in food choice take prominence to influence behaviour: particularly access to shops, affordable food, budgeting strategies, and the need for cultural and social acceptability (see 'Influences on Food choice', Chapter 14).

It has been proposed that 'food deserts', i.e. poor communities where residents cannot buy affordable healthy food, are an important contributor to poor diet. Whilst others have questioned the lack of empirical evidence for this, eradication of food deserts is an integral part of government policy aimed at reducing health inequalities (Food Poverty Eradication Act, 2001).

Dietary and nutritional consequences of poverty

Children

The UK National Diet and Nutrition Survey of young people aged 4–18 years[2] found that children in households of lower socio-economic status have lower intakes of energy, and most vitamins and minerals. When differences in energy intake were accounted for, the following was found:

---

[1] Department of Health (2003). Tackling health in equalities: status report on the Programme for Action. HMSO, London.
[2] Gregory, J., and Lowe, S., et al., (2000). National Diet and Nutrition Survey children aged 4–18 years. HMSO, London.

Boys and girls in households of lower socio-economic status ate less fruit and vegetables, and had lower intakes of vitamin C, calcium, phosphorus, magnesium, and iodine.

Boys in households of lower socio-economic status had lower intakes of pantothenic acid.

Girls in households of lower socio-economic status had lower intakes of riboflavin, niacin, carotene, manganese.

Children <5 y from low income families are also at greater risk of having an unbalanced diet, developing micronutrient deficiency, such as iron deficiency anaemia and faltering growth.

There is convincing evidence that parents make sacrifices so that children have similar foods/snacks as other children, to avoid being teased or ostracized by their peers.

The short-and long-term consequences of poor diet in childhood include: reduced immune status, increased dental caries, reduced cognitive function and learning ability, and increased risk of developing obesity in girls.

Adults

Poverty is associated with poor nutrition in the UK and the *National Diet and Nutrition Survey of adults aged 19–64 years*[3] found that men and women on benefits compared with those in non-benefit households had poorer diets (food sources only) that were:

Higher in non-milk extrinsic sugars;

Lower in protein, non-starch polysaccharides, fruit and vegetables, most minerals and vitamins (but these were all above the RNI except for vitamin A in women)

Intakes of women on benefits were most vulnerable, i.e. intakes were < LRNI for vitamin A, riboflavin and lower intakes of all minerals compared with women living in non-benefit households; particular concern that 53% of women aged 19–50 y in benefit households had iron intakes < LRNI.

The long-term consequences include increased incidence of obesity in lower social economic groups, especially for women, and reduced life expectancy for men and women.

Further information is available at www.statistics.gov.uk/focuson/social inequalities.

Pregnant and breastfeeding women

UK women on low incomes may find it harder to achieve an adequate diet during pregnancy. Nutrients most at risk are: zinc, iron, vitamins A, C, and E, and essential fatty acids (EFAs) needed for fetal neural and vascular system development. EFAs are found in green vegetables, oily fish (e.g. tuna, sardines, mackerel, pilchards, kippers), and certain vegetable oils (e.g. corn, sunflower, and soya oils). There is an increased likelihood of giving birth to a low birthweight baby (<2.5 kg), infant mortality in the first year, and of suffering stillbirth or congenital malformations. See 'Vulnerable groups in pregnancy', Chapter 9.

Hoare, J., Henderson, L., *et al.* (2004), *The National Diet and Nutrition Survey adults aged 19 to 64 years*. Vol. 5. *Summary report*. HMSO, London. Available at www.food.gov.uk/science/0/717/ndns documents.

Breastfeeding rates are less in lower socio-economic groups in the UK and education should target these groups.

Older adults and low income

There is evidence that intakes of a range of nutrients are less in older people living on a low income. Poor access to shops may be one contributing factor. Older people are not a homogeneous group and although the majority are adequately nourished and meet the RNI for most vitamins and minerals, those living in institutions and in lower socio-economic groups tend to have lower intakes of energy, protein, fibre some vitamins and minerals (especially magnesium and potassium in women).

Terminology

Food poverty
Is widely defined as 'the inability to acquire or consume an adequate quality or quantity of food in socially acceptable ways, or the uncertainty that one will be able to do so'

Food security
Is widely defined as meaning that 'people at all times should have physical and economic access to sufficient, affordable, safe and nutritious food necessary and appropriate for a healthy life, and the security of knowing that this access is sustainable in the future'

Refugee
A refugee is a person who (United Nations Convention, 1951) 'owing to a well founded fear of being persecuted for reasons of race, religion, nationality, membership of a particular social group or political opinion is outside the country of his nationality and is unable, or owing to such fear, is unwilling to avail himself of the protection of that country; or who, not having a nationality and being outside the country of his former habitual residence, as a result of such events, is unable to or, owing to such fear, is unwilling to return to it'

Asylum seeker
An asylum seeker is someone who has applied for refugee status in order to be recognized as a refugee in the UK

Statutorily homeless
After assessment by the local authority, the statutorily homeless qualify for permanent council/housing association housing. Includes people with dependent children, pregnant women, and vulnerable single people. They often wait in temporary accommodation such as bed and breakfast, and hostels that have limited cooking and storage facilities

Non-statutorily homeless
The non-statutorily homeless do not qualify for permanent housing; they are usually single men. Often live in temporary accommodation such as bed and breakfast, and hostels that have limited cooking and storage facilities, but many 'sleep rough' on the streets, especially middle-aged, white men

Refugees, asylum seekers, and homeless people

Refugees and asylum seekers in the UK

Refugees' health and nutritional status varies widely, and they should be treated on an individual basis as they are not a homogeneous group. Children may be well nourished or they may suffer from chronic undernutrition with growth stunting. The UK centiles have been complied using data from Caucasian children (see 'Infant growth and development', Chapter 10) and therefore some ethnic groups, e.g. Ethiopians may appear unusually tall whereas others may appear unusually short. It is important to refer children where there is more than a two centile discrepancy between height and weight or where serial measurements of growth fail to show adequate weight or height gain.

However, there are a number of factors indicating nutritional risk.

- **Nutritional status on arrival in UK**. Depends on the nature of their departure from their country of origin, whether time was spent in refugee camps, and exposure to communicable disease, which could all ↓ nutritional status and weight.
- **Poverty**. After arrival in the UK, many refugees live in poor housing, receive limited financial support, and have difficulty obtaining paid work → low income and poor diet. Professional skills may not be recognized.
- **Cultural factors**. Foods eaten, preparation methods, and the social context of eating help define cultural identity. For refugees displaced from their own culture, friends, and family, the symbolic value of food can grow. Certain foods may not be available locally and familiar cooking implements or facilities unavailable. Whilst many refugees adapt, food intake will change by necessity, which may ↑ risk of a nutritionally inadequate diet compared with a traditional diet. Some refugees may have poor cooking skills as they are not used to preparing food, e.g. young men.
- **Communication**. Refugees who do not speak English may have difficulty shopping for food, which is compounded when foods are unfamiliar and ingredients or cooking instructions cannot be read.
- **Psychological issues**. Many have experienced violence, loss, or separation in their country of origin and two-thirds of adult refugees in the UK report anxiety or depression. This could ↓ appetite and interest in eating. Cooking and sharing food has been used as therapy with some refugees.

Homeless people

There are two main groups of homeless people: statutory and non-statutory homeless (see box); these include those living in hostels and bed and breakfast accommodation and those sleeping rough on the streets. Most homeless people have few or no means of buying, storing or preparing fresh food. A number of studies have shown that the health of homeless people is severely compromised due to inadequate diets, e.g. ~50–60% have no daily intake of fresh fruit and vegetables and those who do have usually received a free meal at a day centre. There is idence of a high level of alcohol use among people sleeping rough, ten coexisting with a mental health problem.

Some of the short-term consequences of a poor diet are:

Iron deficiency anaemia due to low intakes of meat, fruit, and vegetables;

↑ susceptibility to infection due to micro-and macronutrient deficiencies;

Constipation due to low dietary fibre intake from fruit and vegetables and higher fibre cereals.

me of the long-term consequences are:

An increased risk of premature mortality from CVD and cancer. The average mortality rate of a homeless man is ~ 42 y compared to the national average of 76 y;

Dental caries and gum disease due to poor oral hygiene and eating patterns. If untreated could → difficulty eating certain 'hard' foods; ∴ ↑ chance of malnutrition.

rategies to improve nutritional status of the homeless

rtnership working between staff and residents at hostels/bed and eakfasts, dietitians, city and borough councils, and health promotion ficers can lead to improvements in the nutritional quality of meals ovided by:

Developing nutrition education, e.g. practical nutrition resources and running cooking classes for residents on preparing healthy, affordable meals with limited cooking and storage facilities;

Lobbying for funding for 'mini-fridges' and microwaves in resident's rooms, locked food storage facilities, and better communal cooking facilities;

Producing a nutrition information pack for catering staff and home leaders that includes nutritional standards for meals provided.

See box below.

Nutritional standards for meals provided in hostels, bed and breakfast accommodation, and day centres for homeless people

- Involve residents in menu planning
- Encourage the social and pleasurable aspects of eating
- Staff and volunteers need to be fully trained in food hygiene procedures
- Plan meals around a healthy eating food model (see 'Balance of good health' in 'Food-based dietary guidelines', Chapter 2)
- Use less salt and saturated fat in foods provided, e.g. ↓ processed foods used with low nutritional value, such as processed meat products, soups, and sauces
- Provide fortified breakfast cereals with a choice of full and lower fat milk
- Provide fruit and vegetables with every meal
- Provide plenty of foods rich in non-starch polysaccharides
- Provide water with meals
- Offer special diets where appropriate, i.e. therapeutic diets, and take into account dietary needs of people from different cultural groups (see 'Minority ethnic communities', this chapter)

Policy options for reducing food poverty

Ideas for local food projects

- Community shops: not-for-profit shop serving isolated shoppers, usually grocery produce. Also adds a social focus to communities.
- Community cafés where people can eat a cheap meal in a sociable setting, e.g. at pensioners clubs, community centre.
- Food cooperatives: a group of people organizing to buy food in bulk direct from wholesalers or farmers to save money.
- Community transport: to help bring shops nearer to the isolated. Could be run by a local supermarket or local authority funded. Especially useful for older people and people with disabilities.
- Links with local shops: to stock and promote healthier food produce, encouraging people to use their local shops.
- Food vouchers and coupons, e.g. provided by local authorities by distributing 'money-off' coupons to local people or national government 'healthy start' vouchers for parents on a low income.
- Farmers' markets, where farmers and growers make up the majority of vendors.
- Cooking club: practical group cooking sessions to improve food skills working with a health professional. Members of the group will cook and taste different recipes.
- Breakfast clubs: providing healthy breakfast choices at school.
- Box schemes: customers receive a weekly box of fresh fruit and vegetables from a farmer that is distributed to a central place in the community. A group of people have to buy food regularly. Prices are more affordable as produce is bought directly from the farmer.
- Lunch clubs and meals on wheels: provide hot meals for older and disabled people; may be run by the local authority or a voluntary organization such as Age Concern or the WRVS (largest provider).
- Food redistribution: surplus food is moved from shops and supermarkets to day centres and homeless facilities to provide free meals.
- Grow your own, e.g. growing food in allotments, on wasteland, schools, parks, and in back gardens.
- School Nutrition Action Groups: multidisciplinary group that develops a whole school approach to better nutrition. See 'Model of a local food policy' in 'Examples of nutrition policy in different settings', Chapter 15.

Using a community development approach

The above local policy options need to be developed using a community development approach.

- Community-based, involving genuine partnerships between local residents, local workers, and professionals.
- Reaffirms community identity and meets local needs.
- Promotes active citizenship.
- Combats age, gender, and ethnic discrimination.
- Encourages community participation.
- Addresses other social and cultural issues as well as eating behaviour.
- Is flexible and responsive.

Useful websites

www.ukfg.org.uk
www.sustainweb.org/poverty_index.asp
www.fareshare.org.uk/whatdo/*food* poverty.html
www.refugeecouncil.org.uk

Chapter 14

Nutrition intervention with individuals

Influences on food choice

Many factors interplay to influence the foods individuals choos
besides a basic physiological need to eat. Factors act on three leve
individual, societal, and national/international level (see Fig. 14.1
Interventions need to bear this in mind, so that they are matched at th
right level. Public health professionals working at a national/internation
level will be working primarily on the wider policy level, so they will nee
to be fully aware of these wider influences on food choice such as legisla
tion, subsidies and taxes, world trade agreements, government polic
production methods and agricultural policy, advertising, plus global publi
health policy (WHO/FAO/UNICEF), global economic bodies (e.g. th
World Bank, IMF, World Trade Organization), intergovernmental agree
ments (International Conference on Nutrition, commercial interest
(International Chamber of Commerce), European bodies (EU, Regiona
offices of WHO/FAO), and networks to promote public health (Health
Cities Network, International Baby Food Network).

Health professionals working at the local level are able to influence
some of the individual and societal/community influences on food choic
(see Fig. 14.2). This could be during one to one consultations wit
patients and when developing appropriate public health nutrition pro
grammes. It is not just 'what' is eaten that is important but understandin
'why' and in which context it is eaten is crucial in helping people ea
more healthily. Health professionals working locally will also need to
have a wider vision of the international context of public health nutrition
to be able to promote health, as there are conventions and internationa
agreements that have an impact on a regional and local level. An exampl
is the rapid increase in obesity, which is related to factors that are muc
wider than those that are modifiable locally. Professionals working ir
public health locally can be involved in advocacy work to try and stimu
late change, e.g. lobbying government for stricter food and drink advertising
regulations, nutrient standards for food procurement.

Further information Pencheon, D. *et al.* (2003). Oxford handbook of
public health practice. Oxford University Press, Oxford.

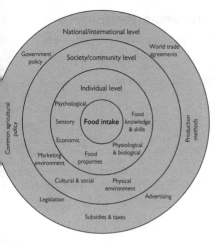

Fig. 14.1 Influences on food choice: individual, societal, and national/international level.

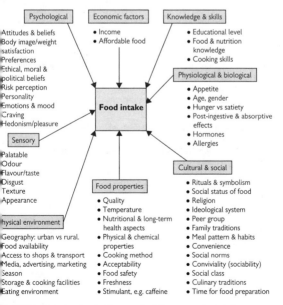

Fig. 14.2 Individual and societal/community influences on food choice.

Nutrition education techniques

Developing effective nutrition education messages

Nutrition education is a component of promoting healthier eating and the process of applying scientific knowledge about diet–health to individuals' dietary behaviour to improve health literacy (nutrition and health related knowledge, attitudes, motivation, behavioural intentions, personal skills, and self-efficacy).

Nutrition education messages are most effective if they are:
- Clear, simple, avoiding technical jargon;
- Use foods rather than nutrients to communicate;
- Consistent with other sources;
- Personally relevant to the audience;
- Sensitive to how consumers perceive the risk of unhealthy eating;
- Positive (eat more fruit), rather than negative (eat less fat);
- Emphasize the benefits of change;
- Acknowledge barriers to change;
- Avoid messages that stigmatize individuals;
- Use persuasion, prompts, and reminders.

Using talks and group work for nutrition education

Where to start
- Think of what you expect your audience to be able to do /to know before attending your session.

Then
- Think of them after they have attended it. What should they now be able to **do** as a result of that? (learning outcomes).
- The key word is **do**; so include active verbs when drafting learning outcomes (see Table 14.1).
- Learning outcomes should be measurable.
- Usually about 5–10 outcomes are sufficient.

Why do we need learning outcomes?
- To help the audience learn more effectively as they know what the goals are.
- To make it clear what the audience can hope to gain from attending a particular teaching session
- To help practitioners to design materials more effectively by acting as a template for them (see 'Designing nutrition education materials', this chapter).
- To help choose an appropriate teaching strategy, e.g. lecture, seminar, group work.
- To assist team work as it is easier to share with colleagues what a particular activity is expected to achieve.

How are learning outcomes structured?

As well as being measurable, learning outcomes need to be matched to the type of learning expected. This is hierarchical with teaching 'knowledge' at a lower level of learning, whereas teaching 'evaluation' skills is the highest level (see Table 14.1).

Knowledge: recalling appropriate previously learned information.
Comprehension: understanding the meaning.
Application: using previously learned information in new situations to solve problems that have single or best answers.
Analysis: breaking down information into its component parts, examining and trying to understand the organizational structure of such information to develop divergent conclusions by identifying causes, making inferences.
Synthesis: creatively applying prior knowledge and skills to produce a new or original whole.
Evaluation: judging the value of material based on personal values/ opinions, resulting in an end product, with a given purpose, without right or wrong answers.

Table 14.1 Possible active verbs for defining learning outcomes

Knowledge	Comprehension	Application	Analysis	Synthesis	Evaluation
arrange	classify	apply	analyse	arrange	appraise
order	locate	operate	differentiate	formulate	judge
define	describe	choose	appraise	assemble	argue
recognize	recognize	practise	discriminate	manage	predict
duplicate	discuss	demonstrate	calculate	collect	assess
label	report	schedule	distinguish	organize	rate
recall	explain	sketch	categorize	compose	attach
list	express	employ	examine	plan	score
repeat	review	solve	compare	construct	choose
memorize	identify	illustrate	experiment	prepare	select
name	select	use	contrast	create	compare
state	indicate	interpret	question	propose	support
relate	translate	write	criticize	design	estimate
reproduce			test	write	evaluate

Increasing learning level

Sample lesson plan*

Session 1: Title, e.g. 'Current dietary recommendations'
Audience: adults in workplace setting
Numbers expected = 20
Duration of session: 1 h
Aim: (general statement of intent): to explain dietary recommendations in food terms
Learning outcomes
- State the 8 nationally agreed guidelines for a healthy diet
- Describe the 5 food groups in the healthy eating food model of the 'Balance of good health'
- List the healthier 'types' of these foods
- Explain the reasoning for the current dietary guidelines in relation to health
- Identify practical examples to help meet the dietary recommendations
- Identify 6 factors that influence their food choice

Time (min)	Activity	Resources
3	Introduction—plan for the session	Verbal & on the board
7	Nutrition and diet quiz: distribute quiz and ask participants to complete	Quiz handout
15	Go through the answers to the quiz to stimulate discussion:	
	Q1: Scientific reports and dietary recommendations	Overhead 1
		Overhead 2
	Q2: Dietary Reference values & terminology	Overhead 3
	Q3: % population eating 5 portions of fruits and vegetables a day	Overhead 4
	Q4: Prevalence of obesity	Overhead 5
	Q5: Public attitudes and beliefs to eating more healthily	Overhead 6
	Q6: Public views on health information	Handout
	Distribute quiz answers	
10	Healthy eating food model	Poster
		Food model leaflet
		Verbal explanation
10	Practical examples of meeting recommendations	Case studies
10	Factors influencing food choice	Brainstorm
	Line exercise on white board	Practical exercise
	Feedback	
5	Sum up—back to original overhead showing plan	

* More information on teaching skills. Rogers, A. (2003). *Teaching adults*, 3rd edn. Oxford University Press, Oxford.

Designing nutrition education materials

When writing a diet sheet, a report, or patients' notes, a practitioner is intent on transmitting information to the reader. How well the practitioner succeeds will depend on several factors, including the readability of the text.

Readability

Readability is concerned with the problem of matching between reader and text. There is often a large discrepancy between readability and the average patient's reading ability. An accomplished reader is likely to be bored by simple repetitive texts. A poor reader will soon become discouraged by texts that s/he finds too difficult to read fluently.

A typical readability index uses an average sentence length and average number of words of 3–4 syllables per sample used (>200 tests exist). Tests do not account for the order of words in a sentence.

A suitable diet sheet/patient information needs to match the reading age of the general public (average of 11 years).

Example of a readability test (Gunning 'FOG')

Select samples of 100 words, normally 3 such samples from 1 piece of writing.
1. Calculate L, the average sentence length (number of words ÷ number of sentences). Estimate the number of sentences to the nearest tenth, where necessary.
2. In each sample, count the number of words with 3 or more syllables. Find N, the average number of these words per sample. Then the grade level needed to understand the material = $(L + N) \times 0.4$.
   So the reading age = $[(L + N) \times 0.4] + 5$ years.

Besides readability, the overall structure and presentation, organization of text, and vocabulary used are important when evaluating the quality of nutrition education materials. See opposite for a checklist for evaluating patient information.

Suggested checklist for evaluating the quality of educational materials for patients and the general public

Content
- Is there a clear description of the purpose and structure of the text?
- Are headings present; if so, are they appropriate?
- Are the facts correct and up to date?
- Is the quality and strength of the evidence discussed?
- Does the material take account of current government policy?
- Are nutrition messages clear, unambiguous, and consistent throughout?
- Are any statements about nutrition placed within the context of a healthy lifestyle and based on the 'Balance of good health?'
- Is the source of information given (e.g. nutrition & dietetic service, BMA)?
- If the use of a branded product can be justified in terms of helping users to identify types of products, is the use sparing and in a relevant context?
- Are references to product names used as examples only, so that single products are not favoured over others?
- Where there is reference to particular foods, are generic groupings used?
- Have contact numbers, addresses, or websites been given for further information, e.g. self-help groups?
- For commercial literature, are logos and brand names used sparingly and in context?
- Is the date of production included?

Is the material appropriate for the intended audience?
- How technical is the vocabulary in the text? Are all acronyms and jargon explained?
- How readable is the text?
- Is it clear who the writer and intended audience are?
- Have users been consulted? Have materials been pretested for comprehension?
- Is the visual layout satisfactory, e.g. layout, font size, large enough for intended audience, visual appeal?
- Is the information adapted for the sociocultural characteristics of target audience in terms of language and food habits?

Communication skills and behaviour change on a one to one level

Practitioners use their communication skills to inform, educate, and facilitate motivation in others by enabling patients to make informed choices about food and lifestyle. Practitioners need to draw on a repertoire of 'helping' skills that enable them to encourage behaviour change. There are a number of theoretical models underpinning this way of working, but essentially it is based on a 'person-centred model' where practitioner and patient agree the plan of action.

Essential practitioner characteristics

A number of specific skills and qualities need to be practised to improve the practitioner's ability to listen, respond, and reflect empathetically.

* **Unconditional acceptance** accepting and respecting patients, not judging.
* **Congruence** genuine, being sincere and not defensive.
* **Empathy** understanding a patient's personal meanings.
* **Open questioning style** (see Table 14.2)
* **Good listening skills** (see Table 14.3): appropriate use of active versus passive listening.
* Awareness of the effect of **non-verbal communication**: posture, gestures, appearance, voice, eye contact, and facial expressions.

A **client-centred approach** to give more control to the patient, rather than the practitioner; build on the patient's expertise about him or her self.

* Recognize that the patient has the **right to decide** if s/he wants to change behaviour or not.

Table 14.2 Asking questions: open vs closed questioning

Open questions	Closed questions
Include 'what', 'how', 'where', and 'when'	Invite a monosyllabic response, such as 'yes or no'
e.g. Tell me about where you do your shopping?	e.g. Have you been to the supermarket this week?
Avoid 'why' questions as patients can become defensive	
Encourage patients to talk in more depth	Hard to establish empathy. Can be useful for clarifying information.
Help the patient keep the control, rather than the helper	The dietitian/helper retains control over the interview

Table 14.3 The process of listening

Active	Passive
Dynamic process includes using:	Sit back whilst the patient talks.
'Minimal encouragers (e.g. 'go on', 'uh-huh', and allowing silence)	
Paraphrasing (repeating back the general content of what was said).	
Reflection (feeding back to show patients that they have been understood)	
Summarizing (condense the substance of what was said).	
Giving full attention (attending): face the patient squarely; adopt open posture; lean towards patient; maintain eye contact	Full attention is not given; may start to think about something else
Boredom less likely for practitioner	Practitioner can feel bored or irritated
The patient feels valued	The patient feels undervalued

Value of counselling skills for motivating dietary change

- Helps establish the current scenario.
- Explores preferred situation and sets appropriate goals with the patient.
- Provides a supportive relationship that may improve adherence to dietary change.
- Encourages the patient to be more 'empowered' to make appropriate choices.
- Helps patients to explore their feelings about changing their eating behaviour.
- Assists patients in the selection of problem-solving strategies to encourage dietary change.

Using these skills for behaviour change

Various models of health behaviour have been developed that make an important contribution to understanding dietary behaviour. Health behaviour models conceptualize the social cognitive variables important in determining behaviour. Such models focus on the idea that the attitudes a person holds can influence their dietary behaviour. They acknowledge that dietary 'knowledge' alone is not necessarily enough to lead to behaviour change. They take account of:

- Whether individuals are fatalistic about their health (locus of control);
- Whether individuals feel able or confident to change certain aspects of health behaviour (self-efficacy);
- The value individuals place on their health (health as a valve);
- The stage in which individuals can be placed in relation to their health behaviour (stage of change).

See ' Behavioural therapy' in 'Treatment physical activity and behavioural therapy', Chapter 17.

Stage of change

One model that is widely used to understand health-related behaviour change is the 'transtheoretical model of change'.[1] This model regards individuals as traversing through 5 phases (Fig. 14.3 and Table 14.4). Movement through the stages is not necessarily linear; individuals may relapse to earlier stages several times, but this does not necessarily mean that they are starting at the beginning. The practitioner's role is to facilitate a natural process of change, matching the support given to the stage where the patient is. It is often difficult to pinpoint which stage a person is in and indeed they can move from stage to stage during the course of an interview, whereas others get 'stuck' in a particular stage. Therefore the model should only be used as a guide.

Table 14.4 stage of change and associated practitioner role

Stage	Practitioner role
Pre-contemplation Not interested in change or 'in denial or immune to their health problems'	Elicit open discussion to assess how the current situation is perceived and to highlight health risks about their unhealthy behaviour to encourage the possibility of change
Contemplation Ambivalent or thinking about change	Help the patient weigh up the pros and cons of changing compared with those for not changing
Preparation Preparing for change	Support in developing their action plan for change. Suggest or give educational material
Action Actively modifying habits or environment	Helping the patient to set clear, realistic goals including rewards. Praise action taken by patients
Maintenance Sustaining new, healthier habits and preventing relapse **Relapse**	Reassuring patients that occasional 'lapses' are normal, so that they are not so discouraged that they give up. However, most patients will go through the stages of change several times before changes become established

How do you know which stage a patient is in?

Assignment of individuals to one of the stages may be done intuitively during discussion with patients or more formally by asking a limited number of mutually exclusive questions and applying a basic algorithm (Table 14.5). However, it is important that assignment of individuals to a particular stage does not get in the way of the helping process. The focus should be on the interpersonal relationship. For example,

[1] Prochaska, J.O. and DiClemente, C.C. (1986). The transtheoretical approach. In the *Handbook of eclectic psychotherapy* (ed. J.C. Norcross), pp.163–200.Bruner/ Mazel, New york.

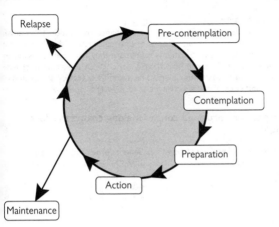

Fig. 14.3 The 'stage of change' model of Prochaska and DiClemente.

Table 14.5 Scoring for stage of change

Stage	Q1	Q2	Q3	Q4
Pre-contemplation	N	N	N	
Contemplation	N	N	Y	
Action	Y			N
Maintenance	Y			Y

- Q1 In the past month, have you been actively trying to lose weight? Yes/No.
- Q2 In the past month, have you been actively trying to keep from losing weight? Yes/No.
- Q3 Are you seriously trying to lose weight to reach your goal weight in the next 6 months? Yes/No.
- Q4 Have you maintained your desired weight for more than 6 months? Yes/No.

Motivational interviewing

Motivational interviewing (MI) is a client-centred, directive method for enhancing intrinsic motivation to change by exploring and resolving ambivalence.

It is not just a set of techniques, but relies heavily on good reflective listening skills.

Decisional balance

Decisional balance is used as a tool to enhance motivation to change. Thinking through the pros and cons of both changing and not making a change is one way to help patients make sure they have fully considered a possible change. This can help them to 'stick' with their plan in stressful/tempting moments. Patients could be asked to reflect on for example, the pros and cons of making changes to lose weight, (see box).

One patient's pros and cons of making changes to lose weight

Benefits/pros of making changes
- Feel better about myself, more confident.
- Fit into all those clothes hanging in the wardrobe!
- Save money as will be eating less.
- Help control my blood pressure.

Benefits/pros of not changing
- Not having to change routine of the family.
- Partner likes me chubby.
- Still being able to eat lots of tasty food.

Cons of making changes
- Will miss tasty food.
- Will be hungry at first.
- Partner might not like it if I am too slim.

Cons of not changing
- Health: could develop diabetes in the future.
- Blood pressure might get worse.
- Will carry on feeling a bit of a failure due to being self conscious about my weight.

Further information

1 Gable, J. (1997). *Counselling Skills for dietitians*. Blackwell, Science, Oxford.

2 Hunt P. Hillsdon, M. (1996). *Changing eating and exercise behaviour. A handbook for professionals*. Blackwell Science, Oxford.

3 Prochaska, J.O., Norcross, J.C., and DiClemente, C.C. (1994). *Changing for good: a revolutionary six-stage program for overcoming bad habits and moving your life positively forward*. Avon Books, New York.

4 Miller, W. and Rollnick, S. (2002). *Motivational interviewing: preparing people for change*, 2nd edn. Guilford Press, New York.

Planning change

Once a patient has made the decision to change, a change plan can be constructed with the help of the practitioner.

Example of an outline change plan for a patient wanting to lose weight

The changes I want to make are:
- List specific areas or ways in which you want to change
- Include positive goals (beginning, increasing, improving behaviour), *e.g. have a healthy snack mid-afternoon so that I eat less food when I return home from work; eat smaller quantities at mealtimes*

The most important reasons why I want to make these changes are:
- What are some likely consequences of action and inaction?
- Which motivations for change seem most important to you, *e.g. to feel better about myself, more confident*

The steps I plan to take in changing are:
- How do you plan to achieve the goals? Are there some specific first steps you might take? When, where and how will these steps be taken, *e.g. have a shower/drink of tea when I get in from work to avoid 'picking' before mealtime; weigh out food quantities at first so that I can see what I am aiming for to be able to lose weight*

The ways other people can help me are:
- List ways that others can help support you in your change attempt. How will you go about getting others' support, *e.g. Ask my partner not to eat snacks in front of me or cook high calorie meals*

I will know that my plan is working if:
- What do you hope will happen as a result of the change?
- What benefits can you expect from the change, *e.g. Lose weight, around 1–2 lbs a week.*

Some things that could interfere with my plan are:
- Anticipate situations or changes that could undermine the plan.
- What could go wrong? How might you stick with the plan despite the changes or setbacks, *e.g. lack of self-control, feeling hungry and tired; could let me have a smaller quantity of the food I am trying to resist or plan what I want to eat beforehand so that I know I can't have the extra nibbles*

Nutrition intervention with populations

National food and nutrition policy

The major causes of mortality and morbidity in the UK are cardiovascular disease, type 2 diabetes, and cancer; all have a strong nutritional aetiology. Both public policy and direct contact with patients present opportunities to reduce risk factors associated with the major non-communicable diseases (poor diet, physical inactivity, smoking, and obesity). Strategies for preventing these diseases are developed at a national and local level in the UK.

Who informs national food and nutrition policy in the UK?

Food Standards Agency (FSA)

Although the FSA is a government agency, it works 'independently' of the government as it does not report to a specific minister. However, it is accountable to parliament via health ministers, and to the devolved administrations of Scotland, Wales, and Northern Ireland for its activities within these areas. Further information, at www.food.gov.uk.

Main roles

- Help people to eat more healthily.
- Promote simple, informative labelling to consumers.
- Reduce food-borne illness by improving food safety throughout the food chain.
- Promote best practice within the food industry.
- Improve the enforcement of food law.

The Scientific Advisory Committee on Nutrition (SACN)

In the past (from 1963 to 2000), the government relied on expert advice on nutrition from COMA (Committee on Medical Aspects of Food and Nutrition Policy), which produced a series of reports that were used to inform nutritional policy.

Since the establishment of the FSA in 2000, the Government has replaced COMA with SACN (www.sacn.gov.uk), which provides independent expertise to the government, primarily through the FSA and the DH. Its remit includes advising on:

- Nutrient content of foods; definition of a balanced diet and nutritional status;
- Nutritional problems that impact on wider public health policy, where nutrition is one of several risk factors, e.g. obesity, cancer, cardiovascular disease, and osteoporosis;
- Nutrition of vulnerable groups, e.g. infants, older people, and disadvantaged groups;
- Nutrition monitoring and surveillance;
- Research needs arising from the above areas.

he Department of Health (DH)

One section of the DH is involved in public health, e.g. the *Choosing health* white paper had a public consultation period before being published by the DH in 2004. In 2005, the Choosing Health delivery plan, *delivering choosing health: making healthy choices easier,* was published, setting out clear objectives in relation to major food policy issues, e.g. possible restrictions on advertising to children, commitment to an obesity awareness campaign, possible signposting on food labels. The interface between the DH and the FSA is sometimes unclear though; for example, both have recently produced infant weaning leaflets (2005).

Other sections of the DH coordinate National Service Frameworks (NSFs) and the National Institute for Health and Clinical Excellence (NICE) provides guidance, e.g. NSFs for CHD, diabetes, children and young people, and maternity services and the forthcoming NICE guidance on obesity prevention and management (due 2007). NICE provides independent guidance on the promotion of good health and the prevention and treatment of ill health (www.nice.org.uk).

What are current governmental public health nutrition policies/strategies in the UK?

argeting the whole population

Since 1990 a series of white papers setting national targets for the prevention of obesity and diet-related disease have been produced by the Department of Health. Starting with *Health of the nation* (1991) → *Saving lives: our healthier nation* (1999) → *Choosing health: making healthier choices easier* (2004).

The most recent national strategy documents are the following:

Choosing Health: making healthier choices easier (DH, 2004). Outlines how health professionals can provide advice on disease prevention and lifestyle advice.

Delivering choosing health: making healthy choices easier (DH, 2005). Sets out clear objectives in relation to major health issues, including those relating to nutrition policy.

Choosing a better diet: a Food and health action plan (DH, 2005). The DH has worked across government, with the food industry, and other stakeholders to establish a national plan to help people in England improve their diets.

Choosing activity: a physical activity action plan (DH, 2005).

The strategy, 'Tackling health inequalities: a programme for action' lays the foundations for meeting the Government's target to reduce the health gap on infant mortality and life expectancy by 2010. *Securing good health for the whole population* 2004, particularly focuses on public health measures and health inequalities.

Front of pack food labelling scheme. The FSA recommends that such a scheme should use red, amber or green color coding to show at a glance whether a food contains high, medium or low levels of fat, saturated fat, sugar, and salt. Nutritional criteria developed by the FSA to determine the color code are proposed. Information on the levels of nutrient should be give per portion of product.

Further information is available at www.dh.gov.uk and www.food.gov.uk

Targeting children

To curb the rising trend in childhood obesity, the national target (set i 2004) is to halt the year on year rise in obesity in children under 11 year by 2010.

The school fruit and vegetable scheme

Under the scheme, all 4–6 year olds in LEA maintained infant, primar and special schools are entitled to a free piece of fruit or vegetable eac school day. It was introduced after the NHS Plan 2000 included commitment to implement a national school fruit scheme by 2004. Th School Fruit and Vegetable Scheme is part of the 5 A DAY programm to increase fruit and vegetable consumption. Further information available at: www.dh.gov.uk/PolicyAndGuidance/HealthAndSocialCar Topics/FiveADay/fs/en; www.5aday.nhs.uk.

Promotion of foods to children: nutrient profiling model

A nutrient profiling model has been developed by the FSA as a tool t help tighten controls relating to the broadcast advertising of foods tha are high in saturated fat, salt, or sugar to children. A stakeholder consu tation assisted the FSA in the development of the model. This model i what is known as a 'simple scoring' system, where points are allocated o the basis of the nutritional content in 100 g of a food or drink.

Further information is available from www.foodstandards.gov.uk healthiereating/nutlab/nutprofmod.

Nutritional standards for school lunches and other school food

The UK Government reintroduced compulsory national nutritiona standards for school lunches in England in April 2001. However, thes standards have been revised. The standards comprise 14 quantitativ nutrient and 9 food-based standards that will be applied to schoc lunches and other school food provision. The standards will b phased in from September 2006 to 2009 and are summarized i Table 15.1 and further information is available from www.dfes.gov.uk consultations/conDetails.cfm?consultationId=1319.

Table 15.1 Summary of nutrient and food standards for school lunches and other school food in England*

Nutrient/food	Recommendation**
Energy	30% of estimated average requirement (EAR)
Protein	≥30% of reference nutrient intake (RNI)
Total carbohydrate	≥50% of food energy
Non-milk extrinsic sugars	≤11% of food energy
Fat	≤35% of food energy
Saturated fat	≤11% of food energy
Fibre	≥30% of the calculated reference value
Sodium	≤30% of the SACN recommendation
Vitamin A	≥40% of the RNI
Vitamin C	≥40% of the RNI
Folate/folic acid	≥40% of the RNI
Calcium	≥40% of the RNI
Iron	≥40% of the RNI
Zinc	≥40% of the RNI
Fruit and vegetables	≥2 portions per day per child, at least one of which should be salad or vegetables, and at least one of which should be fruit
Oily fish	On the school lunch menu at least once every 3 weeks
Deep fried products	Meals should not contain more than two deep fried products in a single week. This includes products that are deep fried when manufactured.
Manufactured meat products	May only be served occasionally.
Bread (without spread)	Available unrestricted throughout lunch
Confectionery and savoury snacks	Not available at school. Only nuts and seeds with no added salt or sugar will be available.
Salt and condiments	Not available at lunch tables
Drinks	The only drinks available should be water (still or fizzy), skimmed or semi-skimmed milk, pure fruit juices, yoghurt and milk drinks <5% added sugar, low calorie hot chocolate, coffee, tea)
Water	Easy access to free, fresh, drinking water

** The figures are for the recommended nutrient content of an average lunch over 5 consecutive school days.
Summary of recommended School meal review panel nutrient and food standards school lunches in England.
* To be phased in from 2008 (primary schools) and 2009 (secondary schools)

The Food in Schools Programme (UK)

The Department for Education and Skills (DFES) and Department O Health (DH) have jointly developed the Food in Schools Programme (FiS) to support the National Healthy Schools Standard, which include tackling rising levels of childhood obesity, as well as proposing means o improving poor diet and lack of activity generally. The programme is developing a whole range of nutrition-related activities and projects in schools to complement and add value to the wide range of other initiatives in schools. The aim is to introduce a programme that follows children throughout the school day, using a whole school approach Further details can be found on www.teachernet.gov.uk/. See example o whole school food policy in 'Examples of nutrition policy in different settings,' this chapter.

Further information: National Food in Schools www.wiredforhealth.gov.uk

National campaigns coordinated by the British Dietetic Association (BDA)

Weight Wise

Weight Wise is a nutrition campaign to increase awareness of the benefits of a balanced and varied diet in achieving and maintaining a healthy weight. It started in June 2002 and each year there will be a focus of activities during the BDA's Food First month (June). Weight Wise is supported by an interactive website www.bdaweightwise.com, which provides free information and support for anyone wanting to reach a healthier weight.

Food First

Overall, the generic aims are:

- To raise the awareness of the importance of diet and health amongst target audiences;
- To promote the delivery of evidence-based nutritional messages to the general public;
- To raise awareness of the role of registered dietitians, their unique skills, and what they can offer to target audiences;
- To develop mutually beneficial partnerships with industry, government bodies, media, other health professional groups
- The BDA and registered dietitians to be seen as a credible and authoritative voice on nutrition, diet, and health.

How is nutritional status monitored in the UK?

Household food consumption surveys

An example is the National Food Survey. In the UK, the National Food Survey (NFS) was established in the 1940s to monitor the diet of the urban 'working class' population during the war years. It was extended to over all households in the general population in the 1950s and to collect data on food expenditure and consumption. For more information see www.statistics.gov.uk/ssd/surveys/national_food_survey.asp.

Individual dietary surveys

The National Diet and Nutrition Survey (NDNS) programme comprises diet surveys for different age groups, also incorporating measurements of weight and height to gather information about the dietary habits and nutritional status of the British population. The NDNS is produced on behalf of the Food Standards Agency (FSA) and the Department of Health (DH) by the Social Survey Division of the Office for National Statistics and Medical Research Council Human Nutrition Research. The results of the survey are used to develop nutrition policy and to contribute to the evidence base for Government advice on healthy eating. Also see Chapter 3.

Surveys are conducted for the following population groups:
Children aged 1½–4½ y;
Young people aged 4–18 y;
Adults aged 19–64 y;
People aged 65 y and over.

Health Survey for England

The Health Survey for England comprises a series of annual surveys beginning in 1991. The series is part of an overall programme of surveys commissioned by the DH and designed to provide regular information on various health topics in England for adults >16 y and children since 1995, including infant feeding practices. Dietary data are qualitative and based on frequency and type of foods consumed with a food record or questionnaire. Weight and height is usually measured, and additionally waist and hip circumference in more recent surveys. For more information see www.dh.gov.uk/PublicationsAndStatistics/PublishedSurvey/HealthSurvey forEngland/fs/en.

Food supply data (to ensure adequacy of national food supplies)

The aims of surveys are to:
Monitor progress towards public health nutrition targets;
Detect nutrient insufficiency;
Identify nutrient excess;
Assess the level of intake of additives/contaminants.

Local food and nutrition policy

Translating government policy into local action

Process of developing national and local food policy

Scientific link between diet and health and disease

⇓

Assessing diet and nutritional status of population

⇓

Development and implementation of national government policies

⇓

Development and implementation of local policies based on national priorities and those of concern locally

Local (regional/city-wide) food and health policies were initiated in th⁣ UK in the early 1980s in response to growing consensus about the ro⁣ of diet in the prevention of disease and by the late 1980s most healt⁣ authorities had their own policy. These usually contained a food safet⁣ component and promoted the nutrition education messages emerging a⁣ that time (less fat, more fibre, and less sugar), primarily in NHS caterin⁣ settings, although some had community activities.

Publication of national public health strategy documents (see 'Nation⁣ Food and nutrition policy', this chapter) stimulated the production ⁣ local health plans from a range of authorities and organizations, whic⁣ widened the focus from NHS settings to multi-sectorial partnership⁣ within the community. This meant that wider perspectives on nutrition⁣ evolved incorporating issues such as food production, biodiversity, an⁣ inequality and food access (see Fig. 15.1). Although the nutrition⁣ messages relating to macronutrients are still relevant, there has been ⁣ shift in focus towards nutritional adequacy. Wider partnerships mean th⁣ the scope for implementation and impact is also much broader.

The Following list expands on the points listed in Fig. 15.1.

1. **Food, health, and nutrition:** to improve the diet of local citizens by providing consistent and appropriate nutrition messages and addressing the potential barriers to achieving a healthier diet.
2. **Food and mental health:** to develop awareness of the emotional and psychological dimensions of food growing and consumption.
3. **Organic production:** to stimulate expansion of production and consumption of local organic food.
4. **Genetically modified food:** to raise awareness about the different perspectives that exist regarding genetically modified organisms.
5. **Food safety:** to reduce the number of cases of food and water borne diseases.
6. **Waste and composting:** to reduce the amount of waste associated with production, consumption, and disposal of food that is sent to landfill or incineration.
7. **Animal welfare:** to promote high standards of animal welfare.

8. *Inequality and food access:* to address issues of social exclusion and ensure people on a low income have access to healthy, affordable food.
9. *Local food:* to increase the local consumption of locally produced food.
0. *Global perspective:* to raise awareness of the effects of the world trade system on small farmers in the developing world.
1. *Food production and biodiversity:* to encourage methods of food production that protects and enhances biodiversity.

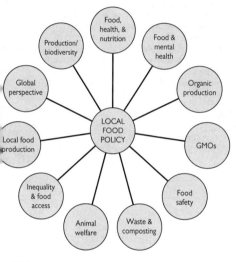

Fig. 15.1 Example of the wide scope of a holistic, sustainable local food policy. (Reproduced with kind permission of the Food Initatives Group, Greater Nottingham.)

The need for local food and nutrition policy

- To provide a political mandate and support for implementation.
- To make available a scientifically accurate document of what constitutes a 'healthy diet' to a wide audience.
- To encourage consistent dietary messages by health professionals and other agencies who have a role in nutrition education.
- To recommend an action plan for implementing the policy in key settings.
- To ensure, by collaboration with other local agencies and employers, that it is easier for citizens to eat a healthy, sustainable diet.
- To use a population-wide approach to try and shift the distribution of risk factors for diet related non-communicable disease.
- To develop strategies that makes healthier behaviour the 'social norm' therefore lowering risk in the whole population.
- To provide nutritional advice for certain groups within the population who have specific nutritional needs, e.g. some hospital patients, children, and older people.
- To facilitate a wider choice of foods in establishments within and outside the NHS, so that a healthier diet can be selected.

Useful websites

www.sustainweb.org

www.groundworkgreaternottingham.org.uk/fig.

www.invo.org.uk (national advisory group funded by the DH aims to promote and support active public involvement in the NHS and health-related local policy development).

Steps in conducting nutrition interventions to promote health

STEP 1 Defining the problem

Needs assessment of nutrition priorities: scale of the problem using epidemiological and sociodemographic information

Analyse possible modifiable determinants, e.g. environmental, behavioural, economic, and social

Identify the main partners from the planning stage

Assess community needs and perceived priorities

Define measurable short and long term nutrition and health goals

⇓

STEP 2 Generating solutions

Aim for inter-sectorial working with a range of stakeholders

Use tacit knowledge (know-how) from practitioners to inform interventions

Review and refer to explicit knowledge sources, i.e. research and evidence based guidelines to build on theoretical principles

Use participatory appraisal methods with the local community to develop sustainable solutions

⇓

STEP 3 Building capacity

Develop an institutional framework in which to act and identify support structures

Determine and mobilize the amount of resources needed: funding, key actors, materials

Training and infrastructure development

Raise public and political awareness

Define the management and operational roles of different partners

⇓

STEP 4 Implementing the intervention

Elaborate an action plan (strategies and activities).

Verify that there are a range of complementary interventions working on:

- *education*, e.g. media, educating patients, school education
- *social mobilization*, e.g. community development, mass communication to influence social, environmental and economic factors that influence health
- *advocacy*, e.g. lobbying for political, organizational, and structural change

Monitor using process measures to help assuring quality in practice, allowing feedback on implementation, participant and practitioner response

⇓

STEP 5 Evaluating if the programme meets its objectives

Health promotion outcomes include: health literacy (knowledge, attitudes & beliefs, self efficacy); social action (community participation, social norms, public opinion); and healthy public and organizational policy (policy statements, legislation, resource allocation and organizational practice)

Intermediate health outcomes include: healthy behaviour (food consumption), healthy environments (urban planning to encourage physical activity), and effective health services (provision of preventive services, access to health services)

Health & social outcomes long-term goals of ↓ morbidity for a group of people, e.g. ↓ obesity, cardiovascular disease, and ↑ quality of life and equity

Case study of a local food and health policy

Case study: Leicestershire food and health plan

The development, implementation, monitoring, and evaluation of a food and nutrition policy within a local health plan in Leicestershire.

Development

To develop an action plan to target people at increased risk of poor nutrition, i.e. lower income groups, minority ethnic groups, and generally increase public awareness of healthier eating. A 'Healthy Eating Group' was established, led by the county's Nutrition and Dietetic Service with membership drawn from a wide range of agencies, i.e. local authorities, universities, school meals service, community health groups, community dental service, public health medicine, health promotion service (physical activity), primary care development, voluntary organizations, occupational health, and environmental health. The group's remit was to develop a public health nutrition strategy by devising a 3-year action plan that would work towards achieving the national public health nutrition targets.

Implementation

The action plan illustrated in Table 15.2 describes how the policy was executed, monitored, and evaluated in a range of settings. This was based on describing current nutrition interventions and prioritizing additional interventions for funding. Further resources were required for many of these activities to be carried out and the priorities for funding were identified and sought within and outside of the local region including the National Lottery. All of the new projects funded had in-built evaluation and none of them could have evolved as they did without working in partnership with several of the agencies represented on the Healthy Eating Group.

Monitoring and evaluation

Methods for monitoring and evaluation were integrated into the implementation strategy (Table 15.2). A combination of quantitative and qualitative research techniques was used to assess programme effectiveness (process, impact, and outcome measures). The evaluation of food policy implementation is based on assessing the effectiveness of interventions in meeting their objectives, e.g. changing attitudes and behaviour, rather than focusing solely on health outcomes relating to disease incidence.

A profile of possible indicators of success and a data collection system that fits into the existing framework of activity were developed. One of the related challenges is how to demonstrate the validity of programmes. It may be that a programme on its own is insufficient but that the 'community of action' is effective in increasing the likelihood of change.

Table 15.2 Example for implementing a local food and nutrition policy for preventing nutrition-related chronic disease by setting and target group

Strategy/action	Partners	Indicators of success
Schools: pupils, teachers, parents, governors		
Fruit in tuck-shops Healthy food awards School nutrition action groups School meals liaison working group School nurse support and training Production of nutrition resources Nutrition in taught curriculum Developing breakfast clubs National School Fruit scheme Cooking skills clubs	• Teachers • Parents • Governors • Pupils • School nurses • Dietitians • Health promotion officers • School meals service • County Council	• ↑ in nutritional quality of school meals using audit • ↑ number of secondary schools with healthy food scheme • ↑ number of schools with nutrition policy • ↑ uptake of healthy choices at breakfast clubs.
General public		
Public exhibitions Healthy food awards Using local media, e.g. radio, TV Availability of healthy food at retail outlets Train local people to work in their communities to promote healthy eating Develop 'cook & eat' sessions Nutrition education in adult leisure classes Support local allotment schemes for fruit and vegetable production Community weight management classes	• Health promotion officers • Health professionals • Dietitians • Public interest • Local media • Environmental health officers • Primary Care Trusts • Community food workers	• Review attendance profile at public exhibitions • ↑ number of healthy food awards in establishments for the public • ↑ media contacts • ↑ availability of healthy food at retail outlets • ↑ number of food workers trained
Workplace: all employees		
Promotion of healthy food awards Weight management groups	• Managers • Dietitians • Environmental health officers • Health promotion officers • Employees • NHS Trusts • Catering managers	• ↑ number of healthy food awards • Evaluating if the scheme changes attitudes and eating habits of target groups
Hospitals: staff and patients, patient groups		
Better hospital food programme Healthy food award for patient and staff meals Support nutritional guidelines in hospital meals	• Dietitians • Catering staff • Hospital management • WRVS	• Audit of nutritional value of delivered meals • Audit of food policy promotion & awareness in hospitals

Strategy/action	Partners	Indicators of success
Primary health care: patients, primary health care teams (PHCTs)		
• Diet sheets and infant feeding policy • Training PHCTs • Production of nutrition resources for patients • Promotion of food policy to patients	• GPs, practice nurses, health visitors, school nurses, district nurses, dietitians, dental practitioners • Primary Care Trusts	• ↑ number of practices working to minimum nutrition standards • ↑ number of trained PHCTs • ↑ nutritional knowledge and practice of PHCTs • ↑ uptake of nutrition resources
Homeless and those living in bed and breakfasts and facilities for the homeless		
• Practical nutrition resources • Nutrition information pack for homes providing meals • Developing nutritional standards for meals provided	• Dietitians • City and Borough Councils • Health promotion officers • Staff at hostels and bed and breakfasts	• ↑ nutritional quality of meals provided • ↑ nutritional knowledge of catering staff and home leaders
Social services & residential homes, e.g. elderly, learning disabilities		
• Food policy for older people • Community mental health team nutrition pack • Lunches at day care centres • Training carers, e.g. Age Concern • Nutrition package to social services/residential homes for healthy food award	• Carers • Dietitians • Social services • Residents • Private home care • Mental health dietitians • Community mental health teams	• ↑ nutritional quality of meals • ↑ nutritional knowledge of carers • ↑ uptake of appropriate nutrition resources • ↑ number of key workers trained • ↑ number of homes applying for healthy food award
Under 5s at day nursery, playgroups, & childminders		
• Nutrition policy for <5s • Training health professionals & nursery staff • Advising on meals at nurseries • Nutrition guidelines for nurseries	• Health visitors • GPs • Midwives • Dietitians • Day nursery staff	• ↑ number of key workers receiving training • ↑ knowledge of workers related to nutrition of <5s • ↑ quality of meals at day nurseries

ips for success in implementing and evaluating local :rategies, e.g. food and nutrition policy, obesity strategy

Good management: a named individual needs to be responsible for coordination.

Clear objectives have to be defined, even though on-going monitoring may mean these evolve and change as the programme develops.

The policy should reflect local priorities and political structures.

Use a population-wide approach to try and shift the distribution of risk factors for diet-related non-communicable disease.

Develop strategies that help make healthier behaviour into the social norm therefore lowering risk in the whole population.

Develop sustainable solutions by combining know-how from practitioners, evidence-based practice, and local community participation.

Use an inter-sectorial approach, as the combined contribution becomes more than the sum of the contributions of individual agencies.

Priorities for funding for new projects should be identified by a multidisciplinary group if they are to represent community needs.

Awareness of the pressures and changes occurring in other organizations that may affect policy implementation is essential.

Identify barriers locally to healthier living and support local action to overcome them.

Link local action to national public health programmes, e.g. five a day, school fruit scheme, 'Choosing health'.

Monitoring techniques need to be realistic and flexible enough to evolve with programmes.

Include means of measuring how effective the intervention is to optimize use of resources and assess the quality of programmes.

Achieve an appropriate balance between expenditure on implementation and evaluation (can be expensive to evaluate).

May be better use of time and resources to carry out in-depth evaluation of key projects/ activities rather than seek to evaluate all activities.

Develop strong links with appropriate university departments to develop the skills for evaluation of ongoing and new work.

Examples of nutrition policy in different settings

Model of a local infant feeding policy for under-5s

The composition of the working party could be as follows.

- Nutrition and dietetic service (especially hospital and community pediatric dietitians working with sick children, community dietitians working with well children).
- Community and hospital pediatricians.
- Health Visitors.
- Community dental health service.
- Midwives.
- Children's hospitals nurses.
- Surestart/Children's Centre representative.
- Representative of local council responsible for nursery schools.
- Community/voluntary groups, e.g. National Childbirth Trust, parent groups.

Suggested topics for a joint local community–hospital based infant feeding policy could be the following.

1. Feeding policy aims.
2. Applying healthy eating guidance to this age group after 2 years.
3. Breastfeeding: diet, drug use, tips.
4. Infant formula milks: types, preparation.
5. Other drinks: goat, sheep, cows, soya milk, juice, bottled/tap water (see 'Weaning' in Chapter 10 for advice on suitability).
6. Weaning: practical guidelines for first year of life.
7. Vitamin and mineral supplements: during pregnancy and lactation, in infancy.
8. Special dietary considerations.
    - Religious and ethnic groups.
    - Vegetarians and vegans.
    - Food allergy and food intolerance.
    - Diarrhoea and constipation.
    - Iron deficiency anaemia.
    - Faltering growth.
9. Faddy eaters and behavioural management.
10. Food safety.
11. Action plans for implementation.
    - Training programme for key staff.
    - Applying guidelines to food provided in nursery schools/units.
12. Regular monitoring and evaluation, e.g. annual updates to infant feeding practice and 5 yearly review.
13. Appendices: tables with growth charts, dietary reference values, and key contacts.

See Chapter 10.

Model of a local school food policy

Suggested topics for a model school food policy incorporating a 'whole school approach' could be the following.[1]

1. Food policy aims.
2. Equal opportunities.
   • Strive to provide equal access of opportunity for all.
3. Curriculum opportunities.
   • Leading by example and staff training.
   • Visitors in the classroom.
   • Resources for teaching.
   • Evaluation of pupils' learning.
4. Food and drink provision throughout the school day.
   • Breakfast.
   • Food & nutrient based standards for school lunches and school food.
   • School fruit scheme (if applicable).
   • Tuck-shop (if applicable).
   • Vending machines (if applicable).
   • Out of hours learning.
   • Use of food as a reward.
   • Drinking water provision.
5. Food and drink brought into school.
   • Snacking.
   • Mobile caterers serving food on school premises.
   • Packed lunches brought to school by pupils.
6. Growing food.
   • Opportunity to see food growing.
   • Discuss where food is produced.
   • Importance of fruit and vegetables as part of a healthy diet.
7. Special diets.
   • Religious and ethnic groups.
   • Vegetarians and vegans.
   • Food allergy and food intolerance.
8. Food safety.
9. Action plans for implementation.
10. Regular monitoring and evaluation, e.g. annual survey of the views of teachers, pupils, and parents about the school eating environment.

NB. Implementation of the government report *Turning the tables: transforming school food—recommendations for the development and implementation of revised school lunch standards* (2005) means all schools will need to develop a food policy.

Further information is available at www.wiredforhealth.gov.uk. Also see Chapter 11.

Adapted from the School Food Action Group, Greater Nottingham Food Initiatives Group.

Policy options for preventing obesity

It is widely recognized that preventing obesity requires more than health or medical perspective; it needs to be viewed from a wider societal and economic context that involves partnership working on a population wide basis, as obesity touches all of society.

There are a wealth of potential environmental strategies for the prevention of obesity, as highlighted in the World Health Organization *Global strategy on diet, physical activity and health* (WHO, 2004, www.who.int/dietphysicalactivity/en/). Developing strategies that will involve structural or environmental change will require the participation of a range of key stakeholders, for example:

- Governmental (departments of: health; nutrition; food; food and agriculture; transport; education; family and social care; advertising control);
- Food production system (producers; farmers; unions; food industry representatives; large retailers: supermarkets; small retailers; catering);
- Health systems (pharmaceutical industry; general practitioners; specialist medics; dietitians; nutritionists; nurses; health promotion specialists);
- Media (advertisers; newspapers; TV and radio; female press);
- Education system (pre-school care; schools and colleges; universities);
- Workplace (unions; large vs small institutions);
- Non-governmental organizations (consumer associations; marginal group associations; low income associations; family groups);
- Local communities.

Possible policy options for obesity prevention

Laws and regulations

Mandatory nutritional information labelling for energy-dense food.
Controls on the advertising and promotion of food and drink products, particularly to children.
Agricultural policy reform to encourage production of cheaper fruit and vegetables.
Incentives to improve nutrient composition of processed food products.

Transport policies and town planning

Provide improved facilities for walking and cycling.
Improve conditions for pedestrian travel to school.
Plan for the use of streets as social spaces rather than just for cars.
Improve public transport.

Economic incentives

Tax changes to alter patterns of food consumption, and to reduce consumption of energy-dense foods.
Public subsidies on healthy foods to improve patterns of food consumption.
Reduce car tax for those who use public transport during the week.

Food and catering standards

Develop nutrition standards and guidelines for institutional catering services, e.g. school meals, workplaces, prisons.

Food production

Encourage use of land in urban areas for growing fruit and vegetables for use by households, e.g. allotments.

Promotion of healthier behaviours

Improve training for health professionals in obesity prevention and diagnosing and counselling those at risk of obesity.
Use the media to promote positive behaviour.
Educate the public about the main causes of obesity so that stigmatization of the obese is reduced.
Raise awareness in the general public about the need for collective action to improve the environment to one that encourages rather than discourages healthy behaviour.

Schools

Encourage training in practical food skills for children.
Ensure provision of healthy, tasty school meals.

Model for a local obesity strategy

Sample strategy for a 'health community' for the prevention and management of obesity

An example of the composition of working party:
- Nutrition & dietetic service: community and hospital;
- Consultant diabetologist and/or diabetes specialist nurse;
- General practitioner;
- Health visitors;
- Health promotion officers specializing in health behaviour;
- Public health specialist;
- Practice nurse;
- Consultant surgeon;
- Pharmaceutical advisor;
- Cardiac rehabilitation nurse;
- Consultant psychiatrist;
- Local authority representatives.

Suggested areas to include in the strategy could be the following.
1. Background: obesity as a health problem nationally and locally; related strategies locally; defining at risk groups locally.
2. Evidence base: models of obesity prevention and management.
3. National and local strategic direction.
4. Aims/objectives of obesity strategy.
   - Primary health care.
   - Wider community.
   - Secondary care.
   - Partnership approaches.
5. Framework for obesity prevention and care pathway for management of overweight and obesity.
6. Action plans for implementation.
   - Training programme for key staff.
   - Timescale.
   - Key areas for action.
7. Regular monitoring and evaluation of key aspects.

NICE guidance on obesity prevention and management is planned for 2007.

Further information
1. IOTF : www.iotf.org/
2. WHO: www.who.int/dietphysicalactivity/en/)
3. EU: Diet, Physical Activity and Health—EU Platform for Action: www.europa.eu.int/com health/ph_determinants/life_style/nutrition/platform/platform_en.htm.
4. Jain, A. (2004). Fighting obesity: evidence of effectiveness will be needed to sustain polic Br. Med. J. **328**, 1327–8.
5. Kumanyika, S., et al. (2002). Obesity prevention: the case for action. Int.J.Obes.Relaf.Met Disord. **26**, 425–36.

Definitions in health promotion

Nutrition intervention programmes draw on health promotion technique. **Health promotion** is almost always concerned with change and has bee defined by the WHO as a process enabling people to exert control ove and improve their health, whilst recognizing that the shaping of a health environment contributes to improving health status. Health is a positiv concept emphasizing social and personal resources, as well as physica capacities. Therefore, health promotion is not just the responsibility c the health sector, but goes beyond healthy behaviour to well-being Participation is essential to sustain health promotion action. The Firs International Conference on Health Promotion was held in Ottawa Canada, in 1986, producing what is now widely known as the Ottawa Charter for Health Promotion.

The Ottawa Charter (1986) identified 3 basic strategies for health promotion.
- **Advocacy** for health to create the essential conditions for health.
- **Enabling** all people to achieve their full health potential.
- **Mediating** between the different interests in society in the pursuit of health.

These strategies are supported by five priority action areas as outlined ir the Ottawa Charter.
- Build healthy public policy.
- Create supportive environments for health.
- Strengthen community action for health.
- Develop personal skills.
- Re-orient health services.

This was taken a step further at the Fourth International Conference or Health Promotion, which was held in Jakarta, Indonesia, in 1997. The Jakarta Declaration on *Leading health promotion into the 21st century* confirmed that these strategies and action areas are relevant for all countries. Comprehensive approaches to health development are the most effective. Those that use combinations of the above 5 strategies are more effective than single-track approaches. It identified five priorities.
- Promote social responsibility for health.
- Increase investments for health development.
- Expand partnerships for health promotion.
- Increase community capacity and empower the individual.
- Secure an infrastructure for health promotion.

Health education is not only concerned with the communication of information, but also with fostering the motivation, skills, and self-efficacy necessary to take action to improve health. Health education includes the communication of information concerning the underlying social, economic, and environmental conditions impacting on health, as well as individual risk factors and risk behaviours, and use of the health-care system. Thus, health education may involve the communication of infor- mation, and development of skills that demonstrate the political feasibility and organizational possibilities of various forms of action to address social, economic, and environmental determinants of health.

Qualitative and quantitative methods for evaluation health education

Basic experimental design and particularly a randomized control design, is well established as the ideal method for evaluation. In the field, it is not always possible to meet the basic criteria for such an experimental design, and doing so can reduce programmes to unreal 'sterile' interventions that are not appropriate to real life situations.

Using multiple methods in health promotion evaluation improves the power of the evaluation and the validity of the conclusions.

A distinction is often made between qualitative and quantitative approaches to evaluation.

Quantitative research examines patterns of behaviour or attitudes by assessing how certain factors influence the expression of these patterns. Particularly useful to estimate net effects of programmes, e.g. whether dietary changes can be attributed to the intervention.

Qualitative methods attempt to determine the meaning and experience of the programme for those involved and to interpret the effects that may have been observed. Particularly useful for measuring the process.

Further information

Naidoo, J. and Wills, J. (2000). *Health promotion: foundations for practice*, 2nd edn. Baillière Tindall, London.

Thorgood, M., and Coombes, Y. (2000). *Evaluating health promotion: practice and methods*, 2nd edn. Oxford University Press, Oxford.

Society of Health Education and Health Promotion Specialists. www.hj-web.co.uk/sheps/

WHO Noncommunicable Disease Prevention and Health Promotion www.who.int/hpr/support.material.shtml.

Nutrition support

Nutrition in the 'non-healthy state'

Whilst it is generally accepted that a healthy, well-balanced diet shoul be based on a low fat, high unrefined carbohydrate diet and include minimum of 5 portions of fruit or vegetables per day ('Balance of Goo Health in 'Food-based dietary guidelines', Chapter 2), some individua who are unwell may require an intake that is higher or, conversel restricted in certain nutrients.

It is ∴ inappropriate to promote a low fat, high carbohydrate diet or portions of fruit or vegetables per day to *some* groups of people whic may include those with:

- poor intake;
- loss of appetite;
- unintentional weight loss;
- infectious disease;
- acute and chronic illness;
- disorders of the gastrointestinal tract, kidney, or liver;
- injuries.

The next part of this book discusses how nutritional intake should b modified in situations of ill health. By its nature, the information given is brief overview and in many cases the reader would be well advised t seek specific advice for individual cases from a registered dietitian.

Nutritional screening

This is routinely undertaken to identify individuals within a population who are at risk from under- or over-nutrition. It differs from nutritional assessment, which is undertaken by a nutrition-trained health-care professional, usually a registered dietitian, and which gives a more detailed nutritional profile of an individual.

The screening procedure should be:
• rapid;
• simple;
• acceptable to patients;
• undertaken at first contact (or soon after);
• carried out by nursing, medical, or other staff;
• provide an outcome that links to an action plan;
• repeated at intervals.

Many different nutritional screening tools are available. The tool of choice should:
• be appropriate for the patient population;
• have validity confirmed by peer reviewed publication;
• have suitable cut-off points to maximize sensitivity and specificity (minimizing false positive and false negative results);
• provide outcomes that can be acted on when appropriate (link to care plans);
• reflect local needs and overcome resistance to implementation;
• be associated with a staff training programme.

Malnutrition universal screening tool (MUST)

The MUST, developed by the multidisciplinary British Association f Parenteral and Enteral Nutrition (BAPEN), is considered the most scie tifically robust, practical, and versatile nutritional screening tool. It h been designed for use:

- in different care settings including:
  - hospital inpatients and outpatients;
  - care homes;
  - GP surgeries and health centres;
  - community.
- with different groups of adult patients:
  - elderly;
  - surgical;
  - medical;
  - orthopaedic;
  - those requiring intensive care;
  - mental health care;
  - pregnancy and lactation (with adaptation).
- by different health-care professionals:
  - nurses;
  - doctors;
  - dietitians;
  - health-care assistants;
  - students.
- to detect
  - undernutriton (malnutrition);
  - overnutrition (overweight/obesity).

Surrogate measures for height

Where height cannot be measured a surrogate measure can be used, e ulnar length, knee height, or demi-span. Ulnar length is the easiest obtain in bed-bound patients.

- The forearm is placed diagonally across the chest with fingers pointing towards the shoulder and palm inwards.
- The distance is measured between the central and most prominent part of the styloid process (bony knobble on outer wrist, little finger side) and the centre tip of the olecranon process (elbow). See Fig. 16.1.
- Estimated height ($_e$Ht) is calculated:
  - Men <65 y: $_e$Ht (cm) = 79.2 + 3.60 × ulnar length (cm).
  - Men ≥65 y: $_e$Ht (cm) = 86.3 + 3.15 × ulnar length (cm).
  - Women <65 y: $_e$Ht (cm) = 95.6 + 2.77 × ulnar length (cm).
  - Women ≥65 y: $_e$Ht (cm) = 80.4 + 3.25 × ulnar length (cm).

The five MUST steps

1	Calculate body mass index (BMI) from weight and height (see 'Anthropometry' in Chapter 4)	
	BMI >20	= 0 (>30 = obese)
	18.5–0	= 1
	<18.5	= 2
2	Determine unplanned weight loss (%) in past 3–6 months.	
	<5%	= 0
	5–0%	= 1
	>10%	= 2
3	Consider the effect of acute disease	
	If patient is acutely ill and there has been or is likely to have been no nutritional intake for >5 days, score 2	
4	Add scores from 1, 2 & 3 together to give overall risk of malnutrition.	
	Total score	= 0–low risk
		= 1–medium risk
		≥2–high risk
5	Initiate appropriate nutritional management.	
	Using local management guidelines, prepare appropriate care plan	

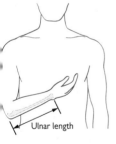

Ulnar length

Fig 16.1 Measurement of ulnar length.

MUST nutritional management guidelines

Low risk—routine clinical care Repeat screening (hospital, weekly; care home, monthly; community, annually for special groups, e.g. those >75 years).

Medium risk—observe Document dietary intake for 3 days if subject in hospital or care home. If improved or adequate intake, little clinical concern; if no improvement, clinical concern: follow local policy.

Repeat screening (hospital, weekly; care home, at least monthly; community, at least every 2–3 months.)

High risk—treat[1] Refer to dietitian, nutritional support team or implement local policy.

Improve and increase overall nutritional intake.

Monitor and review care plan (hospital, weekly; care home, monthly; community, monthly).

Further information

MUST charts, guidelines, and explanatory booklet can be downloaded from http://www.bapen.org.uk/the-must.htm.

---

[1] Unless detrimental or no benefit is expected from nutritional support, e.g. imminent death. In obese patients, underlying acute conditions are generally treated before the treatment of obesity.

Undernutrition

Undernutrition (often referred to as malnutrition) arises as a conse quence of an inadequate intake of energy and macronutrients. In som individuals it may also be associated with frank or subclinical micronutri ent deficiencies.

Classification

There is no single, universally accepted definition or classification c undernutrition although a pattern of < optimum body weight or loss c body weight is the main feature.

Body mass index (BMI)   Cut-off values between 18.5 and 20.0 kg/m^2 ar most often used to identify risk of undernutrition in adults (Table 16.1 However, the use of BMI has its limitations. It cannot be used in childre where height may be stunted as a result of poor nutrition, in the ver elderly where a true height may be difficult to measure, or where unusua body morphology invalidates the ratio of weight to height.

$$BMI = weight (kg)/height^2 (m^2)$$

See 'Anthropometry', Chapter 4 and inside front cover.

Mid–upper arm circumference (MUAC)   Can be used if BMI cannot b calculated due to the absence of an accurate height measurement c because true weight is obscured by fluid retention (Table 16.2). (Se 'Anthropometry', Chapter 4).

Standard deviation score (Z-score)   Calculated from reference popula tion data and used to determine risk of undernutrition in children (Tabl 16.3). No values for height are required and it is independent of ag making it useful in field situations.

$$Z\text{-score} = (patient's weight - median weight for population)/SD$$
$$value for population$$

See 'Anthropometry', Chapter 4.

✒ Malnourished patients are not always thin. They may be overweight o obese but have suffered recent, unplanned weight loss.

✒ Classifying undernutrition is concerned with establishing risk. None c the methods described above are foolproof but they do provide simpl and reproducible means of undertaking this. The consequences of failin to identify and treat undernutrition are potentially serious and ∴ cautio should be used when interpreting results. (For routine nutritional screen ing see 'Malnutrition Universal Screening Tool', this chapter).

Prevalence

The prevalence of undernutrition varies with the population, age grou presence and severity of disease, health, care setting, and the metho used to identify undernutrition. Values cited frequently include:

• 10% of individuals with cancer or chronic disease living in the community
• up to 50% of individuals living in care homes;
• 40–70% of patients admitted to hospital.

These figures show that undernutrition is not a rare event and so health care staff working in all settings should be aware of this and the need t instigate and implement screening, prevention, and treatment policies.

Table 16.1 Categories of BMI for identifying undernutrition in adults

BMI (kg/m^2) (WHO Classification)	Interpretation
≤18.5 (underweight)	Chronic undernutrition probable
18.5–24.9 (health/ normal weight)	
18.5–20	Chronic undernutrition possible
20–24.9	Chronic undernutrition unlikely (low risk)

Table 16.2 Classification of undernutrition in adults using MUAC*

MUAC (cm)	Classification
Males	
≥23	Low risk of undernutrition
<23	Risk of undernutrition
Females	
≥22	Low risk of undernutrition
<22	Risk of undernutrition

* Adapted from *Human Nutrition and Dietetics*. Golden, MNH. and Golden, BE. Severe In, Garrow, JS James, WPT, and. Ralph A Copyright (2000) with permission from Elsevier.

Table 16.3 Classification of undernutrition in adults and children using Z-scores*

Z-score	Type and degree of undernutrition (ICD code)
–1 to +1	No undernutrition
–1 to –2	Mild undernutrition (E44.0)
–2 to –3	Moderate undernutrition (E44.1)
<–3	Severe undernutrition (E43)

* Adapted from Stratton R. J., Green, C.J., and Elia, M. (2003). *Disease-related malnutrition*: Reproduced with permission CABI publishing.

Contributing causes

In most cases, the causes of undernutrition are multifactorial (Fig. 16.2) but an awareness of some specific contributory factors is a valuable first step in prevention. The following is just a brief summary.

Reduced nutritional intake

- Inadequate food availability (quantitative or qualitative):
  - patients nursed in isolation or where meal trays cannot be reached;
  - repeated deliberate starvation, e.g. nil by mouth for multiple tests or treatment;
  - slow motor coordination requiring feeding assistance;
  - culturally inappropriate meals, e.g. providing non-halal or non-kosher food for Muslims or Jews (see 'Minority ethnic communities', Chapter 13).
  - poor quality or unappetizing food.
- Anorexia (loss of appetite):
  - effects of disease, e.g. cancer, infection, inflammation;
  - nausea and vomiting;
  - psychological issues, e.g. depression, anxiety, loneliness;
  - effects of treatment, e.g. chemotherapy.
- Eating problems:
  - poor dentition;
  - changes in taste and smell;
  - dry or painful mouth;
  - breathlessness;
  - disordered swallowing.

Reduced nutrient absorption

- Insufficient GI secretions, including bile and all digestive enzymes, e.g. lack of pancreatic enzymes.
- Damage to absorptive GI surface, e.g. Crohn's disease.
- Gastrointestinal resection ± fistulae.
- Complication of drug therapy.

Increased requirements

- Disease-related hypermetabolism, e.g. liver cirrhosis, some cancers.
- Infection.
- Treatment-related, e.g. post-surgery.
- ↑ Losses, e.g. via GI tract, urine, skin, breath, or drains.
- ↑ Activity, voluntary and involuntary, e.g. Parkinson's disease.

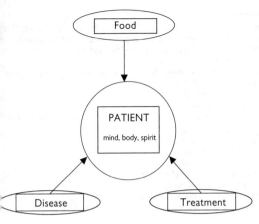

Fig. 16.2 To identify key causative factors of undernutrition, a holistic view of the patient is required.

Consequences

The effects of undernutrition vary from subclinical with no apparent clinical impairment to death, and are dependent on the type, length, and degree of nutritional inadequacy and the age and nutritional and health status of the individual.

Survival in the total abstinence from all nutrient intake (water only) is:
- ~55–75 days in lean adults;
- ~32 days newborn infant;
- ~5 days pre-term infant.

In addition to a significant ↑ risk of mortality, undernutrition is associated with greater morbidity:
- Weight loss (predominantly fat and muscle).
- Impaired muscle function:
  - skeletal muscle—poor mobility, ↑ risk of falls;
  - respiratory—↑ risk of chest infection, ↓ reduced exercise capacity, delayed ventilator weaning;
  - cardiac—bradycardia, hypotension, ↓ cardiac output;
  - GI tract—↓ gut wall integrity increasing potential for micro-organism access.
- Reduced immune function:
  - ↓ phagocytosis, ↓ chemotaxis, ↓ intracellular bacterial destruction, ↓ T lymphocytes;
  - ↑ rates of infection;
  - poor response to vaccination.
- Impaired synthesis of new protein:
  - poor wound healing, ↑ risk of ulceration;
  - delayed recovery from surgery;
  - growth faltering or cessation in children;
  - ↓ fertility in women and men.
- Psychological impairment:
  - depression, anorexia, ↓ motivation;
  - ↓ quality of life;
  - intellectual impairment if malnourished in infancy.
- Increased economic cost:
  - ↑ complications;
  - ↑ length of stay in hospital and intensive care unit;
  - ↑ re-admission rates following discharge;
  - longer rehabilitation;
  - ↑ pharmaceutical cost;
  - ↑ visits to GP.

Treatment of undernutrition

Why bother treating undernourished patients? There is good evidence that nutritional support can increase energy and protein intake, improve body weight and attenuate weight loss, improve functional outcomes (muscle strength, walking distances, activity levels, mental health) and clinical outcomes (mortality, complications, length of hospital stay) in both hospital and community settings.

Pathway of nutrition support for undernourished patients

The following numbered sections correspond to the numbered stages in the algorithm in Fig. 16.3.

1 Assessment

On diagnosis of undernutrition, a full nutritional assessment should be undertaken by a dietitian to identify contributing causes (see 'Undernutrition', this chapter) and provide a basis for treatment.

After assessment, the following steps can be taken. Although they are suggested in a sequential path, it may be appropriate to undertake a number simultaneously and utilize points that are relevant to the individual being treated.

2 Food access

After assessment, it may become apparent that some relatively simple, non-technical measures are needed to help the undernourished individual access suitable food. Examples:
- arranging support through appropriate carers, e.g. shopping, cooking, company whilst eating;
- locating/repairing dentures;
- providing appropriate cutlery, dishes, utensils, etc. Seek expertise from occupational therapy;
- modifying texture of foods provided (see 'Texture modification' in 'Cerebrovascular accident/stroke', Chapter 19);
- requesting suitable meals, e.g. vegetarian, halal, kosher see Chapter 13).

3 Supplementation using food

The modification and/or supplementation of food and drink using ordinary food items can substantially increase energy and nutrient intake in many patients. This is a relatively straightforward step and should be a tried before more complex interventions are initiated. The patient's nutritional status must be monitored regularly. Examples:
- ensuring three or four meals each day;
- offering nutritious snacks between meals, e.g. small sandwiches, cheese and biscuits, yogurt;
- limiting drinks or foods that provide little energy or nutrients, e.g. low calorie drinks, salads, clear soups;
- replacing all low fat items with higher fat alternatives (e.g. full cream milk);
- increasing energy/protein density of meals and drinks by fortifying, e.g. adding butter, margarine, olive oil, grated cheese to mashed potato or savoury sauces or adding sugar, honey, jam, milk powder, cream to desserts, milky drinks, etc.;

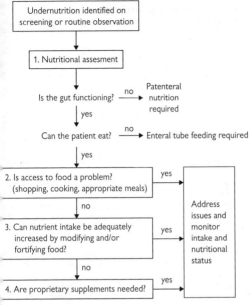

Fig. 16.3 Algorithm showing pathway of nutrition support for undernourished patients.

- 'treats' like cake, biscuits, chocolate, crisps, etc. can provide valuable additional calories but should not replace meals providing protein and range of other nutrients;
- Alcohol, as an aperitif or added to milky drinks, can stimulate the appetite and provide some extra energy.

Advantages include flexibility, palatability, the non-medicalization of eating, and lower cost. Success depends on the patient being able to consume enough food and a dedicated team of carers and/or health professionals.

Disadvantages include the requirement of a high level of motivation and effort ± culinary skill in patient, carers, and health professionals, the limited availability of appropriate ingredients in institutional food production, the difficulty in measuring ↑ intake, and potential need for additional micronutrient supplementation.

4 Supplementation using proprietary oral nutrition supplements

Many ready-to-use oral nutrition supplements, often called sip feeds, are available that can contribute to a nutritionally well-balanced intake. These may be used in conjunction with the food fortification described above or used to make up a deficit if an individual cannot eat sufficient food. Some products are prescribable for patients who are undernourished (Table 16.4; see also 'Prescription of nutritional products', Chapter 8).

Table 16.4 Examples of proprietary oral nutrition supplements available on prescription:

Type	Brand name (manufacturer)
Milk-based drinks	Fresubin Original (Fresenius Kabi)
	Resource Shake (Novartis Consumer Health)
Juice-based drinks	Enlive (Abbott)
	Fortijuice (Nutricia Clinical)
Savoury drinks	Ensure chicken, mushroom, asparagus (Abbott)
	Vitasavoury (Vitaflo)
Desserts	Clinutren Dessert (Nestlé)
	Forticreme (Nutricia Clinical)

These products can also be bought without a prescription but are relatively expensive. Non-prescribable powdered supplements, which need to be mixed with milk or water, provide comparable nutrition and are a cheaper alternative and easier to transport, e.g. Build Up (Nestlé UK), Complan (Complan Foods).

Advantages include known composition, most provide well-balanced intake of energy, macro- and micro-nutrients, availability of ready-to-use form requiring little or no preparation, range of products and flavours, no cost to patient if prescribed.

Disadvantages include the 'quick fix' of readily dispensed products without full evaluation of patient's needs, flavour-fatigue after prolonged use, prescribing cost, medicalization of nutritional intake may further discourage eating, and (ready-to-use only) bulky/heavy and require storage space for patients at home.

Next step

If an undernourished patient is unable to achieve an adequate intake orally using the above suggestions and is considered to need additional support, feeding artificially via the gut see 'Enteral feeding', this chapter or directly into the blood (see 'Parenteral nutrition', this chapter) will be required.

Enteral feeding: introduction

'Enteral' refers to the gastrointestinal tract so theoretically, 'enteral feeding' encompasses all nutrition assimilated via the gut, including eating and drinking. However, in clinical practice the term is often used to describe the administration of nutritional feed into the gut through a tube including via nasogastric, nasojejunal, gastrostomy, and jejunostomy routes. Wherever possible, nutrition should be provided by enteral feeding.

Advantages of enteral over intravenous feeding

- More physiological
- Absorbed nutrients transported via portal circulation directly to liver to support synthesis and metabolic regulation
- Promotes integrity of gastrointestinal tract mucosa
- Reduces bacterial translocation, e.g. bacteria migrating from gut lumen into circulation, so associated with lower risk of sepsis and multiorgan failure
- Stimulates gall bladder emptying so reducing risk of gallstone formation
- Provides (usually) all dietary constituents including some conditionally essential, e.g. glutamine, which may not be added to intravenous formulae
- Provides (usually) dietary fibre which stimulates colonocytes and short chain fatty acid production, optimizing bowel function
- Microbiologically safer than intravenous feeding
- Avoids complications associated with intravenous access including pneumothorax, catheter embolism, etc.
- Cheaper
- Easier (usually) for staff, carers, and patients to manage

Most complications associated with enteral feeding, e.g. diarrhoea, tube dislodgement, can be overcome ± managed by experienced administration and following correct clinical procedures (see 'Complication of enteral feeding', this chapter).

In order to undertake enteral feeding, the patient must have some gastrointestinal tract function. ❶ Absolute contraindications include:
- obstruction;
- prolonged ileus;
- severe gastrointestinal tract bleeding (while bleeding is active and patient is haemodynamically unstable).

The enteral routes available are described in the following section.

Routes for enteral feeding

Nasogastric (NG) feeding

Why feed via the nose ?
- Nutrients can be delivered into the gut more easily through a tube passed via the nose, rather than by mouth, because the tube can be fixed more securely and is less likely to dislodge.
- A nasal tube is less likely to disturb eating, if the patient is able and so will help facilitate transfer back on to oral nutrition.

NG feeding is indicated when:
- the patient is unable to take sufficient nutrition orally, e.g. severe anorexia, dysphagia, mouth/jaw injury;
- nutrition support is predicted to be required for <14–28 days;
- nutrition support likely to be required for >28 days but gastrostomy contraindicated.

Tubes and placement

- Fine bore tubes (French gauge 6–9) should be used in preference. Wide bore tubes or 'Ryles' tubes (French gauge 10–18) are associated with ↑ complications, e.g. nasal/oesophageal ulceration and ↓ patient comfort.
- External tube diameter (Table 16.5) is important for patient comfort; internal diameter influences the flow of feed but varies for a given French gauge—contact tube suppliers for details.
- Tube should be passed via nose with the help of integral guide wire (do not re-insert once removed); if possible, ask the patient to sit rather than lie during insertion; swallowing sips of iced water as tube is inserted helps (providing patient is safe to do so, see 'in 'Cerebro-vascular accident/stroke' in Chapter 19); a confident, trained and practised operator minimizes placement stress.
- Correct placement should be confirmed.
  - Check aspirate using pH sticks or paper (not litmus); pH<5 is indicative of gastric placement in adults.
  - X-ray is not 1st choice but can be used.
  - Injection of air and auscultation is no longer recommended.
  Also see 'Enteral feeding regimes', this chapter.

Nasojejunal (NJ) feeding

NJ feeding enables nutrition to be infused into the gut distally to the pyloric sphincter.
Advantages:
- reduces risk of aspirating feed due to gastroparesis;
- facilitates early post-operative feeding.
Disadvantages:
- placement of tube is more difficult;
- tube may migrate into stomach.

Table 16.5 External diameters corresponding to different French gauges

French gauge	External diameter (mm)	French gauge	External Diameter (mm)
5	1.7	14	4.7
6	2.0	16	5.3
8	2.7	18	6.0
10	3.3	22	7.3
12	4.0	24	8.0

ubes and placement

Fine bore tubes of adequate length (100–120 cm) are required.

Double or triple lumen tubes are available to facilitate simultaneous feeding (postpylorus), aspiration (gastric) ± pressure regulation.

To ensure placement in the jejunum, NJ tubes usually require endoscopic insertion or guidance radiologically or by gastric ECG. Placement beyond the ligament of Treitz, i.e. distal section, will reduce migration into stomach.

For unguided placement, spiral-ended tubes have a higher rate of postpyloric placement than straight-ended tubes.

Correct placement may be obvious, depending on the insertion technique; pH of jejunal aspirate should be alkaline.

ystematic review found no advantages to providing enteral feed postylorically compared to gastrically and found that the difficulty in tube lacement may lead to a delay in the initiation of feeding.[1] The NJ route hould be the first choice only for patients who require short-term nteral feeding when their NG route is precluded.

Also see 'Enteral feeding regimes', this chapter.

Marik, **P.E.** and Zaloga, G.P. (2003). Gastric versus post-pyloric feeding a systematic review. *Crit. are* **7**, R46–R51.

Gastrostomy feeding

A feeding gastrostomy is an artificial route made between the stomac and outside the body. Although this can be made surgically if the patien is undergoing an upper abdominal operation, it is most commonl inserted endoscopically or radiologically.

Percutaneous endoscopic gastrostomy (PEG)

Indication:

- Patients requiring enteral nutrition support >14–28 days. Insertion is minimally invasive and ↑ comfort than an NG tube.

Contraindications:

- Pharyngeal/oesophageal tumour (depending on tumour position).
- Portal hypertension.
- Peritoneal dialysis.
- Coagulopathy.

Advantages

- ↓ Inadvertent removal of tube so fewer disruptions to feeding.
- ↓ Reflux and aspiration of feed (as tube cannot migrate into the oesophagus) so overnight feeding may be safer.
- Cosmetically more appealing, especially for patients who are 'out and about'.
- Discreet fixation devices are available that facilitate tube detachment and are more practical for active patients, especially children.
- Easily removed when no longer needed, either endoscopically or by cutting (internal fixation device passes out through GI tract).

Complications

- Tube blockage (see 'Complications of enteral feeding', this chapter).
- Tube displacement. Reasonable care is needed to avoid inadvertently removing PEG. Those held by an internal balloon device may dislodge if balloon deflates—this should be checked weekly[2] by withdrawing and replacing water within. If the tube is inadvertently removed, the tract will remain patent for ~48 h and a temporary Foley catheter can be inserted until the PEG is replaced.
- Peristomal infection/abscess. This can be ↓ by giving prophylactic antibiotics at insertion and undertaking good clinical practice, e.g. bathe, dry carefully, watch for redness.
- 'Buried bumper syndrome'. This may occur if the internal fixation plate becomes buried within the abdominal wall due to overgrowth. This can be prevented by releasing the tube and rotating it by 360° every week[2]. PEGs held by an internal balloon are not prone to 'buried bumper syndrome' ∴ do not need to be rotated.
- Feed aspiration leading to pneumonia. Regular patient monitoring is required, especially in more vulnerable patients.

---

[2] Or follow local guidance.

Practicalities

PEGs can be inserted as a day-care procedure providing appropriate aftercare is available. Patients remain nil enterally for 4 h, then 50 ml sterile water is infused for 4 h, then commence feed (see 'Enteral feeding regimes', this chapter). Ongoing supplies of feed and consumable items, 'plastics', required for delivery and PEG care need to be organized for patients in the community along with education for them and their carers about how to manage feeding with maximum care and minimum stress.

The most common diagnosis for PEG insertion in adults in the UK is cerebrovascular accident, particularly in patients aged >64 years. A high mortality rate in first 30 days after insertion has been reported; this is likely to reflect the patient population rather than PEG-related complications but it is a reminder that the decision to insert a PEG should be taken holistically and consider *all* aspects of the patient's care and prognosis.

Other types of gastrostomy

- A percutaneous radiological gastrostomy (PRG; radiologically inserted gastrostomy, RIG) may be inserted under X-ray guidance and is more suitable for patients with compromised ventilation if endoscopy sedation is undesirable.
  - Insertion success rate is > PEGs.
  - Longevity of tubes < PEGs (need to plan replacements).
  - Associated with some post-procedural pain.
  - Different after care to PEGs: all except pig-tail type require daily 360° rotation (or follow local guidance).
- A surgical gastrostomy may be placed if an endoscopic insertion is not possible and the patient is undergoing surgery for other reasons. Complications include haemorrhage, skin excoriation from leaking gastric fluid, wound dehiscence, and intraperitoneal leakage of gastric contents.

🅞 Patients with a gastrostomy may be hospital inpatients but many manage their own nutrition in the community, either alone or with the help of carers. Advice on management of both feeding and gastrostomy care, and practical assistance is vital for this nutrition support to be completely successful and not become another burden for the chronically ill person. Dietitians and nutrition nurses with expertise in this area have a vital role to play and their valuable input cannot be overemphasized.

See 'Enteral feeding regimes', this chapter.

Jejunostomy feeding

A feeding jejunostomy is an artificial route made between the jejunum and outside the body; occasionally access will be made into the duodenum (duodenostomy).

The indications are similar to those for gastrostomy, i.e. nutrition support required for >14–28 days, but where post-pyloric feeding required, e.g. in gastric stasis. Contraindications are the same.

Percutaneous endoscopic jejunostomy (PEJ)

This may be placed in patients with a high risk of aspiration pneumonia where a PEG is considered unsuitable. The insertion technique is more demanding. As an alternative, a conversion kit can be attached to an existing PEG to deliver feed into the jejunum although some risks remain.

Surgical jejunostomy

A number of different techniques are available including Witzel and Roux-en-Y procedures and the insertion of a needle catheter jejunostomy, which is the most common and usually placed during abdominal surgery.

See 'Enteral feeding regimes', this chapter.

Enteral feeding regimes

- The patient's nutritional requirements should be estimated (see 'Estimating requirements in disease states', this chapter). Energy and protein are very important and usually take priority but fluid, electrolytes, macro- and micronutrients, and fibre also need consideration.
- The type and amount of feed that will provide the requirements should be calculated—a dietitian will be best placed to advise.
  - Most standard feeds = 100 kcal and 4 g protein/100 ml.
  - Most high energy feeds = 150–200 kcal and 6 g protein/100 ml.
- Method and rate of administration should be determined to ensure all feed is given in a way best suited to the patient's needs. Options include:
  - continuous infusion over 24 h ± regulated by a pump. Often best if patient is unstable or has difficulty tolerating large quantities of feed
  - intermittent infusion over 8–20 h ± regulated by pump. Providing 'rest' periods may facilitate patient activity, eating, and sleeping; alternatively, feeding can be undertaken overnight. Stopping feeding for >4 h is associated with ↓ gastric pH and ↑ antibacterial effect;
  - bolus feeding of 100–500 ml given by gravity feed or syringed in over 10–30 minutes × 4–10 times daily. Time-consuming and may lead to abdominal symptoms especially in sick patients but is more physiological, e.g. resembles 'meal pattern', so can work well for stable patients.
- Initial administration of feeding needs special consideration.
  - There is little evidence that starter regimes are associated with improved feed tolerance, even with hypertonic feeds, but they will result in delayed administration of the full feed volume.
  - Ready-to-feed enteral preparations should not be diluted prior to use when starting a feed as the risk of contamination outweighs potential benefit.
  - If the patient has been eating relatively normally prior to starting enteral feeding and is relatively well, then the rate of administration can be ↑ steadily so that the full amount of feed is given on the first full day of feeding.
  - If the patient has not been eating or taking any oral or enteral nutrition for some days, if intake has been inadequate, or the patient is very sick or has gastrointestinal symptoms, the rate of feeding should be ↑ more slowly to ensure that (1) tolerance to feed is maximized and (2) risk of re-feeding syndrome ❶ is minimized (see 'Re-feeding syndrome', this chapter): 20 kcal/kg for the first 24 h then gradually ↑ within 1 week to full feeding with careful monitoring and the provision of additional electrolytes as indicated. Anecdotal reports suggest that even this cautious approach may lead to re-feeding syndrome in very depleted patients and as an alternative, 50% of basal metabolic rate (see Schofield equations, Appendix 4) should be infused.

Gastric aspirate should be checked to confirm tolerance in critically ill patients and those with known gastroparesis, intestinal pseudo-obstruction, recurrent vomiting, etc. (Fig. 16.4). This is not required in stable patients who tolerate feeding well.

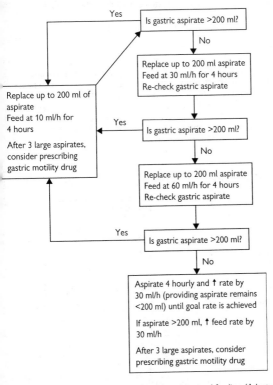

Fig. 16.4 Algorithm for checking gastric aspirate in enteral feeding. (Adapted from p. 17.9 of Todorovic, V E., *et al.* (2004). *A Pocket Guide to Clinical Nutrition*. Reproduced with permission from the British Dietetic Association, London.)

Monitoring enteral feeding

- Monitoring the patient on a regular basis will minimize the risk of developing complications and help ensure that the patient's nutritional requirements are met. It may also contribute to the best use of resources.
- Categories of variables for monitoring include:
  - clinical;
  - nutritional;
  - biochemical.
- Deciding which variables and how often to monitor them depends on the clinical and nutritional status of the patient, the disease process, and the duration of feeding. Obviously, a stable patient who has been fed via a PEG for 18 months and lives at home will require <monitoring than a patient receiving NG feeding on an intensive care unit. It is ∴ impossible to give absolute guidelines about what and when to measure. Table 16.6 is an outline that should be adapted to the needs of individual patients.

Table 16.6 Guidelines for monitoring enteral feeding (for hospital inpatients)*

Type	Until stable	If stable
Body weight	Daily	Twice weekly
Fluid balance	Daily	—
Bowel activity	Daily	—
Plasma		
Glucose	Daily	Twice weekly
Urea	Daily	Twice weekly
Electrolytes	Daily	Twice weekly
Creatinine	Daily	Twice weekly
Magnesium	Daily	Twice weekly
Corrected calcium	Daily	Twice weekly
Plasma phosphate	Daily	Twice weekly
Liver function tests	Daily	—
Temperature, pulse & respiration	Daily	—
Drug-nutrient interactions	Daily	—
C-reactive protein	Twice weekly	—
Mid-arm muscle circumference	Weekly	Weekly

*Adapted from the Enteral Nutrition Policy of Northwick Park and St. Mark's Hospitals. Permision requested.

Plasma albumin is of limited value in monitoring enteral feeding because of its long half-life ($t_{1/2} \sim 20$ days) and because it reflects hydration and clinical rather than nutritional status.

Complications of enteral feeding

Tube blockage (NG, NJ, PEG)

Prevention

- Flush tube with water every 6 hours and at start and end of rest periods. Tap water is suitable, unless patient is immunocompromised or fed post-pylorically (cooled boiled or sterile water is recommended). Use 30–50 ml water in a 50 ml syringe.
- Medication must be in liquid form and not crushed tablets or opened capsules (see 'Enteral feeding and drugs', this chapter). Flush tube with water before and after all medication.
- Low pH (associated with gastric aspirates) encourages protein precipitation. Flush tube with water after each aspiration.

Unblocking

- Never use guide wire—it may pierce tube and injure patient.
- Ensure tube is unkinked and feel external part of tube to identify any lumps. If located, these may be dispersed by squeezing tube gently.
- Use a 50 ml syringe of cold water to apply push/pull pressure.
- Progress on to warm water, again using push/pull technique. Leave water in tube for ~30 minutes and repeat.
- Progress on to fizzy water and repeat as above.
- Leave tube filled with water for up to 4 hours and repeat.
- Numerous other agents, including cola and cranberry juice, are anecdotally recommended but none are licensed in UK for unblocking tubes. Limited evidence suggests the most effective are water, pancreatic enzymes, and a commercial product, Clog Zapper (Merck Pharmaceuticals, Leicester) containing papain and amylase.

Aspiration

- ↑ Risk with ↑ age, ↑ debility, dementia, disordered swallow.
- Occurs in 6–12% neurological patients and up to 30% patients with tracheostomy.
- Feed may be aspirated into the respiratory tract without obvious evidence of vomiting.
- Signs include dyspnoea, cyanosis, tachycardia, hypotension.
- Can lead to pneumonia with associated ↑ morbidity and mortality.
- Treat by stopping feed; try to aspirate feed from lungs; prescribe antibiotics if infection confirmed.
- Prevent by elevating bed by 30–45°; regulate flow with pump, use iso-osmotic feeds (optimize gastric emptying), reduce overnight feeding, consider promotility drugs, e.g. metoclopramide 10 mg tds.

Diarrhoea

- Prevalence ~2–95% of patients receiving enteral tube feeds, depending on patient group and definition of diarrhoea.
- Characteristics of faecal output, e.g. frequency and consistency, are useful in identifying potential abnormality. Numerous, liquid stools will compromise absorption, cause patient discomfort, and present difficulties in care; occasional semi-formed motions are less likely to; ∴ the feed should not automatically be blamed and stopped.

Factors associated with causing diarrhoea and potential solutions

Causes	Potential solutions
Medication, especially antibiotics and sorbitol	Seek expertise from pharmacist to review and modify if possible
↓ Fibre in gut lumen and consequent effect on colonocytes	Consider changing to a fibre-providing feed, e.g. Enrich (Abbott), Isosource Energy Fibre (Novartis)
↓ or ↑ change in bowel microflora	Send stool specimen, e.g. to check for *Clostridium difficile*, *Escherichia coli*, and treat accordingly
	Consider probiotics orally or administered by syringe and flush (do not add to feed)
Rate of continuous feeding	Change to bolus regime if feeding intragastrically, OR ↓ rate if feeding intraduodenally
Hyperosmolar feed	If using high-energy feed, consider changing to standard 1 kcal/ml feed and increasing volume. If using peptide or elemental feed, review osmolarity between brands
Contaminated feed	Ensure good clinical practice; see below
Constipation leading to overflow	Check if colon impacted with faeces; if so, prescribe suppository. Change to fibre feed, ensure adequate hydration, encourage mobility if patient able

Microbiological contamination

- Enteral feeds provide an ideal environment for bacteria to multiply in; the consequences of contamination are potentially very serious.
- All equipment for enteral feeding should be used only once. If bags and giving sets are used, they should be replaced every 24 h and feeding tubes replaced according to the manufacturer's guidelines.
- Sterile feeds should be hung in ward for <24 hours.
- Non-sterile feeds, e.g. re-constituted powder, should be prepared with strict attention to hygiene, covered and stored in a refrigerator for <24 h, and hung in ward for <4 h. Unused feed must be discarded.
- The reservoir of feed (bag, bottle, carton) must not be hung below the level of the patient's stomach.
- If the pump is inadvertently reversed, leading to the stomach contents being infused up into the feed reservoir, feeding should be stopped, all the feed and equipment must be discarded, and feeding re-started with new feed, bag, giving set, etc.

Enteral feeding and drugs

Patients receiving enteral feeding are often unable to take medication orally and ∴ it may need to be administered via the feeding tube. Using this route, or crushing tablets and opening tablets is generally outside the drug's product licence meaning that the prescriber and practitioner accept liability for any adverse effects resulting from their administration. In each case, advice should be sought from a pharmacist and the following considered.

- If the patient can still take the drug orally, this is best.
- Review all medication—is it all still needed ?
- Does the tube deliver the drug distal to the site of absorption ?
- ❶ Drugs have a notorious reputation for blocking feeding tubes, especially antacids, so care must be taken at each dosing.
- Should the drug usually be given before/after or with food ? This may mean that the feed has to be stopped; the feeding regime should be amended to take this into consideration so that the patient still receives the total volume prescribed.
- Drugs should not be added to the feed but should be introduced into the tube using a 50 ml syringe (smaller syringes ↑ pressure in tube and may cause it to split).
- Each drug should be administered separately, unless advised by a pharmacist, followed by 10 ml water. A gap may be required between different drugs.
- Wherever possible, prescribe medication in liquid form or as soluble tablets. Crushing tablets and opening capsules should be considered a last resort.
- Soluble tablets should be dissolved in 10–15 ml water before administration.
- Liquids should be diluted with an equal volume of water and mixed well before administration.
- Tablets that have to be crushed should be ground finely using a pestle and mortar or tablet-crusher. Mix with 10–15 ml water to syringe into tube. Rinse crusher and syringe-in rinsings to ensure full drug dose is given.
- Do not crush tablets that are enterically coated, modified, or slow release.
- Staff should wash their hands and wear gloves to minimize exposure to the drugs. Cytotoxic medication and hormones should not be crushed due to the risk associated with staff exposure.

More information is available at http://www.bapen.org.uk/drugs-enteral.htm

Parenteral nutrition (PN)

PN refers to the administration of nutrients via the intravenous route. It is required when a patient has intestinal failure to a degree that prevents adequate absorption of nutrients via the gastrointestinal tract. Complications associated with the access route and the nutrition formulation frequently occur with PN, so careful patient selection and monitoring are essential.

Indications

PN may be required in the short term where the gastrointestinal tract is temporarily unavailable. It is generally recommended that the patient is fed parenterally for ≥5 days for the benefits of PN to outweigh the complications associated with this form of nutrition support.

- Examples where PN may be used in the short-term:
  - severe pancreatitis;
  - intensive chemotherapy causing mucositis;
  - multi-organ failure where nutritional requirements cannot be met by the enteral route alone;
  - prolonged nil by mouth following excisional surgery;
  - high output or enterococcus fistula.
- Examples where PN may be required long-term:
  - inflammatory bowel disease;
  - radiation enteritis;
  - motility disorders (e.g. scleroderma);
  - extreme short bowel syndrome;
  - chronic malabsorption.

Routes for provision of PN

Patients who require PN in the short term, are fed continuously, and use a regimen of <1200 mosmols may be fed via a peripheral route, e.g. a venflon. The following may minimize the risk of thrombophlebitis.

- Access the largest peripheral vein available.
- Use a small cannula (18Fr).
- Use a GTN (glyceryl trinitrate) patch distal to the exit site.

Where it is anticipated that patients may require parenteral nutrition for >14 days, are to be fed on a cyclical basis, or require a regimen of >1200 mosmols, central catheter insertion may be appropriate. The tip of the catheter is surgically placed to lie in the superior vena cava or right atrium. Examples include:

- Single dedicated feeding line;
- Peripherally inserted central catheter (PICC);
- Multi-lumen using one lumen as dedicated feeding line.

Where PN is anticipated to be required on a more permanent basis, access can be provided by:

- Hickman or implanted port (Portacath);
- Cuffed (Dacron cuff to secure).

Complications

Related to:	Examples
Line insertion	Pneumothorax, haemothorax, air embolism
Access routes	Thrombophlebitis, central vein thrombosis, line infection
PN solution	Fluid and electrolyte imbalance, metabolic disturbances, gut atrophy, impaired liver function (long-term use)

To minimize the risk of infection always feed via a dedicated feeding line.

Parenteral nutrition regimes

- To meet a patient's nutritional requirements PN must contain:
  - fluid;
  - nitrogen;
  - source of energy as a combination of carbohydrate and fat;[1]
  - electrolytes;
  - fat- and water-soluble vitamins;
  - trace elements.
- A pharmacy production unit may provide compounded solutions or standardized fixed feeding regimens.
  - Advantages of compounded regimens—greater flexibility to meet the needs of complex patients whose individual requirements could not be met with a standardized regimen.
  - Advantages of standardized regimens—wide range of formulations available, still some flexibility for adding electrolytes, less cost of having a specialized pharmacy production unit.
- Vitamins and trace elements should always be added to ensure the feed is complete.
- Before introducing PN it is important to check biochemical parameters and the patient's clinical condition. From this the nutritional requirements can be calculated and the appropriate regimen prescribed.

---

[1] Inclusion of fat is not necessary on a daily basis (can be given less often).

Monitoring parenteral nutrition

Patients receiving enteral feeding must be monitored to:
- detect potential complications associated with the feeding and/or their clinical condition;
- evaluate their nutritional status in relation to the nutrients provided and/or their clinical condition.

Table 16.7 Guidelines for monitoring parenteral nutrition.

Type	Rationale
Daily monitoring	
Urea and electrolytes	To prevent electrolyte imbalance
Fluid input and output; patient's weight	To prevent over-or under hydration
Blood glucose	To monitor glucose tolerance and stress response
Temperature; patient's clinical condition	To ensure that regimen meets nutritional requirements
Feeding line	To observe and act on possible signs of infection
Twice weekly monitoring	
Phosphate*, magnesium*, corrected calcium	To ensure regimen meets nutritional requirements
Liver function tests	To monitor hepatic function
FBC and markers of infection e.g. WCC, CRP	To assess for acute phase response and infection
Weekly monitoring	
Anthropometry	To monitor changes in nutritional status
Nitrogen balance	To ensure adequate provision of nitrogen
Triglyceride level	To monitor tolerance of energy provision
Monthly monitoring	
Trace elements	To monitor the need for supplementation due to disease state

* More frequent monitoring may be required with patients at risk of re-feeding syndrome (see 'Re-feeding syndrome', this chapter).

Estimating requirements in disease states

Estimating the nutritional requirements of healthy populations with any degree of accuracy is difficult; it is even more challenging to try to predict the needs of individuals in ill health and disease when substantial change may arise. However, providing appropriate nutrition, i.e. sufficient but no excess, is important to maximize benefits and so every attempt should be made to tailor nutritional intake to the individual.

❶ The following guidelines provide a useful starting point but it must be remembered that:
- they are guidelines and not precise values;
- a carefully calculated estimate of requirements only has the benefit to help the patient if this intake is achieved, i.e. their feed must be given or supplements taken.

Energy

Table 16.8 gives a method of estimating energy requirements which is used in the following examples.

Example 1

Man aged 58 years, weight 81 kg, height 1.72 m, sitting up in bed following cerebral vascular accident. Unable to swallow at present and enteral feed to be started.

1. BMR = 11.5 × 81 + 873 = 1805 kcal
2. Clinical stress factor = 5% of 1805 = 90 kcal
3. Activity factor = 15% of 1805 = 271 kcal

Estimated energy requirement = 1805 + 90 + 271 = 2166 kcal

Example 2

Woman aged 23 years, weight 48 kg, height 1.64, immobile and septic on intensive care unit following complicated intestinal resection 2° to Crohn's disease. Nutrition support instigated.

1. BMR = 13.4 × 48 + 692 = 1335 kcal
2. Clinical stress factor = 60% of 1335 = 801 kcal
3. Activity factor = 10% of 1335 = 134 kcal

Estimated energy requirement = 1335 + 801 + 134 = 2270 kcal

Protein

Requirements should be based on actual body weight except in obesity (if BMI 30–50 kg/m^2 use 75% value; if BMI >50 kg/m^2 use 65% value). Table 16.9 gives an estimation of protein requirements in terms of nitrogen.

Table 16.8 Estimating energy requirements*

1	Estimate basal metabolic rate using the Schofield equation (see appendix 4)

Either:

2a | Add to BMR a stress factor for specific clinical condition (calculated as % of BMR):

Condition	Stress factor (%)
Cerebral vascular accident (stroke)	5
Chronic obstructive pulmonary disease	15–20
Infection	25–40
Inflammatory bowel disease	0–10
Intensive care (ventilated)	0–10
Intensive care (septic)	20–60
Lymphoma	0–25
Pancreatitis (chronic to acute ± abscess)	3–20
Surgery (uncomplicated to complicated)	5–40
Tumour (solid)	0–20
Transplantation	20

Or:

2b | Add to BMR 400–1,000 kcal/d if ↑ in body weight (lean ± fat) is desired or subtract 400–1,000 kcal if ↓ in body fat is desired

3 | Add to BMR an activity factor (calculated as % of BMR)

Activity level	Activity factor (%)
Patient in bed and immobile	10
Patient in bed but able to move and sit up	15–20
Patient mobile on ward	25
Patient living in the community	40–90[†]

* Adapted from pp. 3.1–3.3a of Todorovic V.E., et al. (2004). *A Pocket Guide to Clinical Nutrition*. Permission requested from the British Dietetic Association.
[†] Or use PAL (see 'Energy balance', Chapter 5).

Table 16.9 Estimating protein requirements*

	Nitrogen (g/kg/d)[†]	
	Mean	Range
Normal	0.17	0.14–0.20
Hypermetabolic		
+5–25%	0.20	0.17–0.25
+25–50%	0.25	0.20–0.30
+>50%	0.30	0.25–0.35
Depleted	0.30	0.20–0.40

* Adapted from pp. 3.7 and A15.1 of Todorovic V.E., et al. (2004). *A Pocket Guide to Clinical Nutrition*. Permission requested from the British Dietetic Association.
[†] 1 g nitrogen ≡ 6.25 g protein; 1 g protein ≡ 0.16 g nitrogen.

Carbohydrate

Requirements for healthy and chronically sick are similar: 4–5 g glucose /kg/c
In critical illness, glucose oxidation rate should be considered. Th maximum of 4 mg glucose /kg/minute should not be exceeded.

Lipid

Requirement in health: 1.0–1.5 g/kg/d.
In critical illness: 0.8–1.0 g/kg/d.
Lower levels of fat intake can be tolerated well but ~3.0–4.5% total energ should be provided as lipid to prevent essential fatty acid deficiency.

Fluid

- Basic requirements: 35 ml/kg.
- Pyrexia: add 2.0–2.5 ml/kg for every °C above 37°C.
- Fluid lost via body secretions: replacement should be considered on ar individual basis.

Electroytes Table 16.10 lists the basic daily requirement for electrolytes.

Table 16.10 Basic daily requirements for electrolytes

Electrolyte	Basic daily requirement
Sodium	1.0 mmol/kg
	In pyrexia, add 1.5 mmol to each additional 10 ml fluid given (see above for fluid requirements)
	In hyponatraemia, additional Na^+ (mmol) required = (140 – actual serum Na^+) $\times$ 0.2 $\times$ body weight (kg)
Potassium	1.0 mmol/kg
	In hypokalaemia, additional K^+ (mmol) required = (4.0 – actual serum K^+) $\times$ 0.4 $\times$ body weight (kg)
Calcium	17.5 mmol (700 mg)
Magnesium	Male: 12.3 mmol (300 mg)
	Female: 10.9 mmol (270 mg)
Phosphate	17.5 mmol (equimolar with calcium)

Micronutrients

There is limited evidence about the requirement of micronutrients (vitamins and trace elements) in disease states. In most cases, it is probably appropriate to provide the equivalent to the reference nutrient intake (see Appendix 6). These values are based on providing sufficient for 97% of people in a healthy population, but this may not be adequate for some individual patients if previously depleted. In these cases, it is probably better to provide additional micronutrients in the form of a multi- rather than single-nutrient supplement, unless there is clinical or biochemical evidence of a specific deficiency. This is because of the complex interrelationships between many micronutrients and the potential for competitive absorption and/or biochemical pathways,

Metabolic response to injury

The term 'metabolic response to injury' describes the biochemical and hormonal consequences of major injury, trauma, surgery ± infection and the resulting nutritional changes that may have very significant clinical effects. Traditionally, the response has been described as having two phases, known as the ebb and flow (Table 16.11). Recent studies have shown that good acute clinical management may reduce or possibly eliminate the ebb phase, and that it may not be detectable at all in less severe injury.

Overall effects

- Loss of appetite → ↓ nutrient intake.
- Perturbation of fat and carbohydrate metabolism with apparent inability to use these as metabolic substrates (hence ↑ circulating levels and deposition of lipid in adipose and vital organs). Controlling hyperglycaemia by giving insulin will help ↓ risk of death.
- Lean tissue broken down, may provide amino acids required during inflammatory response, e.g. acute phase proteins, lymphocyte proliferation, glutathione synthesis.
- Protein loss—may be substantial and have clinical consequences (see Table 16.12). In context of 'whole body protein', lean tissue contains ~205 g protein/kg → an average 70 kg man comprises ~10 kg protein. ❶ Most of this protein is 'essential' and cannot be lost without functional implications, i.e. ↓ resistance to infection, ↑ muscle weakness (including respiratory and skeletal muscle) leading to ↓ pulmonary function and ↓ physical activity.

Effect of starvation

Although there are some similarities between the metabolic response to injury and starvation, i.e. both lead to depletion, there are important differences (Table 16.13).

Starvation may interfere with the metabolic response.

❶ Providing nutritional support to patients after injury will not reverse the biochemical effects observed, during the metabolic response to injury, e.g. nitrogen loss. However, it will help to ameliorate the effects of depletion and limit the clinical consequences (see 'undernutrition' this Chapter).

Table 16.11 Simplified model of metabolic response to injury

Metabolic & clinical effects	Ebb phase* (acute)	Flow phase† (hypermetabolic)
Energy expenditure	↓	↑
O₂ consumption	↓	↑
Cardiac output	↓	↑
Body temperature	↓	↑
Circulating levels of		
Glucose	↑	↑
Lactate	↑	↔
Free fatty acids	↑	↑
Catecholamines	↑	↑
Glucagons	↑	↑
Cortisol	↑	↑
Insulin	↓	Insulin resistance
Urinary nitrogen loss	↑	↑

* Occurring immediately after trauma, the ebb phase is the brief 'shock' phase (lasts ~0–8 h)
† The flow phase follows the ebb phase and is a longer 'catabolic' phase (lasts ~5–10 days)

Table 16.12 Estimated loss of protein (g) over 10 day period following trauma and untreated infection

	Tissue loss	Blood loss	Protein catabolism
Muscle wound	500–750	150–400	650
35% burn	500	150–400	600
# Femur	–	up to 200	580–860
Gastrectomy	up to 60	20–180	525–650
Typhoid fever	–	–	675

Table 16.13 Differences between the metabolic response to injury and starvation

	Injury	Starvation
Energy expenditure	↑	↓
Nitrogen losses	↑	↓
Plasma insulin & glucose	↑	↓
Plasma free fatty acids	↑ Turnover	↓ Turnover
Plasma clearance of exogenous triglycerides	↑	↓

Re-feeding syndrome (RS)

❶ Enthusiasm for nutritional support and a desire to replete very under nourished patients rapidly can be fatal unless care is taken to avoid RS.

Definition

Severe fluid and electrolyte shifts and related metabolic complications i malnourished patients undergoing re-feeding.

Pathophysiology

- In starvation, ↓ intake of energy and particularly carbohydrate → ↓ insulin secretion and ↑ catabolism of fat and protein for energy → ↓ intracellular electrolytes and especially ↓ phosphate (↓ intracellular phosphate coexists with normal serum phosphate levels).
- Initiating feeding → change from predominantly fat and protein metabolism to carbohydrate with ↑ insulin secretion → stimulation of cellular uptake of phosphate, potassium, and water → hypophosphataemia, hypokalaemia, and hypomagnesaemia → RS.

Clinical features

- Rhabdomyolysis, weakness, paralysis
- Leucocyte dysfunction, haemolytic anaemia
- Respiratory depression & failure
- Hypotension, arrhythmias, cardiac failure
- ↓ Glomerular filtration rate
- Liver dysfunction
- Diarrhoea, constipation, ileus
- Seizures, coma, sudden death

❶The early features of RS are non-specific and may not be recognized. Awareness and understanding of RS by clinical staff is limited and serum phosphate is often not routinely measured and the significance of depleted levels is not always appreciated. Dietitians who work in nutrition support have an important role in increasing awareness about RS.

At risk patients

- Undernourished patients starting parenteral or enteral feeding who have received inadequate nutrition for >7 days.
- Alcoholism.
- Anorexia nervosa.
- Cancer, especially on chemotherapy.
- Neurological dysphagia, i.e. starting gastrostomy feeding.
- Surgery.

❶ Normal serum values **before** feeding starts do not indicate that the patient is at low risk of RS. In RS, serum levels only fall **after** feeding starts so this is when monitoring must take place.

Treatment   See Fig. 16.5.

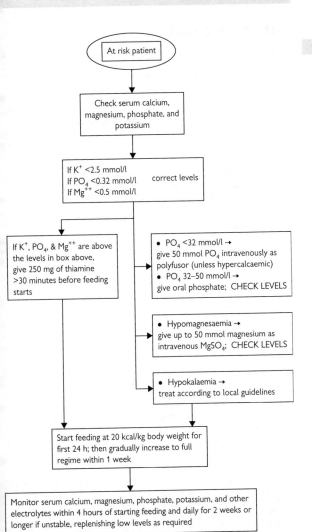

Fig. 16.5 Algorithm for treating re-feeding syndrome. (Adapted from p. 13.7 of Todorovic, V.E., et al. (2004). *A pocket guide to clinical nutrition*. Reproduced with permission from British Dietetic Association, Birmingham).

Critical care (CC)

Defined as patients requiring:
- advanced respiratory support alone *or*
- basic respiratory support together with the support of at least two organ systems;
- includes patients with multi-organ failure.

The aims of nutrition support in CC patients are to minimize nutritional losses and provide basic nutrient requirements to sustain life. Repletion of pre-existing undernutrition during a period of critical care is unlikely to be achieved and should not be a goal because of the ↑ risks associated with overfeeding.

Route of feeding

Access to feeding routes may be limited by the patient's condition, but wherever possible, the gut should be used as first choice (see 'Enteral Feeding', this chapter).

Enteral feeding

There is evidence ♠ to support the early initiation of enteral feeding (<24 h after admission) in CC patients. This will require a standard initial regime to be available to all clinical staff so that feeding can commence as soon as possible.

- Gastric aspirate should be checked every 4–6 hours. Volumes <200 ml with nasogastric feeding and <150 ml with gastrostomy feeding are acceptable and should be returned to the stomach.
- Gastric aspirates above these levels indicate delayed gastric emptying but a single high measurement should not lead to the cessation of feeding unless there is overt regurgitation or signs that the patient is aspirating fluid into the respiratory tract.
- Risk of aspirating feed can be reduced by elevating bed by 30–45°, regulating rate of feeding with a pump, using iso-osmotic feeds (optimize gastric emptying), and considering promotility drugs, e.g. metoclopramide 10 mg tds.
- If absorption is limited and precludes administration of the total volume of enteral feed prescribed to meet requirements, it can be combined with parenteral nutrition. This will facilitate an adequate total nutrient intake but continue the physiological benefits of feeding via the gut.

Parenteral Nutrition (see 'Parenteral nutrition (PN)', this chapter)

- Parenteral nutrition can play an invaluable role where enteral feeding is not possible.
- Avoidance of overfeeding is important (see box).
- Maintaining good glycaemic control (blood glucose 4.4–6.1 mmol/l) and avoiding swings in blood sugar level are associated with lower mortality. Additional insulin may be required to achieve this.

Nutritional Requirements in critical care

ee 'Estimating requirements in disease states', this chapter).

Energy. requirements can be estimated by calculation using standard formulae but ❶ resulting values provide only an approximation and may need adjusting to suit individual patients. Energy requirements are slightly ↓ if patients are ventilated rather than breathing spontaneously but will ↑ as weaning progresses. Patients sedated using propofol will receive additional energy from the lipid emulsion it is carried in (both 1% and 2% propofol contain between 1.06 and 1.10 kcal/ml). The maximum dose recommended for a 70 kg CC patient could ∴ provide as much as 739 kcal/24 h if given as 1% (or 370 kcal/24 h if given as 2%) so care must be given to ensure that adequacy of other nutrients is maintained in the remaining energy provided.

Protein/nitrogen. CC patients have ↑ protein turnover and ↑ nitrogen loss is an unavoidable feature of the metabolic response to injury (see 'Metabolic response to injury', this chapter): nutritional support will not reduce this but will help minimize the accompanying depletion. Evidence suggests that providing >0.2 g nitrogen/kg body weight/day has no additional benefit in septic or trauma patients.

Carbohydrate. In critical illness, glucose administration should not exceed the maximum glucose oxidation rate of 4 mg/kg/minute.

Lipid. In critical illness: 0.8–1.0 g/kg/d (see above *re* propofol). Approximately 3.0–4.5% total energy should be provided as lipid to prevent essential fatty acid deficiency.

Fluid, electrolytes, micronutrients—no evidence is available about specific requirements in CC patients.

Potential consequences of overfeeding

- ↓ Tolerance of feeding, e.g. diarrhoea
- ↑ Physiological stress
- Metabolic acidosis
- Uraemia
- ↑ Respiratory quotient, i.e. ↑ CO_2 produced so weaning harder
- Hyperglycaemia → impaired wound healing
- Hypercholesterolaemia & hypertriglyceridaemia
- Excess lipid → ↓ reticuloendothelial system → ± immunosuppression
- Hepatic steatosis
- Re-feeding syndrome

Surgery

Nutritional depletion is associated with ↑ morbidity and mortality follow ing surgery. Surgery itself is associated with ↑ nutritional losses (se 'Metabolic response to injury', this chapter) and nutritional support is n able to prevent these. However, appropriate nutrition support is capab of minimizing the depletion (i.e. loss of lean body mass) accompanyi major surgical intervention, and is associated with:
• repletion of lean body mass;
• improved skeletal muscle force;
• ↓ fatiguability;
• ↑ ventilatory, cardiac, and gut function;
• ↑ immunity;
• ↑ sense of well-being.

There is less evidence that nutrition support has beneficial effec in relatively well-nourished individuals who have undergone mino moderate surgery indicating that routine nutritional support for surgical patients is inappropriate, especially considering the potential sid effects of feeding and cost implications.

However, it is widely accepted that patients who are critically severely injured, or nutritionally depleted prior to surgery will bene from nutrition support. This raises two issues:
• identifying patients who will benefit (see Chapter 4).
• optimum timing of nutrition support.

Pre-operative nutrition

Feeding undernourished patients 7–10 days prior to surgery is associate with a reduction in non-infectious complications. Shorter periods sho no benefit. Obviously, delaying surgery is clinically inappropriate in son patients, but pre-op feeding should be considered in those who a severely depleted.

Peri-operative nutrition

Overnight fasting prior to surgery may be unnecessary. Evidence sugges that allowing patients to take clear fluids until 2 hours before surge is safe and may have some benefits. Oral carbohydrate (50 g) and flu loading prior to surgery is associated with reduced post-op insulin res tance, improved well-being, and ↓ length of hospital stay.

Post-operative nutrition

Initiating enteral feeding within the first 24 hours after surgery is sa in most patients, even those undergoing abdominal surgery includi major trauma and liver transplantation. It is not, however, risk-free b complications can be minimized by good clinical practice including care monitoring (see 'Monitoring enteral feeding', this chapter).

Spinal cord injury (SCI)

SCI can result in either temporary or permanent impairment of the normal motor, sensory, or autonomic function.

- Tetraplegia—injury to the spinal cord in the cervical region with associated loss of function in all four extremities.
- Paraplegia—injury in the thoracic, lumbar, or sacral segments resulting in loss of function in the lower limbs.

Short-term nutritional issues (<3 months after injury)

- Patients should undergo assessment to determine their nutritional status as soon as possible after injury. Determining body weight may be difficult; estimating requirements may be inaccurate due to variation in individual needs, other coexisting injuries, and reduced mobility.
- Nutritional support may be required if the patient is unable to eat sufficient. Depression, anxiety, and frequent clinical investigations and treatment may also limit intake. Input from a registered dietitian is needed to optimize nutritional care.

Longer-term nutritional issues (>3 months after injury)

- An optimum nutrient intake will help support an active rehabilitation programme. This will include the provision of adequate energy to participate in physiotherapy sessions and sufficient protein and micronutrient to facilitate any continuing healing process and minimize complications associated with limited mobility, e.g. loss of skin integrity
- Constipation is very common and can have a serious impact on quality of life and long-term health. The degree of bowel dysfunction depends on the extent and location of the injury on the spinal cord with complete damage above the 12th thoracic vertebra (T12) associated with loss of anal muscle control. However in most patients, a high fibre diet with ↑ intake of fluid (>35 ml/kg/d) will help to regulate bowel movements and reduce risk of constipation. For those previously unfamiliar with a high fibre diet, sources should be introduced slowly over a 6-week period to optimize tolerance (see 'Constipation' in 'Disorders of the colon', Chapter 21).
- Increasing body weight may become a concern in some people whose level of energy expenditure is curtailed by their lack of mobility. There is also evidence of reduced resting energy expenditure (↓ ~20%), probably 2° to loss of lean body mass. Excessive weight gain may hamper rehabilitation if wasted muscles are overburdened and ↑ the chance of pressure sores (as does underweight). Increasing energy expenditure through limited activity should be encouraged where possible and dietary energy should be tailored to this. If an energy-restricted diet is required to match limited energy expenditure on a long-term basis, care must be taken to ensure that the diet is totally adequate in all other nutrients. A regular review by a dietitian may be appropriate.

Life expectancy ranges after SCI from 70 to 92% of normal. As a consequence and because many SCI patients are young adults, the influence of nutrition on the promotion of long-term good health is important. Advice should be based on the guidance given in the 'Balance of Good Health' (see 'Food-based dietary guidelines' in Chapter 2) accompanied by consideration of energy balance to maintain an optimum weight.

Head injury

Patients sustaining brain damage through external injury to the head or surgery to treat a CVA (see 'Cerebrovascular accident/stroke' in Chapter 19) will require nutritional support in the short- and long-term.

Nutrition is not a priority immediately (<24 hours) after injury as resuscitation and emergency surgery may be required to preserve life.

However, in the following days, patients may become hypermetabolic and hypercatabolic as a consequence of the metabolic response to injury (see 'Metabolic response to injury', this chapter). Requirements should be calculated on an individual basis by a dietitian with experience in caring for the critically ill.

Energy requirements

- Resting energy expenditure may ↑ ~145% of normal although this increase may be moderated by pharmaceutical sedation (↓ ~40%).
- Energy expended through physical activity is usually minimal.
- Most head injured patients are well-nourished at the time of injury although this should not be assumed.
- Accompanying injuries, e.g. after a road traffic accident, must be considered.
- Actual expenditure should be measured using indirect calorimetry if possible.

Protein requirements

- Protein is used as a preferred source of energy and so nitrogen losses increase in the 1st week post-injury and may remain raised for some weeks.
- Reported N losses vary from 0.29 to 0.73 g/kg body weight/d (≡ 125–300 g protein for a 70 kg man). Negative nitrogen balance results.
- Monitoring N losses will give an indication of requirements and, although feeding cannot prevent N loss, it will minimize consequences.
- Providing 0.35 g N/kg body weight is associated with better outcome than lower intakes.

Nutritional support

Systematic review has shown that instigation of early nutrition support (<48 hours) is associated with ↓ 0.67 relative risk of death (95% CI 0.41–1.07). It also suggests that parenteral nutritional support is associated with a more favourable outcome than enteral but this may be confounded by the fact that parenteral feeding usually commences earlier.

Burn injury

Assessment of nutritional requirements

Medical history
- Total % body surface area burn, % full thickness or partial thickness, area of body burn (face, hands, or smoke inhalation injury most significant).
- History and type of injury (flame, hot liquid, contact, chemical, or electrical).
- Previous medical history, e.g. diabetes, GI problems.

Social factors Nutritional status on admission will be affected by physical health, mental health, income, cooking skills, and home circumstances.

Body weight Measured immediately on admission to calculate fluid resuscitation regimen and energy requirements.

Diet history
- Assessment of nutritional intake prior to admission.
- Food preferences/allergies.
- Special dietary requirements.
- Vegetarian ± religious beliefs.

Energy requirements
Thermal injury results in ↑ production of catecholamines producing a hypermetabolic response. This results in accelerated protein and fat breakdown and altered carbohydrate metabolism. Energy requirements are assessed using the specific formulae (see Table 16.14).

Protein requirements
- Adults—give 20% of energy as protein (1.5–2g protein/kg).
- Children—<1 year use reference nutrient intake (RNI) for protein (see Appendix 6); ≥1 year use 2.5–3 g protein/kg.

Trace elements
Patients with total body surface area burns of ≥20% are at risk of copper, zinc, and selenium depletion due to losses through the burn exudates.

Electrolytes
Depletion can result from large losses in exudates, urine, diarrhoea, vomiting, and pyrexia. Replacement should take place intravenously according to biochemical parameters. Hypernatraemia can result from dehydration or high Na^+ loads administered from IV fluids with insufficient free water for excretion.

Minerals and vitamins
↑ Losses of phosphate and magnesium occur through urine and exudates. Vitamins should be given to meet recommended daily intakes.

Table 16.14 Estimating energy requirements in burn injury

Adults

Schofield equations used to calculate basal metabolic rate (see Appendix 4)

Add 10–90% as stress factor per % burn and 10–20% for activity to a maximum of 2 × basal metabolic rate

Children

Galveston formulae:

0–1 years

2100 kcal × body surface area (m²) + 1000 kcal × body surface area burned (m²)

1–12 years

1800 kcal × body surface area (m²) + 1300 kcal × body surface area burned (m²)

>12 years

1500 kcal × body surface area (m²)+ 1500 kcal × body surface area burned (m²)

Feeding routes

Oral feeding In well-nourished patients, with no confusion or facial swelling and <15–20% burn injury, oral nutrition using food and supplementary drinks is usually successful.

Nasogastric or nasojejunal feeding Necessary in patients with burns 20%, the target is to commence within 4 hours of admission. If gastric stasis develops, NJ feeding is usually successful. Total parenteral feeding is rarely used due to risk of infection.

Monitoring

Daily
- Food and fluid intake
- Bowel activity
- Description of wound healing, skin graft take, and % left to heal
- Biochemistry: blood urea and electrolytes

3 × per week
- 24 hour urine collection
- Biochemistry: C-reactive protein, liver function tests, phosphate, magnesium
- Haematology: haemoglobin, white cell count

Weekly
- Body weight
- Biochemistry: trace elements

Clinically functional nutrients

Also referred to as *novel substrates*, these include nutrients that may have some clinical benefits if given in larger than usual intakes in specific medical conditions (see 'Protein' in Chapter 5).

Glutamine

Glutamine (gln) is a conditionally indispensable amino acid:
- an important source of fuel in rapidly dividing cells, e.g. enterocytes and immune cells;
- precursor for antioxidant glutathione;
- becomes indispensable in stress situations, e.g. catabolic patients, as body pool ↓ rapidly to fuel stimulated lymphocytes, etc.;
- standard parenteral solutions do not include gln.

Gln supplementation is associated with clinical benefit including ↓ mucosal atrophy after prolonged parenteral nutrition, ↓ bacterial translocation, and ↑ systemic immune function. Meta-analysis of gln supplementation studies in surgical and critically ill patients shows ↓ risk of mortality (RR 0.78, 95% CI 0.58–1.04), ↓ infection (RR 0.81, 95% CI 0.64–1.00) ↓ length of hospital stay (−2.6 days, 95% CI −4.5 to −0.7).[1] However, benefits have not been universally observed and depend on gln dose (optimum not yet defined), route of administration (oral or IV), and patient population.

Arginine

Arginine (arg) is a conditionally indispensable amino acid:
- plays role in transport, storage, and excretion of nitrogen;
- precursor for nitric oxide;
- becomes indispensable in stress situations, e.g. trauma and sepsis, when arg levels ↓ as it is used for nitric oxide pathways.

Arg supplementation may benefit the microcirculation and protein anabolism and has been associated with ↑ muscle and protein metabolism and intestinal motility. However, there are concerns that ↑ arg intake in septic patients may ↑ nitric oxide production resulting in hypotension, poor perfusion, and ↑ risk of multi-organ failure. This is supported by a review of good quality studies showing ↑ mortality associated with arg-enriched feeding (RR 1.19, 95% CI 0.99–1.43) even though fewer infectious complications were observed (RR 0.53, 95% CI 0.42–0.68).[2] Benefits ∴ may be limited to less sick patients and further studies are needed.

[1] Novak, F., et al. (2002). Glutamine supplementation in serious illness: a systematic review of the evidence. Crit.Care. Med. **30**, 2022–9.
[2] Duggan, C., Gannon, J., and Walker, W.A (2002). Protective nutrients and functional foods for the gastrointestinal tract. Am. J. Clin. Nutr. **75**, 789–808.

Obesity

Classification and prevalence

Classification

The simplest and most widely used classification for obesity in adults is based on body mass index (BMI; Table 17.1 and see Appendix 2). For obesity in children, see 'Nutritional problems of children and adelescents' in Chapter 11.

Table 17.1 Classification of obesity in adults based on BMI*

	BMI (kg/m^2)
Underweight	≤18.5
Healthy/normal weight	18.5–24.9
Overweight (pre-obese)	25–29.9
Obesity moderate (class 1)	30–34.9
severe (class 2)	35–39.9
morbid (class 3)	≥40

* World Health Organization 1998. Obesity. *Preventing and managing the global epidemic. Report of a WHO Consultation on Obesity.* World Health Organization Geneva, Switzerland.

While BMI is simple and quick to use, it has limitations because it is based simply on the ratio of weight to height and does not take account of body composition. For example, lean but well-muscled individuals may have a BMI above 25 kg/m^2 but not have an excess of body fat. However, this is an issue for a relatively small proportion of the population at the boundaries of the categories and BMI remains practical in most situations and is widely used. If clarification is required, waist circumference can be used to identify individuals at ↑ risk (Table 17.2).

Prevalence

UK The prevalence of obesity is the UK has been increasing for decades with ~22% of men and 23% of women in the UK classified as obese (BMI >30 kg/m^2) in 2002[1] compared to 6% and 8% respectively in 1980. ↑ risk of obesity is associated with:
• increasing age;
• lower socio-economic groups, especially women;
• people from Black Caribbean and Pakistani backgrounds, especially women.
Worldwide Prevalence varies greatly from country to country from <0.1% in South Asia to >75% in urban Samoa. Globally, it is estimated that more than 1 billion adults (16%) are overweight and at least 300 million (5%) are obese.[2] Increases in prevalence have been observed in North America, UK, Eastern Europe, the Middle East, the Pacific Islands, Australasia, and China but some of the fastest rates of increase have been observed in urban areas of developing countries where obesity and undernutrition coexist (nutrition transition).

[1] Department of Health (2004). *Health survey for England 2003. Vol. 2 Risk factors for cardiovascular disease.* HMSO, London.
[2] World Health Organization (2004).

Table 17.2 Classification of risk of obesity based on waist circumference*

	Waist circumference (cm)
Men	
↑ risk	94–102
Substantially ↑ risk	>102
Women	
↑ Risk	80–88
Substantially ↑ risk	>88

* World Health Organization 1998. *Obesity. Preventing and managing the global epidemic. Report of a WHO Consultation on Obesity.* World Health Organization Geneva, Switzerland.

Contributing causes and clinical consequences

Contributing causes

Obesity results from an excess of dietary energy intake over energy expenditure and thus both an increase in intake and a decrease in expenditure will lead to excess calories being stored as fat and, ultimately, to obesity.

Increased energy intake

Food has become more accessible and often cheaper in most parts of the world through improved agricultural practices, industrialization of food processing, and introduction of efficient food transport and storage. In addition, energy dense foods are more available and it has become easier and quicker to obtain, prepare, and eat palatable meals. In spite of this trend, it appears that the average total energy intake of the UK has fallen over the last 30 years, a period during which obesity rates have ↑. There is debate over whether this is due to (1) underreporting of food intake or (2) an inadequate evaluation of food consumed outside the home. Although the concentrated calories found in a high fat, high sugar diet undoubtedly contribute to an excessive energy intake, this is not the only factor responsible for the present obesity epidemic.

Decreased energy expenditure

There are no nationally representative data for monitoring energy expenditure in the UK. However, evidence points to a rapid decline in levels of activity when evaluated by participation in manual labour, car ownership, availability of labour-saving devices, hours spent watching television, and computer use. This decline mirrors the rise in obesity and is thus considered a major contributory factor.[1]

Metabolic factors

There is no evidence to support the concept that a low metabolic rate is the major cause of obesity. However, in a very small number of individuals, endocrine disorders such as Cushing's syndrome and hypothyroidism, Prader–Willi syndrome (see 'Conditions associated with obesity', this chapter), and congenital leptin deficiency are the cause of obesity.

Genetic factors

Obesity tends to run in families but shared environmental factors (meals and level of activity) probably contribute more to obesity than common genetic factors and the current, rapid increase in obesity prevalence cannot be explained by the gene pool changing so quickly. However, it is likely that some individuals are genetically more susceptible to the effects of an obesogenic environment.

Fetal programming

The Barker hypothesis proposes that undernutrition during pregnancy may permanently damage the fetus, leading to the programming of ill health, including the ↑ susceptibility to obesity in adulthood.

[1] Prentice, A.M. and Jebb, S. A. (1995). Obesity in Britain: gluttony or sloth? *Br. Med. J.* **311**, 437–9.

Clinical consequences

Obesity is associated with a higher risk of death and morbidity. The life expectancy of men and women with a BMI of >45 kg/m^2 aged 20–30 years is 13 and 8 years lower, respectively, than that of those with a BMI of 24 kg/m^2.

Metabolic   Diabetes type 2 (insulin resistance), hyperlipidaemia, hypertension, stroke, gall stones, breast and colon cancer, infertility (men and women), and polycystic ovary syndrome.

Physical   Osteoarthritis, chronic back pain, respiratory problems, ↓ mobility and accidents, sleep apnoea, skin problems.

Psychosocial   Depression, low self-esteem, social isolation, poor employment status, impaired relationships.

Treatment: Introduction and dietary management

Benefits of weight loss

Losing 10 kg is associated with a reduction of:
- >20% total mortality;
- 10 mmHg systolic and 20 mmHg diastolic BP;
- 50% fasting glucose;
- 10% total cholesterol and rise of 8% HDL cholesterol.

Approach to treatment

The most effective treatment of obesity is a multifactorial approach embracing a number of different strategies which should be individualized for maximum effect. The first essential stage of treatment is to assess the individual by determining:
- history of weight gain and previous attempts at reduction;
- current dietary intake, meal patterns, and food preferences;
- current levels of physical activity;
- degree of motivation and whether the individual is ready to change (see 'Communication skills and behaviour change on a one to one level', Chapter 14);
- treatment preferences.

When this information has been elucidated, a treatment package can be worked out, ideally with the patient's assistance.

Dietary management

A plethora of weight-reducing diets is available to the general public ranging from healthy diets with a modest reduction in energy to questionable, complex single-food regimes. The goal of all dietary management in obesity should be to help the individual to reduce their energy intake to an acceptable level while consuming a diet that is adequate in all other nutrients, compatible with good health, practical to follow and can be reconciled with their life style. The approaches described in this section are an outline from which different elements can be combined.

Modified healthy eating or low fat diets

Based on the 'Balance of Good Health' (see 'Food-based dietary guidelines', Chapter 2), a modest energy reduction can be achieved by reducing or eliminating the intake of concentrated calories particularly from fat (see below), increasing fruit and vegetable intake to a minimum of five portions per day and maintaining intake of whole grain cereals, lean meat or fish, and low fat dairy products.

This regime is ideal for encouraging gentle weight loss of 0.5–1.0 kg/week accompanied by a long-term change in eating habits and is suitable for well-motivated individuals. Although individuals who are looking for a rapid response may find the rate of weight loss and long-term commitment unacceptable, a recent systematic review[1] has shown that low fat diets produce a significant weight loss up to 36 months (–3.55 kg, 95% CI, –4.54 to –2.55 kg).

[1] Avenell, A., et al. (2004). What are the long-term benefits of weight reducing diets in adults? A systematic review of randomized controlled trials. *J. Hum. Nutr. Dietet.* **17**, 317–35.

ow carbohydrate diets

ow carbohydrate diets, also known as protein sparing modified fasts, are efined as providing ≤40 g/d carbohydrate. Recent interest in these egimes has focused on the widespread popularity and apparent success f the Atkins® diet. This advises an initial 2-week reduction in carbohy-rate intake to <20 g per day while eating unrestricted amounts of pro-ein, including poultry, fish, eggs, and red meat, and fats such as butter nd olive oil. The ongoing weight loss and then maintenance programme dvise continued but less stringent carbohydrate restriction.

Low carbohydrate diets are associated with a greater weight loss at months (but not at 12 months) than a conventional low fat diet. ong-term studies are required to evaluate changes in nutritional status, ardiovascular risk factors, and adverse effects.[2]

tructured weight loss plans

hese regimes are designed to be followed for a limited period of time uring which a detailed, prescribed menu is followed. Ideally, this should rovide ~500 kcal per day less than the pre-dieting intake and include dequate nutrients. The advantage for some participants is the comfort f having a structured eating pattern especially if this is accompanied by egular weight loss. Some programmes are associated with regular upport meetings where participants are weighed and motivated by their ader and fellow weight reducers.

he disadvantages can include:
   additional expense;
   rigidity of some regimes;
   hard to follow, particularly in the context of a busy family or work life;
   designed to be followed for a limited period of time;
   no contribution to long-term healthier eating practices (although some have associated weight-maintenance programmes).

xamples include Weight Watchers® (www.weightwatchers.co.uk) and limming World® (www.slimming-world.co.uk).

Concentrated calories—and some alternatives

Fried foods	Grill, roast, or bake without fat or oil
Butter/margarine	Soften and spread thinly or use low fat spreads
Oil/cooking fat	Use non-stick pans and 'dry fry'
Salad dressings	Choose low fat options or use vinegar/mustard
Pastry	Mashed potato or bread crumbs on top of dishes
Full fat milk	Semi-skimmed or skimmed
Double cream	Diet yogurt or fromage frais or custard made from skimmed milk
Sugar/honey	Cultivate a preference for less sweet taste or use artificial sweet-eners
Jam/marmalade	Sugar-free fruit spreads or savoury spreads
Confectionery	Fresh fruit or limited amounts of dried fruit
Sugary soft drinks	Water, low calorie alternatives, tea
Alcohol	Limit intake and use low-calorie mixers

Astrup, A., et al. (2004). Atkins and other low-carbohydrate diets; hoax or an effective tool for eight loss? *Lancet.* **364**, 897–9.

Calorie counting

This is based on the simple concept of reducing energy intake to a level below total energy expenditure—fundamental to weight loss—but is not necessarily compatible with optimum nutritional intake or promoting long-term health. However, some people appreciate the flexibility of being able to plan their own intake and vary this from day to day, including 'naughty' items that conventionally are not encouraged on a weight reducing diet: it is possible but not desirable to construct a low calorie diet based on chocolate, crisps, and beer. Lists of the calorie contents of a wide range of foods are available from most bookshops.

Very low calorie diets (VLCD)

VLCDs are defined as diets providing <1000 kcal/d although some may provide as little as 400 kcal/d. Commercial VLCDs are usually liquid, milk-based drinks or soups, which aim to provide the consumer's total nutrient requirements within a day's limited energy format (Table 17.3). Comparable diets can be made at home from milk but require adequate micronutrient supplementation. A review of studies has shown that VLCDs are effective in bringing about short-term (4–8 week) weight loss and, in some but not all patients, this is maintained over a longer period of time.[3] Concerns have been raised about a reduction in lean body mass associated with rapid weight loss and the absence of re-education about long-term eating habits. VLCDs are contraindicated in individuals who have a history of, or are at risk from cardiac disease, cerebrovascular accident, renal or liver disease, hyperuricaemia, porphyria, or psychiatric disturbances.

Meal replacement

Similar to the 'complete nutrition' concept of very low calorie diets, meal replacement programmes provide the weight reducer with a range of food items that contribute an intake limited in energy but supplemented with micronutrients. The food items vary but include milk shakes, soups, cereal-type snack bars, and pre-prepared meals. Most programmes give the consumer the flexibility to select from interchangeable formats within a total calorie intake and may include one 'normal' but calorie-counted meal. Some also provide lifestyle guidance on increasing physical activity. However, as individuals are able to purchase these from supermarkets, chemists, and by mail order, they frequently do not have input from health-care professionals. The disadvantages of such products include the expense, limited flexibility, and lack of long-term education to support permanent changes in lifestyle.

A recent RCT[4] of four commercial weight-loss diets[5] available in the UK showed all resulted in significant ↓ body fat and weight compared to controls after 6 months with no significant difference in loss between the diets.

---

[3] Jebb, S.A. and Goldberg, G.R. (1998). Efficacy of very low-energy diets and meal replacements in the treatment of obesity. *J. Hum. Nutr. Dietet.* **11**, 219–25.

[4] Truby H *et al* (2006). Randomised controlled trial of four commercial weight loss programmes in the UK: initial findings from the BBC "diet trials". *BMJ* **332**, 1309-1314.

[5] Dr Atkins' new diet revolution, Slim-Fast plan, Weight Watchers pure points programme, Rosemary Conley's eat yourself slim diet and fitness plan.

Table 17.3 Composition of liquid VLCDs

	Cambridge Diet® (3 servings)	Optifast® (3 servings)	Skimmed milk (3 pints)
Energy (kcal)	415	480	594
Protein (g)	43	42	59
Carbohydrate (g)	42	60	90
Fat (g)	8	9	1.8
Micronutrients	supplemented	supplemented	supplementation required

Treatment: Physical activity and behavioural therapy

Physical activity

Increasing energy expenditure is an effective way of reducing weight and preventing weight gain. Additional benefits associated with regular exercise, independent of weight loss, include ↑ sense of well-being and reduced risk of ill health including diabetes, cardiovascular disease, and some cancers. Significant weight loss has been observed after 6–12 month following 2–4 episodes per week of aerobic activity (at 70% maximum physical capacity) each lasting 20–45 minutes.

Physical exercise alone is less effective than dietary modification but ideally both should be used together.

Relatively few side-effects have been reported but range from mild (e.g. minor trauma) to severe (e.g. myocardial infarction) predominantly in individuals with morbid obesity. As the latter have most to gain from losing weight, they require appropriate advice about increasing everyday physical activities, like walking, rather than embarking on an over-taxing exercise programme. The UK-based Walking Health Initiative encourages individuals to take a minimum of 10 000 steps per day monitored using a pedometer: http://www.whi.org.uk.

Behavioural therapy

Strategies to change behaviour relating to weight management include cognitive behavioural therapy. Meta-analysis of studies using behavioural change strategies, either alone or in conjunction with other treatments found the greatest weight loss at 12 months was associated with a combination of behavioural therapy, diet, and sibutramine.[6] 'see Communication skills and behaviour change on a one to one level', Chapter 14 and Table 17.4.

[6] Avenell, A., et al. (2004). What interventions should we add to weight reducing diets in adult with obesity? A systematic review of randomized controlled trials of adding drug therapy, exercise, behaviour therapy or combinations of these interventions. *J. Hum. Nutr. Dietet.* **17** 293–316.

Table 17.4 Examples of behaviour strategies for weight reduction

- Shop for food only after eating and buy items from a list
- Eat all food whilst sitting down in one place and at planned times
- Serve food on a smaller plate; if possible, ask some one else to serve
- Put down fork between each mouthful
- Chew each mouthful thoroughly
- Concentrate on eating and enjoying food
- Do nothing else while eating (e.g. watching TV)
- Leave table as soon as meal is completed
- Differentiate between hunger and the urge to eat
- Identify situations that might lead to a lapse; plan how to cope with these
- Set realistic goals for improved eating and weight loss
- Plan rewards for goals achieved

Pharmacotherapy for obesity

Two drugs are licensed in the UK for the treatment of obesity: orlistat and sibutramine. RCTs show that both are an effective adjunct to dietary treatment and associated with a weight loss of 2–5 kg greater than that of control groups at 2 years.

Orlistat (Xenical®) reduces calorie intake by blocking digestive lipases reducing GI absorption of fatty acids, cholesterol, and fat-soluble vitamins and increasing faecal fat excretion. Side-effects include oily rectal discharge (27%) and faecal incontinence (8%). ↓ Blood fat-soluble vitamins has been observed but no clinical deficiencies have been reported. National Institute for Clinical Excellence (NICE) guidance on use:[1]

- Prescribe only for people who have lost ≥2.5 kg by diet and exercise in last month and have a BMI ≥30 kg/m^2 (≥28 kg/m^2 if significant co-morbidities).
- Arrange concomitant advice on diet, physical activity, and lifestyle change.
- Only continue beyond 3 months if lost at least 5% of body weight since starting treatment.
- Only continue beyond 6 months if lost at least 10% of body weight since starting treatment.
- Treatment should not usually be continued for >12 months and never >24 months.

Sibutramine (Reductil®) reduces calorie intake by inducing early satiety through blocking re-uptake of serotonin and noradrenaline in the brain. Side-effects include increase in heart rate, constipation, sleep problems (>10%), and palpitations, nausea, dizziness, headache (1–10%). On discontinuation, headache and ↑ appetite have been reported in rare cases. NICE guidance for use:[2]

- Prescribe only for people (18–65 years) with a BMI ≥30 kg/m^2 (≥27 kg/m^2 if significant co-morbidities).
- Prescribe only for people who have made previous serious attempts to lose weight.
- Monitor and arrange concomitant advice on diet, physical activity, and lifestyle change.
- Normal starting dose = 10 mg/d. Only continue beyond 4 weeks if lost ≥2 kg but can increase dose to 15 mg/d.
- Only continue beyond 3 months if lost ≥15% of body weight since starting treatment.
- Check BP regularly. Do not prescribe if BP >145/90 mm Hg or if diastolic or systolic BP increases by >10 mm Hg or if resting pulse rate rises by >10 beats/min.
- Treatment should not be continued for >12 months.
- No evidence to support co-prescribing sibutramine and orlistat.

---

[1] www.nice.org.uk/pdf/orlistatguidance.pdf (for review autumn 2006)
[2] http://www.nice.org.UK/pdf/sibutramineguidance.pdf (for review autumn 2006)

Role of the dietitian in weight management

Registered dietitians are well-placed to play a role in weight management programmes having been trained in nutritional science and its application and communication. Their contribution may include the following.

- One-to-one sessions with individuals, evaluating their energy intake and expenditure and readiness to embark on necessary lifestyle changes. Patients can expect practical lifestyle advice (dietary, activity, and motivational) that is tailored to their needs with the dietitian acting as a facilitator or enabler on how to make the necessary behaviour changes.
- Running group programme covering topics such as those in Table 17.5. Sessions can be run for general or specific groups (e.g. men only, over-60s, etc.) and may be open to self- or GP-referred patients.
- Educating other health professionals by running training days for GPs, practice nurses, etc. This might include information about prevalence and effects of obesity, when to refer, weight loss services available locally (NHS, voluntary, and commercial), morbid obesity.
- Obesity prevention through health promotion services and nutrition policy (see 'Example of nutrition policy in different settings', Chapter 15).

Table 17.5 Topics for group weight loss programmes

- Do you want to lose weight — are you ready to change ?
- Realistic goals
- What is a healthy diet ?
- Overcoming temptation
- Stepping up activity
- Supermarket tour — shopping tips to save calories
- Cutting calories in cooking
- Eating out — how to choose sensibly and still enjoy your meal
- Keeping going when things get difficult
- Looking to the future and weight maintenance

Bariatric surgery and alternative treatments

Bariatric surgery

Several different surgical procedures are available for the treatment of obesity and are associated with significant weight loss and reduction in risk factors in individuals with BMI ≥40 kg/m^2.

NICE guidance Surgery is recommended as a treatment option for people with morbid obesity (≥40 kg/m^2 or 35–40 kg/m^2 with significant co-morbidities) providing the individual fulfils the following criteria.

- Has received intensive management from a specialized hospital obesity clinic.
- Aged ≥18 years.
- Evidence that all other available methods of weight loss have been tried and have failed.
- No specific clinical or psychological contradictions to this surgery.
- Fit for anaesthesia and surgery.
- Understands need for long-term follow-up.

Vertical banded gastroplasty Stomach is surgically stapled to create ~30 ml pouch that restricts intake of food at any one time. Associated with weight loss (40–65% of pre-surgery weight lost after 5 years). Re-operation required in 20% within 5–10 years. Fewer serious long-term consequences.

Gastric bypass Small section of upper stomach is formed into a pouch and anastomosed on to proximal jejunum, which limits food intake and bypasses most of stomach and duodenum resulting in some malabsorption. Associated with significant weight loss (50–75% of pre-surgery weight lost after 5 years). Long-term complications include anaemia and incisional hernia.

Gastric banding Formation of stomach pouch using a tight band applied via keyhole surgery. Less invasive than gastroplasty or bypass. Band can be adjusted to change size of pouch using fluid injected via subcutaneous port. Associated with weight loss (mean 37 kg in 58% of patients at 5 years). Fewer short-term complications associated with procedure but long term, 35% of bands required removal due to band slippage, pouch dilatation and erosion.

Other Jejuno-ileal bypass, bilio-pancreatic diversion, and jaw wiring are older procedures that are now rarely undertaken.

Post-surgical dietary management Short term — sips of fluid and small (15–30 g portions), frequent intake of semisolid foods gradually increasing on to a nutrient-dense diet including pured meat, fish, yogurt, mashed potato, fruit juice. Long term—continue on small, nutrient-dense meals with increasing variety determined by trial and error, avoiding concentrated sources of energy or large quantities that may lead to gastrointestinal symptoms. Stop eating when pouch full and drink separately from eating allowing at least 1 hour between. Daily multivitamin supplementation s recommended (adequacy of B vitamins, especially B_{12} is a concern). See www.nice.org.uk/Docref.asp?d=34793.

Alternative treatments

As conventional treatment of obesity is often unsuccessful in the long term, there is considerable interest in novel and alternative approaches to weight reduction. These include acupuncture, herbs, aromatherapy, and hypnosis. A systematic review of 517 published studies drew no conclusions on the effects of alternative treatments for obesity.[1]

Obesity prevention See 'Examples of nutrition policy in different settings', Chapter 15.

[1] Östman, J., Britton, M., and Jonsson, E. (Eds.) (2004). *Treating and preventing obesity: an evidence-based review.* Wiley-VCH, Weinheim.

Conditions associated with obesity

Polycystic ovary syndrome (PCOS)

Approximately 4–10% of women of child-bearing age have PCOS, which is associated with raised androgen levels and an irregular menstrual cycle ± ovarian cysts. Common nutritional features include abdominal weight gain and the characteristics associated with metabolic syndrome (insulin resistance leading to type 2 diabetes, hyperlipidaemia, and hypertension). Reduced fertility and abnormal menstrual cycles are associated with obesity and hyperinsulinaemia and there is ↑ long-term risk of heart disease.

Management

Weight loss in obese women is associated with the resumption of ovulation and ↑ fertility; relatively small losses of ~ 6 kg have been shown to be beneficial. Modification of dietary intake and physical activity is thus considered first-line treatment.

Prader–Willi syndrome

Prader–Willi syndrome (PWS) is a complex, genetic disorder associated with excessive appetite, low muscle tone, emotional instability, immature physical development, and learning disabilities. Although infants with PWS may have feeding difficulties leading to growth faltering, children aged over 1 year often gain weight very rapidly due to hyperphagia. An estimated 3000 individuals in the UK have PWS.

Management

A paediatric dietitian should give individual dietary advice and, ideally, the whole family should be involved. The goal of dietary management is to achieve a nutritionally balanced intake with an appropriate energy intake to treat or prevent obesity. Compliance is often very poor due to an insatiable appetite and sometimes locking fridges and food stores may be required. A number of ethical issues surround the need to protect individuals with PWS as they are incapable of acting independently in relation to food. More information is available from the Prader–Willi Syndrome Association UK, http://pwsa.co.uk/.

Diabetes

Classification and prevalence

Classification

Diabetes is a metabolic disorder characterized by chronic hyperglycaemia with disturbances of carbohydrate, fat, and protein metabolism resulting from defects in insulin secretion, insulin action, or both. See Table 18.1.

- Type 1 diabetes can occur at any age but usually develops in children or adults aged <40 years (previously referred to as insulin dependent diabetes, IDDM). This occurs as a result of lack of insulin production by the pancreatic β cells. It requires treatment with insulin and dietary management.
- Type 2 diabetes is usually diagnosed in older adults but is increasingly seen in younger adults and some children (previously referred to as non-insulin dependent diabetes, NIDDM). It is associated with a lack of insulin function as a result of insulin resistance with or without insufficient production and is strongly associated with overweight and obesity. Dietary management is required, with or without oral hypoglycaemic agents or insulin.
- Gestational diabetes is hyperglycaemia diagnosed during pregnancy that had not been previously diagnosed. Dietary advice is advisable and some patients may also require insulin.

Insulin resistance

There is considerable variation in the cellular response to insulin by different individuals. A lower than normal response is described as insulin resistance. This includes reduced glucose uptake by the skeletal muscles and/or liver, reduced lipolysis in adipose tissue, and altered amino acid metabolism either alone or in combination. As a consequence, blood glucose levels remain high and lead to further stimulation of the pancreas to release more insulin. Insulin resistance increases with overweight and obesity.

Prevalence

Globally, ~ 170 million individuals have diabetes. In the UK, ~ 1.8 million people (3% of population) have been diagnosed with the condition and the majority of these (80–90%) have type 2 diabetes. It is estimated that a further million individuals may have undiagnosed type 2 diabetes. The prevalence increases with age (Fig. 18.1) and lower socio-economic status and varies with ethnicity (~ 20% South Asian community and ~ 17% African Caribbean community). Increasing rates of obesity are closely associated with rising prevalence of diabetes and it is estimated that 3 million people in the UK and 255 million globally will be diagnosed with the condition by 2010.

The overall incidence of diabetes can be reduced by preventing and reducing overweight and obesity, particularly central (abdominal) obesity. Individuals at risk can reduce this by eating a balanced diet, losing weight and increasing their physical activity levels.

Table 18.1 Values for diagnosing diabetes mellitus and other categories of hyperglycaemia*

	Glucose concentration (mmol/l)	
	Capillary blood	Venous plasma
Diabetes mellitus		
Fasting *or*	≥6.1	≥7.0
2 h post-glucose load	≥11.1	≥11.1
Impaired glucose tolerance		
Fasting *and*	<6.1	<7.0
2 h post-glucose load	≥7.8	≥7.8
Impaired fasting glycaemia		
Fasting	≥5.6 and <6.1	≥6.1 and <7.0

* World Health Organization (1999). *Definition, diagnosis and classification of diabetes mellitus and its complications. Report of a WHO consultation. Part 1: Diagnosis and classification of diabetes mellitus* (WHO/NCD/NCS/99.2). World Health Organization, Geneva.

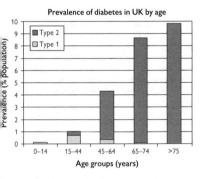

Fig. 18.1 Prevalence of diabetes in UK by age (2003). (Data calculated from figures kindly provided by Diabetes UK, the charity for people with diabetes, from Diabetes UK Report 2004 and from UK population 2003 from ONS: http://www.statistics.gov.uk/statbase/Expodata/Spreadsheets/D8548.xls).

Contributing causes and clinical consequences

Contributing causes

Type 1 diabetes Insulin secretion by the pancreatic β cells is reduced following damage mediated by an autoimmune T-cell reaction. Environmental factors, such as viral infection, may be implicated.

Type 2 diabetes is closely associated with obesity and genetic factors. Approximately 15–25% of first-degree relatives of people with type 2 diabetes develop impaired glucose tolerance or diabetes. However, the substantial contribution made by obesity is particularly important as this is a potentially modifiable risk factor. Excess body fat, stored as lipid in the adipocytes, is associated with ↑ levels of circulating hormones, cytokines, and metabolic fuels (e.g. free fatty acids), which modulate the effect of insulin. Large adipocytes, especially in abdominal fat, are resistant to the lipolytic effects of insulin, which leads to a further release and then increase in circulating free fatty acids. These changes inhibit the insulin signalling cascade resulting in impaired glucose metabolism in skeletal muscle and stimulated hepatic gluconeogenesis with consequent hyperglycaemia.

Clinical consequences

Diabetes is associated with ↑ risk of serious chronic ill health, disability and premature mortality. Long-term complications include macrovascular disease, leading to cardiovascular disease and ↑ risk of stroke, and microvascular disease leading to retinopathy, nephropathy, and neuropathy. People with diabetes also have a greater risk of suffering from infections, cataracts and depression. Many of these complications can be minimized or avoided by earlier diagnosis and more effective treatment (see box).

Benefits of good blood glucose control in type 1 and type 2 diabetes (Diabetes Control and Complications Trial 1993; UK Prospective Diabetes Study 1998):

- New eye disease risk reduced by 76%
- Worsening of existing eye disease reduced by 54%
- Early kidney disease risk reduced by 54%
- More serious kidney problems reduced by 39%
- Nerve damage risk reduced by 60%
- Heart disease risk reduced by 56%
- Stroke risk reduced by 44%
- Kidney disease risk reduced by up to 33%

Goals and principles of dietary management

Goals of dietary management

- To maintain or improve health through the use of appropriate and healthy food choices.
- To achieve and maintain optimal metabolic and physiological outcomes including:
  - reduction of risk for microvascular disease by achieving near normal glycaemia without undue risk of hypoglycaemia;
  - reduction of risk of macrovascular disease including management of body weight, dyslipidaemia, and hypertension.
- To optimize outcomes in diabetic nephropathy and in any concomitant disorder such as coeliac disease or cystic fibrosis.

Dietary advice should be placed within a holistic context of care which includes supporting patients to manage their diabetes and make decisions; it should also complement other treatment including pharmacological, physical activity, behavioural, and smoking cessation programmes. If it is to be effective, dietary advice must take account of the individual's personal preferences, cultural background, and lifestyle.

Principles of dietary management

People with diabetes do not need to follow a 'special diet' or comply with narrow restrictions and measured portions of food that were considered central to dietary advice in previous years (but see DAFNE, in 'New approaches to diabetes education', this chapter). However, eating well is important for good diabetes control and can contribute to improved well-being. The optimum healthy choice of food for people with diabetes is the same as for the general population (see 'Balance of Good Health' in 'Food-based dietary guidelines', Chapter 2) and ideally should be low in fat, sugar, and salt, include plenty of fruit and vegetables, and base meals on starchy foods such as bread, potatoes, and rice (Table 18.2). Patients with newly diagnosed diabetes should be referred for individual advice to a dietitian and afterwards receive an annual dietetic review.

Eight steps to healthy eating in diabetes[1]

The composition of optimum diet above must be translated into practical advice which gives patients guidance about what they should eat. This should be facilitated on an individual basis by a registered dietitian. The following guidelines provide a rough starting point:

1. Eat regular meals based on starchy carbohydrate foods such as bread, potatoes, rice, pasta, and chapattis. Choose wholegrain foods where possible, e.g. wholemeal bread, oats, and whole grain cereals.

---

[1] © Diabetes UK. This information has been reproduced from the Diabetes UK website (July 2006) (www.diabetes.org.uk) with the kind permission of Diabetes UK.

Table 18.2 Composition of the optimum diet in diabetes*

Protein	≤1 g/kg body weight
Total fat	<35% of energy intake
Saturated & transunsaturated fat	<10% of energy intake
n-6 polyunsaturated fat	<10% of energy intake
n-3 polyunsaturated fat	Eat fish, especially oily fish, once or twice weekly. Supplements not recommended
cis-monounsaturated fat	10–20% of energy intake[‡]
Total carbohydrate[†]	45–60% of energy intake[‡]
Sugar	Up to 10% of energy provided eaten in context of healthy diet
Fibre	No quantitative recommendation. Soluble fibre has beneficial effect on glycaemic and lipid metabolism. Insoluble fibre also has health benefits
Vitamins and anti-oxidants	Encourage foods naturally rich in vitamins and antioxidants. Supplements are not recommended
Salt	≤6 g NaCl per day

* Adapted from World Health Organization (http://www.who.int) (1999) *Definition, Diagnosis and Classification of Diabetes Mellitus and its Complications.* Report of WHO Consultation Reproduced with permission.

[†] See 'Glycaemic index', this section and in 'Carbohydrate', Chapter 5.

[‡] 60–70% of energy intake should come from combined monounsaturated fat and carbohydrate.

2. Reduce intake of fat, especially animal fat. Eat less butter, margarine, cheese, and fatty meat and instead choose low fat dairy foods like skimmed milk and low fat yogurt. Replace fried foods with grilled, steamed, or oven baked items. Use small quantities of mono-unsaturated oil, e.g. olive oil or rapeseed oil.
3. Eat more fruit and vegetables—aim for five portions per day.
4. Reduce sugar and sugary foods. Following a strict sugar-free diet is not necessary—sugar can be used as an ingredient in foods, e.g. in many wholegrain breakfast cereals. Sugary drinks can be replaced by sugar-free or diet alternatives.
5. Cut down on salt. Herbs and spices can be used as an alternative.
6. Limit alcohol to two units per day for women and three units per day for men. Avoid drinking alcohol on an empty stomach as it may contribute to hypoglycaemia.
7. Lose weight if overweight by trying to reduce at a rate of 0.5–1.0 kg/ week (See 'Weight management', this chapter). Avoid crash diets.
8. Diabetic food products are not necessary and do not contribute to a healthy diet.

Glycaemic index

The glycaemic index (GI) aims to quantify the blood sugar response after eating specific foods. This has potential significance in diabetes where fluctuations or rapid increases in blood sugar are undesirable. However, the issue is complex and GI values vary considerably depending on the exact nature of the food (e.g. method of processing or cooking, degree of ripeness, or strain of plant) and whether they are eaten alone or accompanying a meal providing mixed macronutrients. At present, it is recommended that using GI values to provide a broad guide to a food's glycaemic effect may be a helpful adjunct to other dietary issues, but that it should not be relied upon as the most important feature of food-related advice (see 'Glycaemic index' in 'Carbohydrates', Chapter 5).

Lower GI	Oats and oat products, pulses, peas, beans, legumes, pasta, unripe fruit, milk, and plain yogurt
Moderate GI	Rice, granary, pitta, and rye bread, new potatoes, muesli
Higher GI	White and wholemeal bread, wheat- and corn-based breakfast cereals, old potatoes, mashed potatoes, fruit juice, honey

Diet and insulin

The hypoglycaemic action of injected insulin should be balanced against the glycaemic effects of consuming carbohydrate. Ideally, the insulin prescribed should be selected on the basis of the compatibility of its timing and mode of action with each patient's lifestyle and meal habits rather than the other way round.

The availability of short-, intermediate-, and long-acting insulin and the ability to administer these via a pen-like injection device increases the flexibility of insulin regimes to meet most meal patterns. However, individuals with very erratic lifestyles and eating habits will benefit from more regular intake of food although this does not need to follow a rigid, clock-watching meal pattern. Rapid-acting analogue insulin starts to work within 5–15 minutes of injection and ∴ eating some carbohydrate within this time period is necessary (see Tables 18.3 and 18.4). All patients taking insulin, but particularly those taking analogue insulin, must be aware of the possibility of hypoglycaemia (see 'Hypoglycaemia' in 'Diet and oral hypoglycaemic dugs', this chapter).

As insulin is anabolic, increasing the dose to control the glycaemic effects of excessive food intake may lead to weight gain and potentially to a cycle of worsening blood sugar control. It is important ∴ that dietary advice to people taking insulin does not simply focus on the short-term glycaemic effects of food and the need to balance the effects of insulin but also incorporates other aspects of the diet described above.

Table 18.3 Analogue insulins

Non-proprietary name	Proprietary name
Insulin aspart	NovoRapid
Insulin detemir	Levemir
Insulin glargine	Lantus
Insulin lispro	Humalog

Table 18.4 Examples of commonly used insulins*

Proprietary name (manufacturer)	Source	Form†	Injection‡	Effect§		
				Onset	Peak	End
Rapid-acting analogue						
Humalog (Lilly)	Analogue	CPV	−15 to +5	0.1	0.2–2	4
NovoRapid (Novo Nordisk)	Analogue	CPV	−15 to +5	0.1	0.2–3	4.5
Short-acting insulins						
Actrapid (Novo Nordisk)	Human	CPV	−30	0.1	0.5–2.5	8
Humulin S (Lilly)	Human	CV	−45 to −20	0.1	0.5–2.5	7
Medium & long-acting insulins						
Hypurin Bovine PZI (Wockhardt UK)	Beef	V	−30	4	10–20	36
Insulatard (Novo Nordisk)	Human	CDV	−30	0.1	1–12	24
Insuman Basal (Sanofi–Aventis)	Human	CPV	−60 to −45	0.1	1.5–4	20
Mixed insulins						
Humulin 3M (Lilly)	Human	CP	−45 to −20	0.1	1–8	22
Hypurin Porcine 30/70 (Wockhardt UK)	Pork	CV	−30 to −15	0.1	4–12	24
Mixtard 30 (Novo Nordisk)	Human	DPV	−30	0.1	0.5–8	24
Analogue mixture						
Humalog Mix 25 (Lilly)	Analogue	CP	−15 to +5	0.2	0.5–2.5	22
NovoMix 30 (Novo Nordisk)	Analogue	CP	−15 to +5	0.1	0.5–4	24
Long-acting analogues						
Lantus (Sanofi-Aventis)	Analogue	CPV	1 × daily	0.1	—	24
Levemir (Novo Nordisk)	Analogue	CP	1–2 × daily	0.1	—	24

* © Diabetes UK. This information has been reproduced from Balance, July–August issue 2005: p 44–45, with the kind permission of Diabetes UK.
† C, Cartridge; D, pre-filled insulin doser; P, pre-filled pen; V, vial.
‡ Optimum time (minutes) of injection in relation to food or, for medium-and long-acting insulin, in relation to bedtime.
§ Approximate time (hours) after injection for effect on blood sugar.

Dietary management of adults treated with insulin analogues[1]

- Dose of insulin should be adjusted primarily on the basis of the CHO content of the meal and in response to blood glucose monitoring before and 2 hours after meals
- If blood glucose increases by >3 mmol/l after meals, review ratio of insulin to CHO
- Post-prandial injection should be considered if a meal will provide a variable CHO load, e.g. buffet or carvery, or if it will result in a reduced post-meal blood glucose, e.g. a low GI or high fat meal
- Pre-prandial injection is preferable if blood glucose >8 mmol/l even if meal will provide slowly absorbed CHO
- Consider splitting dose of rapid-acting analogue if meal is low GI or high fat to avoid delayed hypoglycaemia
- Consider reducing dose of rapid-acting analogue if meal is low GI or high fat but be aware this may result in post-prandial hyperglycaemia
- Late-evening snacks are usually unnecessary with long-acting analogues but should be based on blood glucose levels and patient preference after 2-week adjustment period
- Late-evening snack may be necessary with long-acting analogues if large amounts of alcohol are consumed
- An extra bolus of rapid-acting analogue may be necessary in patients treated with long-acting analogues if between meal snacks provide >15 g CHO
- Dose of rapid-acting analogue may need to be reduced for exercise depending on CHO intake and strenuousness, duration, and timing of exercise
- No additional insulin bolus should be given if extra CHO has been taken to compensate for effect of exercise
- If long-acting analogues result in increases in blood glucose towards end of 24-hour period, consider changing timing of injection

[1] Adapted From Vaughan, L., *et al.* (2005). *Suggested good practice for dietitians involved in the dietetic management of adults with type 1 diabetes treated with insulin analogues.* Reproduced with permission from the Diabetes Management and Education Group of the British Dietetic Association

Diet and oral hypoglycaemic drugs and hypoglycaemia

Diet and oral hypoglycaemic drugs

If fasting blood sugar concentrations cannot be maintained below 7 mmol/l by diet alone in type 2 diabetes, oral hypoglycaemic drugs may be prescribed. Taking this medication does not change the goals or principles of the optimum diet described above but patients should be aware of the potential for weight gain if prescribed sulphonylurea or thiazolinediones and of the small possibility of hypoglycaemia.

Hypoglycaemia

Acute hypoglycaemia should be treated with 10–20 g of glucose orally in conscious patients. If this is not available, regular sugar (sucrose) or sugary drink can be given, although this will not be effective in patients taking the α-glucosidase inhibitor, acarbose.

On recovery, a further 10–20 g of slower-acting carbohydrate (see box) should be given unless the next meal or snack is due, in which case this should be eaten as usual.

Frequent episodes of hypoglycaemia may be resolved by eating smaller quantities of food more frequently but, if ongoing, the treatment regimen should be reviewed.

Suitable snacks after initial recovery from 'hypos'

- Sandwich—ideally made from wholegrain bread
- Bowl of wholegrain or oat-based cereal
- Banana and glass of semi-skimmed milk
- Oat cakes

New approaches to diabetes education

DAFNE The Dose Adjustment For Normal Eating trial was initiated in the UK in 1999 using a 5-day structured training programme in intensive insulin therapy and self-management. The principles are to teach flexible insulin adjustment to match carbohydrate in a free diet on a meal-by-meal basis with an emphasis on self-management and independence from the diabetes care team. Nutrition education sessions cover how to identify macronutrients in the diet and estimate carbohydrate portions, weight control, and healthy eating. Although this intensive programme has only been undertaken in a limited number of centres, initial results suggest improved glycaemic control and quality of life and the programme is being expanded to more areas in the UK.

DESMOND The Diabetes Education and Self-Management for Ongoing and Newly Diagnosed programme is a similar, multicentred, structured educational approach but designed for people with type 2 diabetes. An evaluative randomized controlled trial is currently being undertaken.

Weight management and monitoring glycaemic control

Weight management

More than 80% of people diagnosed with type 2 diabetes are overweight. Weight management in both type 1 and type 2 diabetes is important to help to reduce insulin resistance, control blood glucose levels, and lower the risk of long-term complications. Although preventing weight gain and/or reducing excess body weight can be very challenging, it is central to optimizing diabetes care and is a cornerstone in the dietary management of diabetes. A multifaceted approach utilizing dietary and physical activity advice, drug therapy, and behavioural support is required (see Fig. 18.2).

Monitoring of glycaemic control

Glycosylated haemoglobin (HbA1$_c$) should be measured at least annually. Values ≤7% are considered a desirable target for most patients with type 1 and type 2 diabetes, and are associated with a reduced risk of complications.

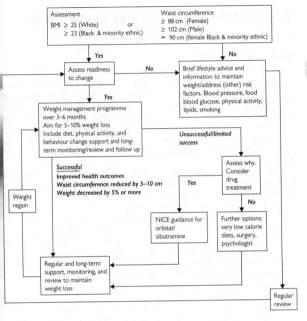

Fig. 18.2 Algorithm for weight management in diabetes. Figure kindly provided by Diabetes UK, the charity for people with diabetes.)

Gestational diabetes and diabetes in children and adolescents

Gestational diabetes

Gestational diabetes (GDM) is a common (~4% of pregnancies) but usually asymptomatic form of intolerance of carbohydrate leading to hyperglycaemia with onset or first recognition in pregnancy. A standard oral glucose tolerance test resulting in 2-h glucose concentration ≥11.1 mmol/l in either capillary blood or venous plasma confirms diagnosis. In most cases it resolves spontaneously after delivery but it is associated with adverse pregnancy outcomes including large-for-gestational-age babies, congenital abnormalities, and the long-term risk of type 2 diabetes in the mother.

Most cases are treated with nutritional management alone although some women also require insulin. However, few studies have evaluated the efficacy of dietary management. In the absence of firm evidence, it is reasonable to recommend a diet providing:

- adequate nutrition for the mother and fetus (see 'Diet before during pregnancy' Chapter 9). This should meet all the nutrient requirements of pregnancy through the provision of regular meals that include a large component of slowly absorbed carbohydrate;
- energy intake that limits unnecessary maternal weight gain. The minimum recommended pregnancy weight gain in women with gestational diabetes is shown in Table 18.5.
- ◆ Limiting weight gain in pregnancy is controversial but in obese women with GDM is associated with ↓ risk of hypertension, Caesarean section, and large for gestational age babies but no increase in risk of pre-term delivery or small for gestational age babies.

Blood sugar levels should be monitored regularly and insulin dose and frequency adjusted to maintain capillary values between 4.4 and 6.1 mmol/l before meals and <8.6 mmol/l after meals.

Diabetes in children and adolescents

Young people with diabetes should be seen in a designated diabetes clinic by a team who operate both in the hospital and the community and who liaise closely with primary healthcare and school. The team should include a dietitian with expertise in childhood diabetes. Among the dietary management issues that must be considered on an individual basis are:

- the need to provide the nutritional requirements associated with growth as well as the optimum diet for diabetes;
- the psycho-social aspects of dietary intervention in a young person.

Table 18.5 Recommended pregnancy weight gain in women with gestational diabetes

BMI (kg/m^2)	Weight gain (kg)
<25	10–12.5
25–30	7–11.5
30–34	7
>34*	0

*See 'Vulnerable groups in pregnancy', Chapter 9.

Further information on diabetes

1. Dornhorst, A. and Frost, G (2002). The principles of dietary management of gestational diabetes: reflection on current evidence. *J. Hum Nutr. Dietet.* **15**, 145.
2. Jensen, D.M, *et al.*, (2005). Gestational weight gain and pregnancy outcomes in 481 obese glucose tolerant women. *Diabetes Care* **28**, 2118.
3. Nutritional Subcommittee of the Diabetes Care Advisory Committee of Diabetes UK (2003). The implementation of nutritional advice for people with diabetes. *Diabetes Med.* **20**, 786.
4. ▣ DAFNE programme http://www.dafne.uk.com.
5. ▣ Diabetes UK http://www.diabetes.org.uk.
6. ▣ SIGN (2001). Management of diabetes. A national clinical guideline, number 55. Edinburgh: www.sign.ac.uk.

Metabolic syndrome

Metabolic syndrome (MS) is also known as syndrome X and the insulin resistance syndrome. It comprises interrelated factors including obesity (particularly central), insulin resistance, glucose intolerance/diabetes, hyperlipidaemia, and hypertension, all of which predispose to cardiovascular disease.

Consensus diagnostic criteria for metabolic syndrome[1] are:
- central obesity defined as a waist circumference above gender- and ethnicity-specific cut-off values (see Table 18.6); *and*
- two of the following four factors:
  - serum triglycerides ≥1.7 mmol/l or treatment for hypertriglyceridaemia;
  - HDL cholesterol <1.0 mmol/l or treatment for dyslipidaemia;
  - systolic BP ≥130 mm Hg or diastolic BP ≥85 mm Hg or treatment for previously diagnosed hypertension;
  - fasting plasma glucose ≥5.6 mmol/l or previously diagnosed type 2 diabetes.

The individual components of metabolic syndrome can be treated by a healthy diet based on the 'Balance of Good Health' (see 'Food-based dietary guidelines', Chapter 2) and incorporating specific advice relevant to the factors present (e.g. diabetes or dyslipidaemia). The fundamental clinical message is that, to avoid this syndrome, people should avoid excessive weight gain and stay physically active.

[1] Taken from the *IDF consensus worldwide definition of the metabolic syndrome*. Available online at www.idf.org. Reproduced with permission from the International Diabetes Federation.

Table 18.6 Cut-off values for identifying central obesity[*]

Country/ethnic group	Waist circumference (cm)	
	Male	Female
Europids	≥94	≥80
South Asians & Chinese	≥90	≥80
Japanese	≥85	≥90
South & Central Americans	Use South Asian data[†]	
Mediterranean & Middle Eastern	Use European data[†]	

[*] International Diabetes Federation (2005). *Rationale for new IDF worldwide definition of metabolic syndrome.*
Available at: http://www.idf.org/webdata/docs/metabolic_syndrome_rationale.pdf. Accessed Sep 7, 2005.
[†] Until specific data available.

Cardiovascular disease

Classification, prevalence, and contributing causes

Classification

Cardiovascular disease (CVD) includes the following.

- Coronary heart disease—narrowing of the lumen of arteries supplying blood to the heart muscle as a result of atheromatous plaque on the arterial walls. This limits the blood supply to the heart muscle causing pain (angina) and breathlessness on exertion. Damaged plaque leads to a clotting response, which may result in a thrombus detaching from the artery wall and occluding the lumen with subsequent heart muscle death (myocardial infarction).
- Cerebral infarction—thrombus occlusion of an artery supplying blood to the brain leading to irreversible damage to brain tissue (stroke or transient ischaemic attack). The thrombus may arise from atheromatous plaque from within the brain or another blood vessel and the risk of occlusion is ↑ in narrowed arteries.
- Peripheral vascular disease—atheromatous plaque leads to narrowing of peripheral blood vessels, most commonly in the legs. This results in poor blood supply and pain on exertion (claudication).

Prevalence

Globally, CVD is the greatest cause of death, ~ 18 million (33%) per year. The prevalence is increasing rapidly in most countries with the highest rates reported in those with a Western diet and lifestyle although rates are also rising in developing countries in parallel with obesity. Countries in the former Soviet Union are currently among those with the highest standardized death rates from coronary heart disease (Fig. 19.1).

The CVD mortality rate (Table 19.1) has fallen in the UK since peak levels in the early 1970s, probably because of improvements in management and treatment of risk factors, although CVD remains the most common cause of death.

CVD prevalence is higher in men than women before the menopause and increases with age. It is higher in Scotland and the north of England compared to the south of England and is higher than average in lower socio-economic groups and South Asians.

Table 19.1 Deaths and morbidity from cardiovascular disease in the UK

	Number(%)		
	Total	Male	Female
CVD deaths all	238 000 (39)	113 000	125 000
CVD deaths, ≤75 years	68 000 (31)	45 000	23 000
Myocardial infarction*	1 200 000 (2)	838 000	394 000
Angina*	1 920 000 (3)	1 000 000	920 000

*Ever experienced, all ages.

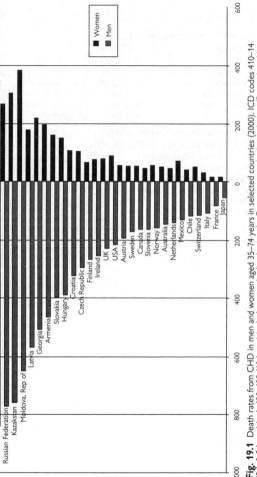

Fig. 19.1 Death rates from CHD in men and women aged 35–74 years in selected countries (2000). ICD codes 410–14 (8th & 9th revision), 120–125 (10th revision). Age-standardized using the European standard population. (Reproduced by permission from the British Heart Foundation, coronary heart statistics at http://www.diabetes.org.UK/infocentre/inform/downloads/riskchrt.pdf. Accessed 2 January 2006.)

Contributing causes

Confirmed risk factors/markers include

- Increasing age
- Male gender
- Females (post-menopause)
- ↓ Socio-economic status
- Ethnic background
- Physical inactivity*
- Smoking*

- Diabetes
- Obesity*
- High blood pressure*
- ↑ Serum total cholesterol*
- ↑ Serum LDL cholesterol*
- ↓ Serum HDL cholesterol*
- ↑ Serum triglycerides*

Other probable risk factors/markers include

- Other lipid-related factors (not cholesterol)*
- Vascular endothelial dysfunction
- Oxidative stress*
- Coagulation factors
- Inflammation factors
- Blood homocysteine*
- Maternal/fetal undernutrition

* Factors that are or may be potentially amenable to modification by intervention.

Cardioprotective diet

Primary prevention

Nutritional recommendations for the general population, including those with CVD risk factors, are given in Table 19.2. Translated into practical food-based dietary advice these can be summarized as follows.[1]

- Eat oily fish at least once per week, e.g. sardines, salmon, fresh tuna.
- Eat five or more portions of fruit and vegetables per day.
- Reduce amount of all fat eaten, e.g. select lean meat and lower fat dairy products, use less oil and fat in cooking, reduce use of full fat spreads, eat less fried food and high fat foods such as cakes, biscuits, pastries, and savoury snacks.
- Choose oils/spreads that are higher in monounsaturates and lower in saturates, e.g. olive oil and rapeseed oil.
- Reduce salt intake by using less at table, in cooking, and salty foods.
- Eat more starchy foods, e.g. bread, potatoes, pasta, rice, etc.
- Drink alcohol sensibly, e.g. 2–3 units/day for women and 3–4 units/day for men.

Secondary prevention

Recommendations based on systematic review of randomized controlled trials show that providing dietary advice to **all** individuals who have had myocardial infarction (MI), and probably others with CVD, will save more lives than targeting dietary advice to only those with raised serum lipids or who are overweight.

The dietary advice that saves lives and improves the health of people who have had an MI is the following.[2]

- ↑ n-3 fat intake from dietary or supplementary fish oils (see Table 19.3). One recent study has shown that this may not be suitable for men with angina and is subject to debate.
- ↓ Saturated fat and total or partial replacement by unsaturated fats, e.g. rapeseed or olive oil.
- Mediterranean dietary advice, which includes ↑ n-3 fats, fruit and vegetables, and fresh foods, ↓ saturated fats and processed food.

Ideally, this advice should be provided by registered dietitians but where access is limited, their workload should be prioritized to:

- optimize the advice provided by other health professionals, e.g. cardiac rehabilitation nurses, practice nurses, etc.;
- support individuals who are struggling with dietary advice or who have other medical conditions, e.g. diabetes;
- provide high quality written information to all people with CVD.

[1] Stanner, S. (2005). Cardiovascular disease diet, nutrition and emerging risk factors, p. 24. Blackwell Publishing, Oxford.
[2] Hooper, L., et al. (2004). Dietetic guidelines: diet in secondary prevention of cardiovascular disease. J. Hum. Nutr. Dietet. **17**, 337–49.

Table 19.2 Nutritional recommendations for the general population*

Nutrient	Recommendation
Fat	
Total fat	Reduce to 35% food energy
Saturated fat	Reduce to 11% food energy
Monounsaturated fat	Increase to 13% food energy
n-6 polyunsaturates	Maintain at current 6.5% food energy; concern if intake >10% food energy
n-3 polyunsaturates	Increase intake to 0.45 g/day
Trans fatty acids	Reduce to < 2% energy intake
Carbohydrates	
Starch, intrinsic & milk sugars	Increase to 39% food energy
Non-milk intrinsic sugars	Restrict to 11% food energy
Non-starch polysaccharides	Increase to 18 g/day (adults)
Sodium	Reduce salt intake from 9 to 6 g/day
Potassium	Increase intake to 3.5 g/day

* Adapted from p. 247 of Stanner, S. (2005). *Cardiovascular disease: diet, nutrition and emerging risk factors*. Permission requested from Blackwell Publishing.

Considering that the prevalence of CVD is higher in lower socio-economic groups and in certain ethnic groups and geographical regions, the advice given must be tailored to the target individual or group's needs so that it is practical and culturally appropriate.

Individuals who have either recently suffered from an MI or other CVD event or have a close family member who has, are often more amenable to acting on dietary advice.

Other lifestyle interventions

Dietary advice should be given in conjunction with guidance/support about other aspects of life including:

- promotion of physical activity, e.g. adults should achieve at least 30 minutes of moderate activity (brisk walking) on at least 5 days per week. Children and young adults should aim to undertake this for at least 60 minutes every day;
- smoking cessation;
- stress management.

Table 19.3 Oily fish providing *n*-3 fatty acids[*]

• Mackerel, fresh or frozen	Very high source
• Kippers, fresh or frozen	
• Pilchards, canned in tomato sauce	
• Tuna, fresh or frozen	
• Trout, fresh or frozen	↓
• Mackerel, smoked	
• Salmon, fresh or frozen	
• Sardines, canned in tomato sauce	
• Salmon, canned in brine	Moderate source
• Salmon, smoked	
• Swordfish	
• Tuna, canned in oil	
• Fish paste, e.g. crab, salmon, sardine	↓
• Cod, fresh or frozen	
• Haddock, fresh or frozen	
• Fish fingers	
• Tuna, canned in brine	Low source

[*] Adapted from UK Heart Health and Thoracic Dietitians Specialist Group. *Heart disease and omega-3s*. (2003) BDA. Reproduced with permission.

Congestive cardiac failure

Heart failure results when damage to the heart leads to reduced efficiency in pumping blood around the body with the consequent symptoms of fluid retention, breathlessness, and fatigue. Medical treatment including the prescription of diuretics and ACE (angiotensin-converting enzyme) inhibitors, may be supported by dietary management.

• Sodium ± fluid restriction. Limiting sodium intake will help maximize the effects of diuretics and thus moderate the workload on the heart by reducing the circulating volume. Low sodium diets can be very unpalatable so a compromise between avoiding an excessive salt intake while maintaining an adequate nutritional intake is required. A 'no added salt' diet should exclude high sources of dietary sodium by avoiding salt added at table (use just a pinch in cooking), stock cubes, meat and vegetable extracts, cured meat, tinned fish and meat, tinned and packet soup, salted nuts and crisps, soy sauce, monosodium glutamate (see 'Low sodium diets' in 'Ascites and oedema', Chapter 23).

• Nutritional adequacy. In more advanced cases, appetite can be very poor and food intake limited by symptoms. Ensuring a nutritionally adequate intake by encouraging small, frequent, nutrient-dense meals may help maintain body weight. This may conflict with the principles of the cardioprotective diet so advice must be given holistically to take into account the likely prognosis.

Dyslipidaemia

↑ Concentrations of total and LDL-cholesterol and triglycerides and ↓ concentrations of HDL-cholesterol are CVD risk factors (Table 19.4).

Cholesterol ratio Some health professionals use the ratio of total cholesterol to HDL-cholesterol but others find absolute values are more useful for determining management. However, as a crude guide, the optimum ratio is serum total cholesterol to HDL-cholesterol = 3.5:1.

Specific lipid profiles

Whilst the cardioprotective diet described above should provide the basis for food-related advice in all forms of dyslipidaemia, additional guidance is appropriate for specific lipid profiles.[1]

- ↑ Total & LDL-cholesterol; normal HDL-cholesterol & triglycerides:
  - reduce saturated fat intake;
  - partially substitute monounsaturated fat;
  - encourage soluble fibre, e.g. fruit, vegetables, oats, pulses;
  - limit dietary cholesterol intake if high.
- ↑ Triglycerides; normal total, LDL, & HDL-cholesterol.
  - if obese, reduce weight;
  - reduce refined carbohydrate;
  - reduce or avoid alcohol.
- ↑ Total & LDL-cholesterol; ↑ triglycerides:
  - if obese, reduce weight;
  - reduce total and saturated fat intake;
  - partially substitute monounsaturated fat;
  - replace refined carbohydrate with complex carbohydrate;
  - reduce or avoid alcohol;
  - limit dietary cholesterol intake if high.
- ↓ HDL-cholesterol:
  - encourage regular aerobic exercise;
  - moderate alcohol, e.g. 1–2 units per day;
  - ensure total fat intake is not reduced too low, e.g. replace saturated fat with monounsaturated fat.

[1] Reproduced from Thomas, B (2001), *Manual of Dietetic Practice*, Table 2.18, p191. Permission requested from Blackwell Publishing.

Table 19.4 Ideal fasting blood lipid concentrations

	Recommended concentration (mmol/l)
Total cholesterol	<5.0
LDL-cholesterol	<3.0
HDL-cholesterol	>1.0
Triglycerides	<2.3

Drug treatment for dyslipidaemia

In addition to dietary modification, patients with a 3% absolute risk of a cardiac event in the next year should be prescribed lipid-lowering drugs, statins, which together with *n*-3 fatty acids have the most favourable effect on reducing cardiac mortality. Individuals at lower risk (e.g. 10–15% risk of cardiac event in next 10 years) can buy statins over-the-counter at a cost of ~£170/year. Concern has been raised about the lack of evidence to support this and that the sum of money could be better spent on following a cardioprotective diet.

A Coronary risk prediction chart is available at the back of the *British National Formulary* or online at: http://www.diabetes.org.uk/infocentre/inform/downloads/riskchrt.pdf.

Refsum's disease (RDis)

RDis is a rare autosomal recessive disorder of lipid metabolism where the presence of a defective enzyme, phytanoyl-coenzyme A hydroxylase, results in the accumulation of phytanic acid leading to neurological symptoms.

Treatment is based on restricting the dietary intake of phytanic acid from a usual intake of 50–100 mg/day to between 10 and 20 mg/day.

- *Rich sources of phytanic acid:* avoid in RDis, e.g. beef, lamb, meat from ruminant animals (e.g. venison), dairy products (including cows' and goats'), fish and fish oils, baked products with unknown sources of fat.
- *Foods containing little phytanic acid:* (or in bound form): acceptable in RDis, e.g. poultry, pork, fruit, vegetables, sea-food with very low fat content, e.g. crab and prawns, cereal products (unless prepared with dairy or fish oil), eggs, soya milk, vegetable oils, and margarine made exclusively from vegetable oils.

The nutritional adequacy of the diet must be checked to ensure sufficient energy and all other nutrients are provided. A low energy diet will lead to weight loss and the accompanying lipolysis will mobilize endogenous phytanic acid.

The dietary restrictions should be followed for life.

Cerebrovascular accident/stroke

Cerebrovascular accidents (CVA) are the third most common cause o death in the UK, the second most common cause of dementia, and th most important single cause of severe disability in people living in thei own homes. The incidence in the UK is ~125 000 per year and increase with ↑ age.

Causes:

- 80% cerebral infarction;
- 15% primary intracerebral or subarachnoid haemorrhage;
- 5% cause uncertain.

Nutrition has two key roles to play:

- Public health, i.e. *prevention*—a healthy, well-balanced diet can help reduce risk.
- Clinical, i.e. *treatment*—an appropriate, modified diet may be required to help maintain adequate nutritional intake.

Prevention of CVA

Risk factor	Nutritional link
Hypertension (major risk)	Associated with obesity, ↓ physical activity alcohol, ↑ Na$^+$ intake, ↓ K$^+$ intake
Hyperhomocysteinaemia	Associated with ↓ fruit and vegetable intake
Oxidative stress	Improved by dietary antioxidants
Endothelial dysfunction	Improved by n–3 fatty acids

Dietary advice

- Reduce weight in obesity. A reduction of 3–9% in body weight is associated with a 3 mm Hg reduction in systolic and diastolic BP. Ideally this should be accompanied by an increase in regular, low intensity activity such as walking.
- Avoid binge drinking of alcohol. A J-shaped curve of ischaemic CVA against alcohol intake suggests that there may be benefits from consuming up to 1–2 units of alcohol/day.
- Reduce excessive salt intake. Cutting salt intake from 9 to 6 g/day is estimated to reduce systolic BP by 3 mm Hg. This could be achieved by avoiding adding salt to food at the table, using just a pinch of salt in cooking, and limiting processed foods including stock cubes, meat and vegetable extracts, cured meat, tinned fish and meat, tinned and packet soup, salted nuts and crisps, soy sauce, monosodium glutamate.
- Increase fruit and vegetable intake. A minimum of five portions per day, including green leafy vegetables, will help increase potassium and folate intake (to counter homocysteinaemia) and provide the antioxidants, vitamin C, carotenoids, and flavonoids.
- There is conflicting evidence over the use of antioxidant supplements and food sources are recommended in preference. In addition to the fruit and vegetables, vitamin E can be obtained from vegetable oil including olive oil and flavonoids from tea.

- Eat oily fish once a week to provide n–3 fatty acids. This has an antithrombogenic effect but without exacerbating bleeding tendency. There is some evidence that a moderate intake from food may be better than high dose supplements.
- In people with diabetes, ensure good blood sugar control.

In summary, this is a general, well-balanced healthy diet that is appropriate for all adults.

Changes in food intake typically associated with older people, including a reduced food intake due to difficulty in shopping, cooking, eating, or lack of appetite, often lead to a reduced intake of fruit and vegetables and ↑ consumption of nutrient-poor, processed foods. Efforts may be required to counter this with an adequate, well-balanced diet.

Treating CVA

Free radical damage may play a role in brain damage after infarction/reperfusion. This suggests that antioxidant therapy may have a role to play although current evidence is unclear. Although a well-balanced, antioxidant-rich diet may have potential value, many patients are unable to eat following CVA. Nutrition support may ∴ be required and it is essential that this provides not only adequate energy and protein but is also complete in all micronutrients so that it can meet a potential ↑ requirement for antioxidants.

Neurological damage after CVA varies with the following losses of function that may impact on eating:
- altered levels of consciousness, 30–40%;
- difficulty in swallowing, 30%;
- motor weakness, 50–80%;
- slurred speech, 30%;
- dysphagia/aphasia, 30%;
- visual field defects, 7%.

As a result, inadequate intake and consequent undernutrition is a common problem, especially in altered states of consciousness, and becomes significantly worse as hospital stay continues and is associated with ↑ morbidity and reduced survival. Evidence from feeding studies has shown that nutritional status, length of hospital stay, and mortality can be influenced by nutrition intervention.

Dysphagia

Dysphagia (discomfort, difficulty, or pain when swallowing) is common following stroke. Swallowing has four stages:
- preparation—transfer of food into the mouth, sealed with lips.
- oral—chewing, mixing with saliva, bolus formation, and transfer toward pharynx.
- pharyngeal—complex stage where bolus is involuntarily transferred towards oesophagus with simultaneous closure of larynx and pause in respiration.
- oesophageal—transfer to stomach by peristalsis and gravity.

⚠ Impaired swallow leads to high risk from aspirating food or liquid into the respiratory tract.

Assessment

All patients should undergo:

- nutrition screening (see 'Malnutrition Universal Screening Tool', Chapter 16) within 48 hours of admission following a stroke and, if risk of malnutrition is detected, should be referred to a dietitian for full nutritional assessment;
- their swallow should be assessed using validated bedside protocol (Fig. 19.2) and, if compromised, they should be referred to a speech and language therapist.

Dietary management should then be based on the findings of these two assessments, ensuring that the patient's nutritional requirements are met in an appropriate format or texture, e.g. soft food, thickened drinks, tube feeding, etc. Patients should be re-assessed according to local guidelines.

This should be carried out by a professional skilled in the management of dysphagia

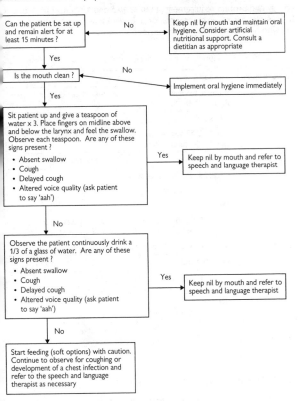

Fig. 19.2 Example of SIGN 78 (2004) algorithm for Screening Swallow. Reproduced with permission. *Management of patients with stroke: identification and management of dysphagia*, Guideline 78. SIGN, Edinburgh.)

Nutritional requirements

Energy and protein requirements (Tables 19.5 and 19.6) may be ↑ due to hypermetabolism, which persists for 4–8 weeks, and in frail elderly people who have pre-existing undernutrition.

Table 19.5 Estimating energy requirements*

Step number	Method	
1	Estimate basal metabolic rate using the Schofield equation (see Appendix 4)	
	Either:	
2a	Add to BMR a stress factor: (calculated as % of BMR) for specific clinical condition	
	Condition	**Stress factor(%)**
	Cerebral vascular accident	5
	Cerebral haemorrhage	30
	Or	
2b	Add to BMR 400–1000 kcal/day if ↑ in body weight (lean or fat) is desired. Subtract 400–1000 kcal/day if ↓ in body fat is desired	
3	Add to BMR an activity factor (calculated as % of BMR)	
	Activity level	**Activity factor (%)**
	Patient in bed and immobile	10
	Patient in bed but able to move and sit up	15–20
	Patient mobile on ward	25

* Requirements should be based on actual body weight except in obesity (if BMI 30–50 kg/m² use 75% value; if BMI >50 kg/m² use 65% value).

Table 19.6 Estimating protein requirements*

Protein	Nitrogen (g/kg/day)	
	Mean	**Range**
Normal	0.17	0.14–0.20
Hypermetabolic (+5–25%)	0.20	0.17–0.25

* Requirements should be based on actual body weight except in obesity (if BMI 30–50 kg/m² use 75% value; if BMI >50 kg/m² use 65% value).

Texture modification

f swallowing is impaired, modifying the texture of food may facilitate safe
ɔral intake. The standardized categories in the box are used.

Standardized categories of food texture*

Fluids	• Thin fluid: still water, tea, coffee without milk, diluted squash, spirits, wine
	• Naturally thick fluid: liquid leaving a coating on an empty glass, e.g. full cream milk, commercial sip feeds
	• Thickened fluid:
	1 Can be drunk through a straw or from a cup if advised/preferred. Leaves thin coat on back of spoon
	2 Cannot be drunk through a straw. Can be drunk from a cup Leaves thick coat on back of spoon
	3 Cannot be drunk through a straw or from a cup. Needs to be taken by spoon
Food texture	(a) Smooth pouring, uniform consistency; pureed and sieved; cannot be eaten with fork. Examples: tinned tomato soup, thin custard
	(b) Smooth, uniform consistency; pureed and sieved; cannot be eaten with fork; drops rather than pours from spoon. Examples: soft whipped cream, thick custard
	(c) Thick, smooth, uniform consistency; pureed and sieved; can be eaten with fork or spoon; holds own shape on plate; no chewing required. Examples: mousse, smooth fromage frais
	(d) Moist food, with some variation in texture; not pureed or sieved; may be served with thick gravy/sauce; easily masked with fork; requires little chewing; meat prepared as (c). Examples: flaked fish in sauce, stewed apple and thick custard
	(e) Soft, moist food; broken into pieces with fork; comprises solids and thick gravy/sauce; avoid foods that cause choking hazard (see following box). Examples: tender meat casseroles, sponge and custard
Normal food	• Any food, including those from choking hazard list.

*Adapted from BDA and RCSLT. *National descriptors for texture modification in adults.* (2002) BDA. Reproduced with permission.

Choking hazard—high risk foods*

- Stringy, fibrous texture, e.g. pineapple, runner beans, celery, lettuce
- Vegetable and fruit skins, e.g. peas, baked beans, broad beans, grapes
- Mixed texture foods, e.g. muesli, mince in thin gravy, soup with lumps
- Crunchy or crumbly foods, e.g. toast, dry biscuits, crisps, flaky pastry
- Hard foods, e.g. boiled and chewy sweets, nuts and seeds
- Husks, e.g. sweetcorn, granary bread

* Adapted from BDA and RCSLT. *National descriptors for texture modification in adults.* (2002) BDA. Reproduced with permission.

Tube feeding

Patients with dysphagia who are unable to achieve their nutritional requirements orally and those who are unconscious may require tube feeding. This may raise ethical issues, depending on prognosis. The decision to undertake feeding should be made by the multidisciplinary team in consultation with the patient and their family or carers; the method of feeding should be based on the estimated length of time over which feeding will be required:

- 0–4 weeks, nasogastric (NG) tube;
- >4 weeks percutaneous enteroscopic gastrostomy (PEG).

If nasogastric feeding is going to be instigated, it should start within the first 2–3 days after admission. Although inserting a PEG is an invasive procedure, and ethical consideration must be given to the associated risks and management issues, feeding via a PEG has a much lower risk of aspiration and is associated with better clinical outcome in some studies.

Longer term

The patient's nutritional status and ability to swallow should be regularly monitored and adjustments made to their nutritional management accordingly. Dysphagia frequently resolves in the first 6 months following a CVA although it may persist. Switching to overnight tube feeding to encourage oral intake during the day may facilitate a return to normality. Patients may continue to need assistance with meals and, most of all, time to maximize their ability to eat an adequate diet.

Further information

1. Garibaila, S. (2004). *Nutrition and stroke*. Blackwell Publishing, Oxford.
2. Royal College of Physicians (2004). *National clinical guidelines for stroke* 2nd edn. Prepared by the Intercollegiate Stroke Working Party. RCP, London.
3. SIGN (2004). *Management of patients with stroke: identification and management of dysphagia*, Guideline 78. SIGN, Edinburgh.
4. British Dietetic Association and Royal College of Speech and Language Therapists (2002). *National descriptors for texture modification in adults*. BDA, Birmingham.

Hypertension

Hypertension (HT) is defined as a systolic blood pressure (SBP) above 140 mm Hg, a diastolic blood pressure (DBP) above 90 mm Hg, or when levels below this are maintained by antihypertensive medication.

It is a significant health problem in the UK with an estimated prevalence of 32% and 30%, respectively, for men and women in England. Prevalence increases with age and is higher in Black and south Asian communities.

HT is a major risk factor for cardiovascular disease (especially stroke, angina, myocardial infarction, heart failure, and left ventricular failure), renal disease, and retinopathy.

Factors contributing to HT include:

- obesity, especially if central adiposity;
- insulin resistance;
- diabetes mellitus;
- low levels of physical activity;
- psychosocial stress;
- high salt intake;
- high alcohol intake, especially if regular heavy or binge drinking.

Management

Lifestyle advice should be offered as the first line of treatment. This should include the promotion of a healthy diet, regular exercise, smoking cessation, and relaxation therapies. Those with diabetes or previous coronary heart disease should receive additional advice.

Dietary intervention

- Reduction of excess body weight. Losing 3–9% body weight is associated with 3 mm Hg reduction in SBP and DBP.
- Limit alcohol intake to maximum of 21 or 14 units per week for men and women, respectively. Structured intervention to reduce excess intake is associated with a mean reduction of 3–4 mm Hg SBP and DBP with a third of patients achieving >10 mm Hg reduction in SBP.
- Limit salt intake to <6 g/day (2.4 g or 100 mmol Na^+). This could be achieved by not adding salt to food at the table, using just a pinch of salt in cooking, and limiting processed foods including stock cubes, meat and vegetable extracts, cured meat, tinned fish and meat, tinned and packet soup, salted nuts and crisps, soy sauce, monosodium glutamate.
- Eat more fruit and vegetables. Five portions per day should be the minimum target.
- Calcium, potassium, and magnesium supplements are not recommended at present although there is some evidence that an adequate intake provided through food may be beneficial.
- Overall, a cardioprotective diet is appropriate for individuals with HT (see 'Cardioprotective diet', this chapter).

Further information

See DASH studies (Dietary approaches to stop hypertension).

Svetkey, L. P., et al. (1999). Effects of dietary patterns on blood pressure. Subgroup analysis of the DASH randomized clinical trial. *Arch. Intern. Med.* **159**, 285–93.

Obarzanek, E., et al. (2003). Individual blood pressure responses to change in salt intake: results from the DASH sodium trial. *Hypertension* **2** 459–67.

🖥 http://www.actiononsalt.org.uk/

Cancer and leukaemia

Cancer: Introduction and dietary guidelines to minimize risk

Cancer is a major cause of morbidity with more than 270 000 new cas
diagnosed in the UK each year and one in four deaths cancer-related.
Nutrition plays an important role in both the aetiology and treatment
many different cancers.

Incidence See Tables 20.1 and 20.2

Aetiology

Dietary factors are responsible for ~25% of cancer deaths in the U
attributed to environmental factors. Only use of tobacco is high
(~30%). The strength of evidence linking specific elements of the diet
different cancers varies (Table 20.3).

The link between food and cancer causation is very complex becau
the variation in what people eat and the interrelationships betwee
different foods, nutrients, lifestyle and environmental factors make unra
elling the connections very difficult. However, a number of current
ongoing, large epidemiological studies may contribute more informatic
and although some links have only been tentatively established at prese
(see Table 20.3) there is sufficient information to make dieta
recommendations.

Dietary guidelines to minimize cancer risk

The UK 'Balance of Good Health' guidelines (see 'Food-based dieta
guidelines', Chapter 2) are compatible with those made by the Wor
Cancer Research Fund.[1]

- Choose a diet rich in a variety of plant-based foods.
- Eat plenty of vegetables and fruits.
- Maintain a healthy weight and be physically active.
- Drink alcohol in moderation, if at all.
- Select foods low in fat and salt.
- Prepare and store foods safely.

[1] Reproduced with kind permission from the World Cancer Research Fund websi
(www.wcrf.org)

Table 20.1 Most common cancers in UK (excluding non-melanoma skin). (2001 data collated by Cancer Research UK)

Men		Women	
Type	Number(%)	Type	Number(%)
Prostate	30 140 (22)	Breast	40 790 (30)
Lung	22 700 (17)	Large bowel	16 040 (12)
Large bowel	18 500 (14)	Lung	14 740 (11)
Bladder	7 580 (6)	Ovary	6 880 (5)
Total	135 370 (100)	Total	135 410 (100)

Table 20.2 Most common cancers in the world (excluding non-melanoma skin). (2002 data from Cancer Mondial: http://www-dep.iarc.fr/)

Men		Women	
Type	Number(%)	Type	Number(%)
Lung	965 000 (17)	Breast	1 151 000 (23)
Prostate	679 000 (12)	Cervix	493 000 (10)
Stomach	603 000 (10)	Large bowel	473 000 (9)
Large bowel	550 000 (9)	Lung	387 000 (8)
Total	5 802 000 (100)	Total	5 061 000 (100)

Table 20.3 Strength of evidence linking specific elements of the diet to different cancers

Level of evidence	Decrease risk		Increase risk	
	Dietary element	Type of cancer	Dietary element	Type of cancer
Convincing			Obesity	oesophagus, bowel, breast, endometrium, kidney
Probable	Fruit & vegetables	Upper GI tract, stomach, bowel	Very hot drinks Salt & salt-preserved foods Preserved & red meat	Upper GI tract, Stomach, Bowel
Insufficient	Fibre, soya, fish, n–3 fats, vitamins, minerals, non-nutrient plant constituents	—	Animal fats, heterocyclic amines, polycyclic aromatic hydrocarbons, nitrosamines, acrylamide	—

Key, T.J., et al. (2004). Diet, nutrition and the prevention of cancer. *Public Health Nutr* **7**, 187–200

Effects of cancer on nutritional status

Whilst the above guidelines are appropriate for healthy adults, those who have been diagnosed with cancer may require different and more specific dietary advice because of the negative nutritional effects of cancer or treatment.

- Reduced intake due to:
  - anxiety/depression/pain;
  - taste changes/dry mouth;
  - nausea;
  - nil by mouth (investigations and treatment).
- Reduced digestion/absorption:
  - ± specific to site of cancer.
- Altered metabolism:
  - ↑ gluconeogenesis ± ↑ insulin resistance;
  - ↑ lipolysis and ↑ fatty acid and glycerol turnover;
  - ↓ muscle protein synthesis;
  - ↑ metabolic rate 2° to tumour growth;
  - secondary infections;
  - loss or gain of weight.
- Increased losses:
  - vomiting;
  - diarrhoea;
  - fistulae.
- Effects of treatment:
  - surgery (see 'Surgery', Chapter 16);
  - chemotherapy (see 'Chemotherapy and radiotherapy', this chapter);
  - radiotherapy (see 'Chemotherapy and radiotherapy', this chapter).

Nutrition goals in anticancer treatment

Nutritional management can play an important role during each of these goals.

- Cure—to obtain a complete response.
- Control—to extend life and quality of life if cure not possible.
- Palliation—to provide comfort where cure and control not possible, to relieve symptoms, and maximize quality of life.

Nutritional stimulation of tumour growth

Could restricting nutritional support to cancer patients reduce tumour growth by withholding the nutrients required for proliferation ? There is little evidence to support this theory. However, there is good evidence that providing nutritional support can maximize the patient's nutritional status and limit cachexia, enabling the patient to better withstand anticancer treatment. Anticancer treatment is most effective when cancer cells are vulnerable during their proliferative phase suggesting that provision of nutrients will not have an adverse effect. There is ∴ no rationale for limiting nutritional intake in cancer patients in order to 'starve' the tumour.

Nutritional assessment

The effects of cancer on nutritional status vary depending on the site of the tumour, the stage of the disease, treatment, and potential complicating factors. Each patient should be assessed as the first step of nutritional management; this should include evaluation as:

- nutritional status (see Chapter 4);
- nutrient intake and dietary preferences;
- clinical diagnosis;
- treatment received or proposed;
- energy and nutrient requirements (see 'Estimating requirements in disease states', Chapter 16 and Appendix 6).

Cancer cachexia

Up to 82% of patients with advanced cancer have some degree of weight loss, known as cancer cachexia, characterized by loss of lean tissue including muscle and organ mass, and most report anorexia. Loss of appetite contributes to the loss of weight but does not totally explain it. Hypermetabolism associated with cytokines released by the immune system in response to the cancer also plays a role.

Not all patients suffer from cachexia. Some may be well-nourished on diagnosis, eat well throughout treatment, and have no food-related problems. However, those who do may require general or specific dietary advice.

Nutrition support

General nutrition support should be given by ensuring that the patient has access to suitable food when they are able to eat, supplementing intake using ordinary food products or proprietary products or a combination of both (see 'Treatment of under nutrition', Chapter 16). If an adequate oral intake cannot be achieved and it is clinically appropriate (see Chapter 29), feeding artificially via the gut (see 'Enteral feeding', Chapter 16) or directly into the blood (see 'Parenteral nutrition', Chapter 16) should be undertaken.

Suggestions to alleviate nutrition-related side-effects

- Anorexia—try to maximize intake by taking high-energy/high-protein foods; gentle exercise/fresh air before meal may promote appetite
- Taste changes—try food chilled; eat more of the foods that still taste good; if red meat doesn't taste right, try poultry, fish, eggs instead; stronger flavours like ginger, lemon or spices may help; maintain regular mouth care
- Dry mouth—sip cool drinks; try using a drinking straw; suck ice chips; sharp tastes like grapefruit or lemon may stimulate saliva; serve meals with sauce or gravy
- Nausea & vomiting—avoid off-putting smells; plain foods in small quantities may be better tolerated; avoid lying down after eating (a gentle walk may help); sip drinks throughout day but wait for 15 min after eating before taking more fluid; try ginger flavours, mints, and plain biscuits
- Mucositis (sore mouth ± oesophagus)—try soft, smooth foods with plenty of sauce; avoid spicy and salty foods and sharp, citrus tastes; chilled or warm foods may be less painful than hot; coarse/crumbly food like toast, crackers, and pastry may be better avoided
- Diarrhoea—avoid irritating foods that exacerbate, e.g. pulses, onions, strong spices; consider reducing fibre-rich foods (including whole grains, fruit and vegetable intake if intake is already high); ensure fluid intake is adequate and try and keep eating even if small quantities of smooth foods; reducing fat intake and milk products is often suggested: this may have a negative effect on nutrient intake so individual advice from a dietitian is required
- Constipation—this may arise 2° to cancer, treatment, or analgesia or simply from a poor intake and inactivity; eating more and gentle exercise may help; increase fluid intake ~2 litre/d; increasing intake of fruit, vegetable, and wholegrain cereals may help if tolerated; prunes and prune juice; a little hot water on waking may stimulate the bowel
- Tiredness—ignore the clock and eat when you feel more awake; a variety of well-balanced snacks can be as nutritious as a main meal; ask for help with food preparation or use ready meals or home-delivered food.

Examples of side-effects related to specific cytotoxic drugs

- Cisplatin—severe nausea & vomiting but little mucositis
- Doxorubicin—severe mucositis (dose-dependent)
- 5-fluorouracil—severe mucositis plus taste alterations
- Vinblastine sulphate—mild–moderate nausea & vomiting plus constipation

Chemotherapy

The nutrition-related side-effects associated with chemotherapy depend on the regime and dose prescribed. Chemotherapy regimes often comprise repeated cycles of cytotoxic drugs repeated at regular intervals over several months. Eating well during the 'good times' between doses may help to maintain nutritional status even if intake falls during and immediately after the infusion period.

Radiotherapy

The nutrition-related side-effects associated with radiotherapy depend on site of the cancer and dose prescribed.

- General effects include anorexia, nausea, tiredness, and depression. Some of the suggestions in the box on previous page may be of help. If the course of radiation includes a prolonged programme of regular sessions requiring daily hospital visits, assistance with the practicalities of food shopping and preparation may be required.
- Local effects arise from the impact of the radiation on healthy tissue near the cancer site. This may have little nutritional impact if it is a discrete, non-systemic area, e.g. limb. However, severe problems can arise with radiotherapy to:
  - Head and neck—includes cancer of mouth, tongue, salivary glands, throat, and face. Damage to the mucosal cells breaches the surface potentially leading to infection, inflammation, and severe pain. A dry mouth, taste changes, loss of taste, and difficulty swallowing may also occur and the combined effects often severely limit food intake leading to a rapid decline in nutritional status. Regular nutritional assessment is required; the suggestions in the box on previous page may help.
  - Abdominal/pelvic area—includes cancer of the cervix, colon, pancreas, prostate, and rectum. Irradiation damages the gastro-intestinal mucosa leading to a reduction in epithelial surface and impaired absorption of nutrients. Diarrhoea, bloating, and cramping pains may result and, in severe cases, ulceration, strictures, and perforation. Reducing dietary fibre, fat, and lactose may help some patients but should *not* be advised routinely to all; individual advice from a dietitian will help identify the dietary components that exacerbate symptoms and facilitate the construction of a nutritional adequate intake compatible with avoiding these.

Other dietary approaches to cancer treatment

There is a considerable amount of information about food and cancer that is available to the general public and some includes dietary advice that is based on limited or questionable scientific evidence. Whilst some is compatible with what is generally regarded as a healthy, well-balanced diet, other advice is not. These include regimes recommending intakes that are nutritionally inadequate and/or unpalatable or advocating complex eating patterns that require either the sourcing of unusual or hard-to-buy items or complicated preparation regimes. Focusing on food can be a valuable and positive activity for a patient and his/her carers and alternative approaches should not automatically be regarded as 'bad'. However, it is essential that unproven benefits are balanced against any potential nutritional inadequacy and negative emotional consequences, e.g. denial of favourite foods, guilt at non-compliance and despair if cure does not occur.

Patients who are interested in following complementary or alternative dietary regimes should be encouraged to discuss this with their doctor and dietitian so that the potential benefits and/or detrimental effects can be evaluated with respect to their individual needs. Consideration can be given to combining such approaches with conventional nutritional support.

Examples of less conventional dietary approaches to cancer

Bristol Cancer Help Centre diet

Promotes healthy eating and recommends eating a wide variety of fresh vegetables, fruit, wholegrains, beans, pulses, nuts, seeds, cold-pressed plant oils, and plenty of water. Foods perceived as undermining health include sugar and refined carbohydrates, dairy products, red meat, processed foods, smoked/cured foods, caffeine, alcohol, and salt.
Comment. This complementary diet can be nutritionally adequate in patients who are eating well. Those whose intake is comprised would benefit from some of the high energy/high protein foods that are discouraged.

Gerson Therapy

Based on stimulating the immune system to rid the body of cancer-related toxins. The diet is a very strict low salt one that includes large quantities of organic fruit and vegetables taken in the form of juice. Associated with other treatments known as 'metabolic therapy'.
Comment. This regime is recommended as an alternative to conventional treatment. The diet is expensive and potentially nutritionally inadequate. Coffee enemas have been associated with infection and inflammation of the bowel. No adequate scientific trials have confirmed efficacy.

Macrobiotics

A philosophical approach to life that includes balancing yin and yang elements. The dietary element is based on predominantly vegetarian, high carbohydrate, low fat food with regular consumption of soya and sea vegetables.
Comment. The high phytoestrogen content of the diet may offer some benefits but there is no firm scientific evidence to confirm this. A low energy and protein density is a concern in patients with a poor appetite.

Plant Programme

Advises the complete avoidance of milk and dairy products because of a perceived aetiological link, particularly with hormone-mediated cancers, e.g. breast and prostate.
Comment. Published epidemiological studies do not support the proposed link. Milk and other dairy products provide useful nutrients in a palatable form and, although avoidance may not comprise intake in relatively well patients, it may be detrimental in those who are eating poorly.

Leukaemia

Patients with leukaemia tend to have a better nutritional status at diagnosis than those with solid tumours. However, this can deteriorate rapidly in response to treatment, including chemo- and radiotherapy (see 'Chemotherapy and radiotherapy', this chapter) and nutritional support is often required to optimize well-being and nutritional status.

Bone marrow transplantation (BMT)

BMT (or stem cell transplantation) is used to treat patients with leukaemia, lymphoma, and other haematological disorders including aplastic anaemia, some solid tumours, and some inherited metabolic disorders. Although most patients embarking on this course of treatment are relatively well-nourished, there are nutritional implications.

- Mucositis of gastrointestinal tract usually occurs within 7–10 days of high dose chemo-/radiotherapy before BMT and continues for 2–3 weeks afterwards. Leads to ↓ oral intake due to nausea, vomiting, pain of eating, and malabsorption and is worse in donor grafts where a greater degree of immunosuppression is required than for autologous grafts. Feeding via the gut, either orally or via a tube, should be attempted but, if this is unsuccessful, parenteral nutrition should be instigated. There is insufficient evidence to confirm that either enteral or parenteral nutrition is better in BMT patients.
- Immunosuppression is a necessary prerequisite for successful grafting of new bone marrow tissue. The unwanted side-effect is ↑ susceptibility to infection, and patients are nursed in isolation and protected from potential sources of pathogens. In some units this includes the provision of a 'clean diet' (see Table 20.4).
- Graft versus host disease (GVHD) arises between 10 and 20 days after BMT from the response of the graft tissue to the leukaemia (a positive outcome) and host cells (a negative complication). This may affect different organs including the intestine which can lead to severe abdominal pain and malabsorption. Dietary manipulation may be required to maximize absorptive function in patients who are able to eat. Parenteral nutrition may be required in severe cases.
- Energy and protein requirements increase following BMT. Studies suggest that energy requirements increase to 130–150% of predicted basal requirements and that protein needs are met by 1.4–1.5 g/kg/d.
- Intravenous lipid, once controversial, has been shown to be safe in parenteral regimes, is a useful source of energy and essential fatty acids, and is not associated with an increase in bacterial or fungal infections.
- Studies have shown that the immunomodulating effects of n–3 fatty acids may have benefits after BMT by reducing GVHD and the potentially fatal complication, veno-occlusive disease. Further studies are needed.
- Parenteral glutamine supplementation is associated with a shorter hospital stay and a reduction in +ve blood cultures in BMT patients.

Clean diets

Ideally, BMT patients should eat a well-balanced and nourishing diet provided by food with a minimum risk of bacterial or fungal contamination. Sterile diets that were implemented 25 years ago are no longer used because they compromise nutrient intake unduly. Although practice varies between centres, most BMT patients are advised to follow a 'clean' diet (Table 20.4) while they are neutropenic and, after their cell count increases, to continue on a 'safe food' (see box) diet for at least 6 months after discharge from hospital.

Table 20.4 Clean diet for patients with neutrophil count <1000/ml[3*]

Allowed	Not allowed
Most hot, freshly cooked food	Take-away meals
Tinned meat/fish (newly opened)	Meat if still red/pink after cooking
Ready meals if cooked properly and within sell by date	Cold meat and fish
	Shell fish
Pasteurized/UHT milk, stored in 'fridge and used <24 h of opening	Unpasteurized milk or any milk opened >24 h
Pasteurized yogurt & cream	Bioyogurt, nut yogurt
Butter, individual wrapped portions	Large packets butter
Cooked or vacuum packed cheese	Soft & blue cheeses
Eggs, well cooked >10 minutes	Raw or lightly cooked eggs
Bread, fresh and wrapped	Bread, unwrapped
Cakes & biscuits, wrapped and eaten <48 h	Cakes with cream, unwrapped or >48 h old
Breakfast cereals: individual packs	Cereal containing fruit & nuts
Fruit & vegetables, hot & freshly cooked or canned or washed & peeled	Raw, unpeeled fruit & vegetables
	Dried or bruised fruit
Wrapped/sealed confectionery & crisps	Ice cream, confectionery with fruit & nuts
Jams, sauces, etc. from individual portions used <48 h of opening	Uncooked spices & black pepper
Wine, spirit, canned beer, lager	Real ale

* Adapted from information provided by Dept of Nutrition and Dietetics, Hammersmith Hospital, London. Reproduced with permission.

Safe food diet for BMT patients with neutrophil count >1000/ml^3 until 6 months after discharge from hospital*

- Food consumed should be bought from clean, reputable shops
- All food should be used within the 'sell by'/'best before' date
- Raw and cooked food should be kept separately (raw food on lower shelves in 'fridge)
- Use only undamaged cans
- Avoid the following foods:
  - Soft and blue cheeses, e.g. Brie, Camembert, Danish blue, Stilton
  - All paté unless tinned
  - Raw or undercooked poultry or meat products
  - All take away meals unless sure freshly cooked—rice is particularly risky
  - Raw eggs or food containing, e.g. fresh mayonnaise
  - Shellfish
  - Cold, unwrapped food eaten without heating, e.g. quiche, sausage rolls
  - Uncooked food eaten without heating, e.g. ready prepared salad

* Adapted from information provided by Dept of Nutrition and Dietetics, Hammersmith Hospital, London. Reproduced with permission.

Nutrition in gastrointestinal diseases

Mouth disorders

Injury or disease in the mouth (including lips, oral cavity, tongue, and nasopharynx) can rapidly compromise nutritional status by inhibiting eating and drinking. To counter this, nutrient intake can be optimized through the modification of food texture or by instigating nutritional support via tube feeding.

Cancer of the mouth and pharynx

Mouth and pharyngeal cancers account for ~6% cancers worldwide but are much more common in developing countries; all head and neck cancers represent only about 3% of total malignancies in the UK. Associated risk factors include the consumption of salted fish (nasopharyngeal cancer) and chewing betel nut or tobacco (oral cancer). High alcohol intake and smoking are associated with ↑ risk and this is multiplied in individuals who undertake both activities. Treatment includes surgery, chemotherapy, and radiotherapy and must include individual dietary advice to maximize nutrient intake (See 'Nutrition goals in anticancer treatment', Chapter 20).

Salivary gland disorders

Disorders include saliva deficiency, inflammation secondary to infection, and calculi. Inflammation can hinder chewing and reduce the flow of saliva, further impeding food intake. Treatment of the underlying condition is required and nutrient intake should be supported by providing moist food that requires little chewing (see 'Texture modification' in 'Cerebrovascular accident/stroke', Chapter 19). Xerostomia (dry mouth) relating to lack of saliva is also associated with Sjögren syndrome, diabetes mellitus, and taking anticholinergic, antihistamine, and decongestant medications as well as some anticancer treatment. Artificial saliva substitutes are available on prescription as gel, spray, and tablets and may help both food intake and promote oral hygiene. Dentures incorporating a refillable reservoir have been devised to facilitate delivery of saliva substitutes.

Jaw wiring

Fixation of the maxilla/mandible may be undertaken following a fractured jaw, oral surgery, or (rarely) in the treatment of obesity. The procedure may accompany complex maxofacial surgery in the presence of severe trauma or may be relatively straightforward in elective jaw wiring for obesity.

- A liquid or semi-liquid diet is required (Table 21.1). This can be based on a combination of supplemented drinks, both homemade and commercial, that can be sucked through the gaps between the jaws.
- Consideration must be given to the total nutrient intake to ensure adequacy for the duration of the fixation (usually 3–8 weeks following fracture); a higher protein intake may be required by patients who have suffered a traumatic fracture while energy should be limited in the treatment of obesity.

- Including some soluble fibre, e.g. pureed porridge or lump-free lentil soup, may help alleviate constipation that is common due to the preclusion of most fruit, vegetable, and wholegrain items. Alternatively, the bulk-forming laxative, ispaghula husk, may be given but care must be taken to ensure an adequate fluid intake.
- Mouth hygiene should be maintained by gently brushing the exterior tooth surfaces and fixtures and using saline or antiseptic mouthwash on waking, before retiring to bed, and after every meal and snack.

Table 21.1 Example of liquid diet

	Volume (ml)	Energy (kcal)	Protein (g)
Orange juice	250	110	2
Porridge, pureed with milk & sugar	300	200	7
Milky coffee with sugar	250	180	8
Drinking yogurt	200	190	8
Tomato juice	250	50	2
Proprietary nutrition supplement*	200	200	8
Mug of tea	300	20	—
Ice cream	100	180	4
Creamy lentil soup (lump free)	200	130	5
Proprietary nutrition supplement*	200	200	8
Pureed fruit with very thin custard	250	220	6
Banana smoothie	250	180	2
Hot chocolate with milk	250	240	10
Approximate total	3000	2100	70

▶ Vitamin and mineral supplementation may be required, depending on the duration of liquid diet.

* Volume and composition vary with brand. See Table 16.4 in 'Treatment of under nutrition', Chapter 16 for examples of proprietary oral nutrition supplements

Dental health

Healthy teeth and gums contribute to overall health and well-being.
- Efficient, pain-free mastication facilitates the intake of a varied and well balanced diet.
- Good oral hygiene is associated with a lower risk of coronary heart disease.
- Complete and decay-free teeth contribute to psychosocial well-being by enhancing facial appearance and speech.

Dental caries

Definition Caries (cavities, tooth decay) are holes in the structure of the tooth.

Prevalence In the UK has ↓ greatly since the 1970s when fluoride toothpaste was introduced. In 2005, a 12-year old child has on average <1 decay, missing, or filled tooth and the percentage of adults with no teeth of their own has fallen from 37% to 12% in last 40 years. However, there are considerable inequalities between socio-economic groups with children from deprived backgrounds experiencing most poor dental health.

Pathogenesis Bacteria living in the dental plaque ferment dietary carbohydrate into acid, which dematerializes the tooth enamel, initiating the cariogenic process (see box). The pH of the mouth determines the extent of decay as this only takes place if <5.7.

Prevention In addition to reducing plaque bacteria by regular brushing and flossing and regular dental visits, dietary prevention includes:
- minimizing effects of fermentable carbohydrate;
- maximizing oral pH.

Dental erosion

Definition Erosion is the acidic destruction of the tooth surface. It does not include the abrasion and attrition associated with normal wear and tear on the biting surface of the teeth.

Prevalence In the UK it is increasing and associated with the rise in consumption of acidic and/or carbonated soft drinks and herbal teas. Severe erosion has been observed in ~1% of 14-year olds in UK study while it is estimated that 6–10% have pathologically unacceptable levels. It is more common in boys than girls and in children from socially deprived backgrounds.

Pathogenesis The acid eroding tooth enamel is not derived from the bacterial fermentation of dietary carbohydrate but from acidic fluid in the mouth, either from dietary intake or regurgitation of stomach contents (reflux or vomiting).

Prevention is based on reducing acid contact. Reflux or vomiting (spontaneous or self-induced, e.g. in bulimia nervosa) require investigation. Dietary prevention includes:
- limiting acidic food and drink to mealtimes;
- finishing meal with alkaline food, e.g. cheese or milk;

Fermentable carbohydrate

- Type of carbohydrate determines cariogenicity: sucrose > fructose, glucose, maltose > lactose, galactose > maltodextrins, polysaccharide > sorbitol, xylitol
- Frequency of exposure: regular ingestion of small quantities of carbohydrate is more damaging to teeth than one larger intake because repeated exposure prevents oral pH from increasing above the 5.7 threshold, thus perpetuating tooth demineralization
- Texture of foods: sticky/chewy food leaves residue on teeth that prolongs exposure to carbohydrate and leads to a lower oral pH. Toffees and dried fruit have a greater potential to contribute to dental caries than the same quantity of carbohydrate taken as fruit juice which rapidly leaves the mouth

Maximizing oral pH

- Milk and dairy products are alkaline and contain protein, calcium, and phosphate which play a role in re-mineralizing dental enamel following acid exposure
- Saliva can be stimulated by chewing sugar-free gum for 10 minutes after meals. Freshly secreted saliva has a pH of >6.3, i.e. above critical threshold and ∴ protective
- Using a drinking straw with acidic drinks (fruit juices and carbonated beverages) can reduce the fall in pH compared with drinking from a cup

- avoiding acid food or drink last thing at night;
- drinking acidic drinks through a straw and minimizing sipping, swishing, and frothing in the mouth;
- beware acidic medication, e.g. chewable vitamin C tablets;
- avoiding brushing teeth immediately after acidic food;
- ⚠ using a baby feeder filled with fruit juice or other acidic drink as a comforter leads to prolonged contact with teeth and potentially very severe erosion.

Oesophageal disorders

After chewing and swallowing, food is transported via the oesophagus (or gullet) to the stomach. Although food passes rapidly through the oesophagus compared to other parts of the gastrointestinal tract, disorders that restrict food intake can have a major detrimental influence on nutritional status (see 'Digestion', Chapter 1).

Achalasia

Leads to food being retained in the oesophagus due to reduced peristalsis and incomplete opening of the lower oesophageal sphincter.

Treatment includes balloon dilatation, surgery, or injection of botulinum toxin to relax the sphincter.

Nutritional management may also help and includes small frequent meals, avoiding foods that exacerbate dyspepsia and very hot or cold foods, and not eating late at night or before lying down. Eating in an upright position (rather than reclining or slumped) may facilitate the passage of food into the stomach. Nutritional assessment should be undertaken to ensure that weight loss through an inadequate intake is prevented.

Dysphagia

Dysphagia (discomfort, difficulty, or pain when swallowing) is common in oesophageal disorders. Inflammation or occlusion of the oesophageal lumen impairs the final stage of swallow as food passes from the pharynx to the stomach by the combined effects of peristalsis and gravity. Patients with oesophageal dysphagia are less at risk from aspirating food or liquid into the respiratory tract than those with dysphagia 2° to stroke where the oral and pharyngeal stages of swallow may also be impaired.

Nutritional management should include assessment of the swallowing problem (see Fig.19.2, in 'Cerebrovascular accident/stroke', Chapter 19) and an evaluation of the optimum texture of foods and liquids (see 'Texture modification' in 'Cerebrovascular accident/stroke', Chapter 19). In general, patients with more severe oesophageal disorders will require more liquids and thinner textures than those with milder dysphagia. The complete nutritional adequacy of the intake should be determined and progress monitored in the context of the underlying condition.

Oesophageal cancer

Approximately 7500 cases are diagnosed in the UK annually, making this the ninth most common malignancy. It is more common in men than women and in people aged >60 years. Smoking, heavy alcohol intake, and consuming caustic substances are risk factors.

Treatment may include surgery, chemotherapy, radiotherapy (see 'Chemotherapy and radiotherapy', Chapter 20), and the insertion of a stent (see below).

Nutritional management should include assessment of nutritional status and aim to provide an adequate energy and nutrient intake in a format that can be swallowed and is acceptable to the patient (see 'Texture modification' in 'Cerebrovascular accident/stroke', Chapter 19). Patients with oesophageal cancer are often undernourished on diagnosis as a result of an inadequate intake due to symptoms; depletion may be exacerbated by treatment. Appropriate nutritional support is ∴ essential. Tube feeding may be required, particularly if surgery is undertaken and a gastrostomy tube, possibly inserted at theatre, may provide valuable access.

Oesophageal stricture

May arise from benign causes (e.g. gastro-oesophageal reflux, damage secondary to intubation) or secondary to malignancy and results in increasing difficulty swallowing.

Treatment is aimed at the underlying cause and attempting to limit the occlusive effects of the stricture including balloon dilatation and stenting.

Nutritional management should ensure an adequate intake. Small, frequent meals comprising moist, semi-solid food and nourishing liquids may be tolerated but, if not, tube feeding should be instigated before severe depletion or dehydration occurs.

Oesophageal varices see Chapter 23.

Oesophagitis

Inflammation of the oesophagus is associated with acid reflux from the stomach and hiatus hernia. Prolonged oesophagitis can lead to thickening and hardening of the mucosal cells, known as Barrett's oesophagus.

Nutritional management See gastro-oesophageal reflux disease/hiatus hernia (in 'Stomach disorders', this chapter).

Stents

The endoscopic insertion of a metal stent into a strictured oesophagus may prevent total occlusion and help the patient to maintain their oral intake. Stents are mainly used as palliation in oesophageal cancer but can also play a role in the management of benign strictures and oesophageal fistulae. Complications include haemorrhage, migration, tumour over-growth, and food-related blockages.

Nutritional management should include dietary advice about maintaining an adequate energy and nutrient intake and how to minimize the risk of tube blockage (see box). Even though this treatment is seen primarily as palliative, 75–90% of patients resume a near-normal diet after stent insertion and improvements in nutritional status and survival have been reported.

Dietary advice after oesophageal stent placement[*]

Fluids

- Prescribe a fluid-only diet for first 24 hours after insertion
- Once food is introduced, advise frequent consumption of any type of liquid after eating food in order to wash away any debris
- There is no evidence to support the use of fizzy drinks. These may cause problems with acid reflux if stent is placed distally
- If the stent becomes blocked following eating, drink warm water to flush through

Food

- Advice given should be modified to take account of the patient's tumour, their ability to chew, continuing dysphagia, and posture/position
- Texture modification should reflect individual patient needs (see 'Texture modification' in 'Cerebrovascular accident/stroke', Chapter 19) and appropriate written advice should be given
- If no texture modification is required, patients should be advised to:
  - take small mouthfuls and chew all food well
  - sit upright when eating
  - eat slowly and without rushing
  - drink plenty of fluid
- Patients are often advised to restrict foods considered potentially stent-blocking. However, experimental evidence suggests that few items need to be totally avoided.
  - Foods causing occlusion: dry meat, fruit with pith, skins of capsicum peppers and tomatoes, >7 sultanas, dried apricots
  - Foods able to pass through stent if taken in small mouthfuls and chewed for twice the usual time: sandwiches, dry toast, apple, tinned pineapple, fresh orange segments with pith removed, ≤6 sultanas, chopped dried apricots, boiled egg, muesli, meat and poultry
  - Controversial items like nuts and vegetables including lettuce caused no occlusions

Nutritional support

Most patients continue to need nutritional support and their nutritional status should be regularly assessed

[*] Adapted from British Dietetic Association (2003). *Dietetic advice post oesophageal stent placement.* BDA, Birmingham; Holdoway, A., et al. (2003). Palliative management of cancer of the oesophagus—opportunities for dietetic intervention. *J. Hum. Nutr. Dietet.* **16**, 369.

Stomach disorders

Nausea and vomiting

Nausea and vomiting can have a significant effect on nutritional status b greatly reducing intake or preventing the digestion and absorption of food consumed. These symptoms may relate to a gastrointestinal disorder, food poisoning, other systemic condition, e.g. uraemia, or treatment e.g. chemotherapy (See 'Chemotherapy and radiotherapy', Chapter 20). Treatment of the underlying cause or self-limitation may bring resolution but, in many cases, managing the situation may help maintain an adequate nutritional intake.

Nutritional management

Try:
- chilled foods as these may be more acceptable than hot items;
- plain foods in small quantities may be better tolerated;
- sip drinks throughout day but wait for 15 min after eating before taking more fluid;
- ginger flavours, mints and plain biscuits.

Avoid:
- off-putting smells (food or others);
- foods that don't appeal—may include spicy or greasy items;
- lying down after eating—a gentle walk may help;
- extreme hunger by eating small amounts regularly.

In severe cases, dehydration may be a concern and oral rehydration solution or intravenous fluids may be required.

Indigestion, heartburn, gastro-oesophageal reflux disease (GORD), and hiatus hernia

This spectrum of gastric disorders is common with an estimated 20–25% of adults in the UK and USA experiencing symptoms of GORD. Although diet has been implicated in the aetiology (erratic eating habits, obesity, alcohol, and other specific food items), there is little firm evidence to confirm this.

Symptoms range from post-prandial discomfort to sharp burning pain below the sternum or between the shoulder blades, regurgitation of acidic stomach contents into oesophagus and possibly mouth, and, in severe cases, mucosal damage.

Nutritional management (in addition to proton pump inhibitors and H_2 blockers) should include review of diet and lifestyle with the aim of introducing a regular and well-balanced eating pattern based on the 'Balance of Good Health' (see 'Food-based dietary guidelines', Chapter 2). Specific dietary advice is mostly anecdotal but usually compatible with a healthy diet and includes reducing intake of alcohol, caffeine, fatty, spicy and other irritating food and reducing excess body weight. Practical suggestions about eating include:
- small, regular meals in place of occasional large meals;
- eat earlier in the evening and avoid late night meals;

Is it necessary for people with stomach disorders to avoid spicy food ?

- There are few clinical studies that confirm that spicy food exacerbates the symptoms or progression of gastritis or gastric ulcers
- Limited evidence, including *in vitro* and animal work, suggests spices play a complex role in influencing gastrointestinal health.
  - Extract of turmeric appears to both inhibit and promote DNA mutation in mucosal cells *in vitro*.
  - Animal studies show chilli extract protects against gastric mucosal injury; a high chilli intake in humans is an independent risk factor for gastric cancer
  - Spice, garam masala, is associated with more rapid gastric emptying in humans
  - Spice extracts (including clove, ginger, and nutmeg) inhibit *Helicobacter pylori* growth *in vitro*, possibly explaining low rates of gastric disease in countries like Thailand
- Conclusion: inadequate evidence for advice—more research required.

Helicobacter pylori—are there any nutritional implications?

H. pylori is a bacterium commonly found in the stomach. Infection may be asymptomatic but is associated with gastritis, ulceration and ↑ risk of stomach cancer. Prevalence of infection ↑ with age and is highest in developing countries and people of lower socio-economic status. In the UK, ~30% of people born in 1930s are infected compared with <5% born in 1970s.

- Acquisition of infection is by person-to-person transmission (oral–oral and faecal–oral) and possibly also via food. Overcrowding and poor hygiene practices are implicated. Good personal and food hygiene may ↓ risk of transmission
- Oral probiotics may act as a beneficial adjunct to antibiotic eradication therapy. Further studies are needed to clarify optimum dose and population
- There is limited evidence that dietary factors, e.g. spices, alcohol, antioxidant intake, may alter the susceptibility to *H. pylori* infection. However, this is insufficient to make recommendations

- sit upright rather than slumped while eating and avoid bending, lifting, or lying down immediately after meals;
- elevate the head-end of the bed to facilitate a semi-upright position while sleeping;
- avoid foods that are known to cause discomfort to individual.

Gastritis and peptic ulcers

Gastritis is the inflammation of mucosal surface of the stomach. It can range from a mild, asymptomatic form to severe ulceration, which if untreated may lead to perforation. Peptic ulcers include lesions in the stomach and duodenum. 80% of gastritis and peptic ulcers are associated with *Helicobacter pylori* infection (see box) but a high intake of alcohol and nonsteroidal anti-inflammatory drugs is also implicated.

Symptoms include nausea, vomiting (possibly blood-stained), and pain.

Nutritional management In severe cases, patients have no desire to eat and 'resting' the stomach from food for 1–2 days may help alleviate pain; adequate fluid including sugar and electrolytes will minimize risk of dehydration. Nutrient intake should be gradually ↑ over 1–3 days by providing other nourishing fluids and then bland, non-irritating foods. There is little clinical evidence about specific foods to avoid, but most individuals are aware of items that exacerbate symptoms (often spicy, highly flavoured foods with a high fat content) and thus should decide whether or not to risk eating them (see box). Fruit and juice with perceptible acidity have traditionally been avoided on the grounds that these exacerbate gastric pH; there is no evidence for this and the antioxidants provided by these food items play a valuable role in promoting healing so they should not be avoided unnecessarily. Some people may find plain, bland food is tolerated best and that milk and milky foods are most agreeable; again, there is no evidence to support this and patients should be encouraged to eat a wide range of foods. Ultimately, a varied and well-balanced diet should be the goal.

Stomach cancer

Approximately 9000 cases are diagnosed in the UK annually, making this the seventh most common malignancy. It is more common in individuals with *Helicobacter pylori* infection and those eating a high intake of smoked, cured, and salted food as, for example, in Japan where such food is eaten regularly.

Symptoms include heartburn, anorexia and bloating progressing to vomiting (sometimes blood stained), pain on eating and severe weight loss.

Treatment is surgical resection (see 'Gastrectomy and stomach surgery', this chapter) if the tumour is operable. Chemotherapy and radiotherapy (see 'Chemotheray and radiotherapy', Chapter 20) may be used in conjunction or as alternatives.

Nutritional management depends on treatment but should aim to maintain an optimum nutritional intake whether by mouth or through artificial nutrition support. Each patient should be individually assessed and their requirements evaluated and nutrition support planned on the basis of these and the access available for feeding. Specific advice is required after surgical resection.

Gastrectomy and stomach surgery

The type of surgical resection of the stomach, e.g. for cancer, perforation following severe ulceration or traumatic injury, varies depending on the degree and position of the lesion to be removed but can be briefly summarized as (see Fig. 21.1) follows

- Total gastrectomy—resection of complete stomach with anastomosis of oesophagus to the small bowel and reconnection of the duodenum to the small bowel (Roux-en-Y reconstruction). Cardiac and pyloric sphincters removed.
- Partial gastrectomy—resection of distal (pyloric) end of stomach by anastomosis of remaining part of upper stomach to duodenum or, more commonly, small bowel (Bilroth 2 reconnection). Pyloric sphincter removed.
- Oesophago-gastrectomy—resection of proximal (cardiac) end of stomach and lower oesophagus by anastomosis of lower stomach to upper oesophagus. Cardiac sphincter removed.
- Vagotomy—cutting the vagus nerve, to reduce acid secretion also causes a decrease in peristalsis and alters the emptying patterns of the stomach. It is often undertaken with gastrectomy or a pyloroplasty, a procedure to widen the outlet from the stomach to the small intestine.

The type of surgery, anastomosis, and removal of sphincter muscles have nutritional relevance because they influence eating-related symptoms after surgery. Evidence from studies of total gastrectomies suggests that a Roux-en-Y anastomosis and reconstruction including some form of pouch is nutritionally and symptomatically optimum.

Nutritional management Recommencing oral intake, usually in the form of clear fluids, should be undertaken as soon as possible after surgery. Gradually increase from liquids to solid food so that in most cases some solid food is being taken 1 week post-op. Food-related complications include the following.

- Feeling full after very small quantities of food is common, particularly following total gastrectomy, so very small meals eaten frequently (~ hourly, initially) will help to maximize nutrient intake and thus contribute to healing. Bulky foods and fizzy drinks may be best avoided at first as these may exacerbate feelings of fullness. Drinking separately from eating may also help.
- Dumping syndrome is caused by the rapid movement of dietary sugar/refined carbohydrate into the intestine. Early post-prandial symptoms include dizziness, faintness, sweating, and a sudden drop in blood pressure. Later symptoms can occur ~2 hours after eating including weakness, cold, and faintness associated with hypoglycaemia resulting from excessive release of insulin in response to rapidly absorbed dietary carbohydrate. Both early and late symptoms can be controlled by eating small meals regularly, limiting refined carbohydrate, including small quantities of high fibre foods if tolerated, and drinking liquids separately from meals. The intensity of symptoms may resolve within 3 months of surgery.

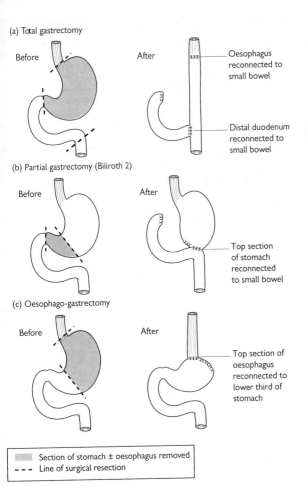

(a) Total gastrectomy

Before   After
Oesophagus reconnected to small bowel

Distal duodenum reconnected to small bowel

(b) Partial gastrectomy (Biliroth 2)

Before   After
Top section of stomach reconnected to small bowel

(c) Oesophago-gastrectomy

Before   After
Top section of oesophagus reconnected to lower third of stomach

Section of stomach ± oesophagus removed
--- Line of surgical resection

Fig.21.1 Gastrectomy and stomach surgery.

- Diarrhoea is relatively common in the first 1–2 months after gastric surgery. Dietary modification is not required but antimotility medication, e.g. codeine phosphate or loperamide hydrochloride, may help.
- Vomiting of bile and other digestive juices may occur after partial gastrectomy, particularly in the morning. No dietary modification is required; antacids or motility stimulants, e.g. domperidone or metoclopramide, may help but some patients require reconstructive surgery to alleviate the problem.
- Indigestion may be relieved by peppermint oil. Foods that exacerbate should be avoided.

Supplementation of nutrients is not routinely required by all patients but should be determined on an individual basis depending on the patient's underlying disorder, extent of surgery, and oral intake.

- Energy and macronutrients. Weight loss may indicate an inadequate intake or a recurrence of malignant disease; intake should be assessed and, if necessary, supplemented.
- Vitamin B_{12}. Prophylactic vitamin B_{12} supplementation by intramuscular injection is mandatory following total gastrectomy due to loss of stomach-derived intrinsic factor required for absorption. In patients with partial gastrectomy, vitamin B_{12} absorption test should be checked to identify requirement.
- Iron and folate. Regular blood tests are required to identify anaemia and iron and\or folate supplemented as necessary.
- Calcium and vitamin D. Bone disease is common after gastrectomy and supplementation may help prevent this.

Small intestine disorders: introduction

The small intestine comprises ~7 m of the gastrointestinal tract running from the pyloric sphincter of the stomach to the ileo-caecal valve and comprises:

- duodenum;
- jejunum;
- ileum.

Its main function is to digest and absorb energy, nutrients, and water from the partially digested food passing through its lumen. As a consequence, any disorders of the small intestine that result in impaired function will potentially have a significant influence on absorption and ∴ on nutritional status.

Disorders with nutritional implications include:

- malabsorption (including steatorrhoea and lactose intolerance);
- inflammatory bowel disease (Crohn's disease and ulcerative colitis);
- coeliac disease;
- intestinal failure and short bowel syndrome;
- fistulae.

Malabsorption: introduction

Symptoms Diarrhoea, abdominal distension, and flatulence due to intestinal gas production, weight loss.

Aetiology Multifactorial, (see box).

Treatment

The underlying cause of malabsorption should be treated wherever possible, e.g. treating infections, prescribing pancreatic lipase in insufficiency, avoiding gluten in coeliac disease. If this cannot be done, the effects of malabsorption can be partially ameliorated through dietary manipulation.

Nutritional management

- Individual patients should be assessed and advised by a dietitian with expertise in treating patients with malabsorption.
- Consideration must be given to the cause of malabsorption in order to identify the specific section of the small intestine that is affected and thus which nutrients are likely to be inadequately absorbed, e.g. disaccharides are absorbed in the proximal jejunum, vitamin B_{12} in the ileum (see 'Digestion', Chapter 1).
- The consequences of inadequate absorption of some specific nutrients, e.g. fat and lactose, must be considered as these will result in generalized malabsorption of most other nutrients because of the effects of interaction with other unabsorbed components and\or bacterial action.
- In addition to dietary manipulation which may resolve symptoms, consideration must be given to overall nutritional adequacy and, in patients who have become nutritionally depleted by malabsorption, restoration of nutritional status.

Main causes of malabsorption

Anatomical
- Surgical resection
- Fistulae

Luminal factors
- Altered pH, e.g. Zollinger–Ellison syndrome
- Bile salt insufficiency

Enzyme insufficiency
- Pancreatic insufficiency, e.g. lipase
- Lactase deficiency, $1°$ or $2°$

Mucosal insufficiency
- Villous atrophy
- Coeliac disease
- Crohn's disease
- Radiation enteritis
- Impaired transport
- Lymphangiectasia

Infection
- Bacterial overgrowth, e.g. in blind loops
- Parasitic infections

Systematic conditions
- Scleroderma
- Lymphoma

Drugs
- Antibiotics
- Excessive laxative use

Steatorrhoea

Untreated fat malabsorption is potentially very serious because undigested fat forms complexes within the gastrointestinal lumen with calcium and other minerals preventing them and a wide range of other nutrients from being absorbed.

If steatorrhoea arises from pancreatic lipase insufficiency, this should be remedied by prescribing pancreatic enzymes (see 'Pancreatic enzyme replacement therapy', Chapter 22). However, bile inadequacy cannot be so readily treated and a low fat diet may be required.

Low fat diet The amount of fat tolerated varies between individuals and it is recommended that a very low fat diet of ~20 g /day (Table 21.2) is instigated temporarily (days only) until symptoms resolve and then small amounts of additional dietary fat are added to the diet to tolerance. Most patients with malabsorption can tolerate a diet providing ± 40 g fat and there is no benefit from advising a lower level of restriction than one that ameliorates symptoms. Attention must be given to the following:

- Total energy content of the diet. 40 g fat provides <20% of the energy requirements of most adults (in a healthy diet, fat provides 30–35%) so the deficit must be made up by increasing carbohydrate or protein intake or by supplementing with medium chain triglycerides (see box).
- Fat-soluble vitamins, A, D, E, and K. If absorption is in doubt, vitamin status should be assessed. Supplements should be given orally or by intramuscular injection depending on the degree of malabsorption (Table 21.3).
- Calcium. Supplements, e.g. 1600 mg/40 mmol daily, should be given if steatorrhoea is prolonged or there is evidence of bone thinning.
- Essential fatty acids. The limited dietary fat consumed should include some linolenic and linoleic fatty acids.

Table 21.3 Vitamin supplements*

| Vitamin | Route of administration | |
	Oral	Intramuscular
A	25 000 IU daily	100 000 IU 3-monthly
D	400–4000 IU daily	100 000 IU monthly
E	α-tocopherol acetate 50–200 IU daily†	DL-α-tocopherol 1–2 IU/kg daily then at intervals
K	2.5–5.0 mg daily	10 mg monthly

* Reproduced from p.415 of Thomas, B. (2001). *Manual of Dietetic Practice*, Table 2.18, p191. Permission requested from Balckwell Publishing.
† Paediatric dose.

Table 21.2 Sample menu for temporary very low fat diet (20 g). Fat intake should be ↑ to tolerance according to individual needs—most patients will tolerate ~40 g/day[*]

	Weight (g)	Energy (kcal)	Fat (g)
Orange juice	250	110	—
Cereal with sugar	55	210	0.5
Skimmed milk for whole day	600	210	0.6
Toast, 2 slices	75	180	1.7
Marmalade	20	50	—
Coffee with skimmed milk + sugar	250	40	—
Low fat yoghurt	150	170	1.7
Dates	40	120	0.2
Sandwich, 4 slices bread	140	330	2.2
½ tsp polyunsaturated margarine[†]	3	20	2.4
Lean ham	80	80	2.2
Sliced tomatoes	60	10	—
Banana	110	90	0.4
Tea with skimmed milk + sugar	250	40	—
Toasted tea cake with honey	45	120	0.9
Roast chicken, no skin	120	120	3.7
Boiled potatoes, large serving	200	170	0.2
Carrots and peas	200	60	0.4
Thin gravy	80	—	—
Tinned fruit in syrup	100	70	—
Low fat custard	75	70	1.1
Low-fat chocolate drink	250	40	1.4
Marshmallow or jelly sweets	30	90	—
Approximate total	—	2400	19.6

[*] Supplementary fat-soluble vitamins ± calcium supplements should be prescribed.
[†] Source of essential fatty acids.

Medium chain triglycerides (MCT)

- MCT comprise fatty acids with 6–12 carbon atoms (long chain triglycerides (LCT) have fatty acids with >12 carbons)
- Partially water-mixable so more easily emulsified than LCT—useful if inadequate bile
- More easily hydrolysed than LCT—useful if inadequate lipase
- Absorbed directly into portal circulation—chylomicrons transport via lymph not required
- Provide 8.4 kcal/g (compared to 9.0 kcal/g with LCT)—a useful source of energy if ordinary fat cannot be taken
- Available as:
  - oil (Alembicol D, Alembic; MCT Oil, Mead Johnson; MCT Oil, SHS)
  - emulsion (Liquigen, SHS)
  - powder, with carbohydrate (Duocal MCT Powder, SHS)
  - complete or partially complete feeds (MCT Pepdite, SHS; Monogen, SHS; Nutrison MCT, Nutricia Clinical; Peptisorb, Nutricia Clinical)
- Indications include steatorrhoea, lymphangiectasia, and ketogenic diets for epilepsy
- MCT should be introduced into the diet gradually (<15 ml oil per dose) to avoid diarrhoea
- In cooking, the oil has a low flash point so very high temperatures can give food a burnt taste
- Emulsion can be added to low fat milkshakes to increase energy

Lactose intolerance

Insufficiency of lactase is the most common cause of carbohydrate-related malabsorption (sucrase and maltase deficiency is very rare except in Greenland).

- 1°—due to autosomal recessive disorder where lactase production is ± normal in children <4 years but declines in older children and adults leading to lactose intolerance. Prevalence varies with ethnicity: African-Caribbean >80%, Indian >50%, White Europeans <10%. 1° lactose intolerance may also occur at birth (but is rare) due to a hereditary total lactase deficiency.
- 2°—due to loss of lactase production as a result of damage to the intestinal villi, often after infection. This is usually temporary (~weeks) and lactase production may slowly resume spontaneously when the damage resolves.

Nutritional management This is based on a low lactose or lactose free diet. This is relatively straightforward in adults and older children providing that the rest of the diet includes sufficient variety to meet all nutrient needs including calcium. However, more expertise is required to plan a regime for infants and younger children, because of the important nutritional role milk usually plays, to ensure that their intake is sufficiently free from lactose and yet remains otherwise nutritionally adequate.

Diet for lactose intolerance Individuals vary in the amount of lactose they can tolerate without experiencing symptoms of malabsorption (diarrhoea, bloating, and discomfort). There is no benefit in avoiding more lactose than is necessary to control symptoms. Although milk should be avoided or reduced by most individuals, a diet for lactose intolerance is *not* the same as a milk-free diet which is required for milk protein allergy (see box).

Lactose tolerance may be maximized by consuming small amounts of lactose in the diet; this allows colonic bacteria to adapt to and metabolize lactose. Lactose in 'hard' foods that also contain dietary fat, e.g. cheese, chocolate, ice cream, is often better tolerated than in milk.

Dietary calcium intake may be compromised in individuals avoiding milk and other dairy products. This is particularly a concern for children, teenagers, pregnant women, and those with a family history of osteoporosis. Good sources of non-milk calcium include: oily fish, e.g. sardines, white or brown bread, calcium-fortified soya drinks (see 'Calcium' in Chapter 5 and discussion of calcium in 'Vegetarians', Chapter 13).

Infants and children <5 years with confirmed lactose intolerance should be given an appropriate lactose-free milk substitute (e.g. Enfamil Lactofree, Mead Johnson; SMA LF, SMA Nutrition) under the advice of a registered dietitian.

Foods usually free from lactose	Foods containing lactose[*]
Soya milks Rice milk drinks Non-dairy creamers (check label) Most hard cheese contains very little lactose so is well tolerated, e.g. Cheddar, Brie, Edam	Milk: skimmed, semi-skimmed, & whole (cow's, goat's, sheep's) Cheese spread, cream, & cottage cheese Cream & sour cream Evaporated & condensed milk Yogurt
Breads made without milk Breakfast cereals made without milk Pasta, noodles, macaroni Potatoes, rice, other cooked grains Rice cakes	Breakfast cereal with milk Instant mashed potato mixes Prepared breads, muffins, biscuits, or rolls made with milk Pancakes or batter made with milk
Margarine without whey (check label) Non-dairy creamers (check label) Oils Some salad dressings (check label)	Butter Margarines with butter or milk
All fresh fruits & vegetables Cooked fruit or vegetables made without milk products Fruit & vegetable juices	Creamed vegetables, e.g. mashed potato Fruit smoothies made with yogurt Fruits or vegetables cooked with milk Vegetables coated in batter
All fresh cooked, plain meat & fish Cooked dried peas & beans Eggs cooked without milk Peanut butter, nuts, & seeds Soya cheese & tofu products	Breaded or battered meat or fish Main dishes with white sauce such as macaroni cheese, fish in parsley sauce Meats in cream sauces Omelette or soufflés with milk
Broth, bouillon, consommé Vegetable or meat soups without milk Gravies made with water Plain herbs & spices	Cream soups Soup mixes with milk products White sauces & gravies
Fruit ices & sorbets Honey, sugar, syrups, molasses, & powdered sweeteners Jellies, jams, preserves Pies & other baked foods without milk	Custard or sauce made from milk Cream or cheese filled cake or pastries Fudge, coated candies, & chocolates Ice cream unless lactose-free Toffee, butterscotch, or caramels

[*] Many people with lactose intolerance can eat some of these foods and a very strict, lactose-free diet is required by very few individuals. It is recommended that very intolerant individuals and carers of small children check labels of food products and proceed with caution if the following ingredients are listed: milk powder, milk protein, milk solids, non-fat milk solids, whey, whey solids or protein.

Inflammatory bowel disease

Inflammatory bowel disease (IBD) includes two major disorders, Crohn disease and ulcerative colitis, which both involve chronic inflammation of the gastrointestinal tract, sometimes with acute episodes. IBD should not be confused with irritable bowel syndrome (IBS).

Crohn's disease (CD)

Prevalence Approximately 1 in 1500 people in the UK have CD. It is less common in Africa, Asian, and Central and South America. All ages can be affected but diagnosis is most frequent in children and young adults.

Aetiology The cause has not yet been identified but dietary origins have not been substantiated.

Symptoms Inflammation can affect any part of the gastrointestinal tract but is most common in the ileo-caecal region of the small intestine and colon. Abdominal pain and diarrhoea (with mucus and blood) feature. Recurrent episodes of inflammation lead to deep ulceration, strictures and fistulae; surgical resection may be required, sometimes repeatedly. Patients often lose weight and feel very unwell.

Nutritional management
Assessment
- A registered dietitian with IBD expertise should undertake a nutrition assessment and provide individual advice.
- Weight (and height in children and adolescents) should be monitored and documented at all outpatient appointments and weekly during admissions.
- Vitamin B_{12} status should be measured annually in patients with ileal CD.

Preventing/treating undernutrition
- Patients with CD are often undernourished (up to 85%) as a result of inadequate intake and ↑ losses through malabsorption. Undernutrition includes energy and protein depletion and, in some patients, specific micronutrient deficiencies.
- Nutritional support is a high priority and should be an integral part of management. The form/degree of support will depend on current severity, i.e. in exacerbation or remission.
- Those most likely to require nutritional support include children and adolescents (who are still growing), patients with existing undernutrition, and those with an exacerbation of symptoms, partial obstruction or recovering from surgery.
- Although patients may avoid specific foods, wherever possible restricted items should be minimized and a 'normal' diet encouraged including energy- and protein-dense foods.
- Patients with strictures or partial obstruction should avoid fibrous foods that may lead to an obstruction, e.g. stringy beans, citrus fruit pith, meat gristle, nuts.
- Limiting dietary fat (~40 g/d or to tolerance) may help reduce proven fat malabsorption but should not be routinely advised.

- Oral nutritional supplements should be offered if insufficient food is consumed (see 'Treatment of undernutrition', this Chapter 16). Most commercial products (except powders that are mixed with milk) are low in lactose so acceptable even if 2° lactose intolerance is suspected (see 'Lactose intolerance', this chapter).
- Enteral feeding is the preferred route if oral intake is inadequate and should be considered early before nutritional depletion is allowed to progress.
- Standard micronutrient supplementation should be given.
- The anti-inflammatory effects of n-3 fatty acids (from oily fish, see box in 'Cardioprotective diet', Chapter 19) may have a beneficial effect on remission. Further evidence is required before a recommendation can be made.

Dietary versus other treatment
- Elemental (amino acid based) or polymeric (containing whole protein) diets are less effective than corticosteroids but may have a role in inducing remission in patients with active CD who have a contraindication or preference not to use this medication. Therefore, elemental or polymeric diets are considered appropriate adjunctive therapy. Elemental diets are less palatable than polymeric diets and consideration should be given to compliance if patients are advised to consume these over a long period.
- Total parenteral nutrition (see 'Parenteral nutrition', Chapter 16) is an appropriate adjunctive therapy in patients with fistulae.

Ulcerative colitis (UC)

Prevalence Approximately 1 in 1250 people in most Western countries have UC. It is less common but increasing in Africa and India. Men and women are equally affected and diagnosis is most frequent between the ages of 20 and 40 years.

Aetiology The cause has not yet been definitively identified but a combination of dietary and colonic microflora origins has been implicated.

Symptoms Inflammation affects the rectum and may extend continuously towards the caecum. The small intestine is not involved. Abdominal pain, diarrhoea (with blood and mucus), and anaemia feature in a chronic, relapsing pattern. Acute episodes may occur and complications include strictures, perforation and toxic megacolon. Surgical resection may be required leading to the formation of colostomy or ileo-rectal pouch.

Nutritional management

Severe nutritional depletion is less of a problem in patients with UC compared to those with CD, probably as a result of inflammation affecting areas of the gut distal to the site of absorption of most nutrients. However, UC patients frequently have a poor appetite or consume a restricted diet in an effort to relieve their symptoms and poor nutritional status is common. Nutritional management should ∴ focus on the adequacy of patients' intake and their nutritional status.

- No dietary restrictions should be routinely advised (there is no evidence to support the use of low residue diets).
- Patients should be encouraged to eat as normally as possible.
- There is no evidence that elemental or other dietary interventions have a specific therapeutic impact on the condition.
- 'Bowel rest' has no proven benefits in UC.
- Patients undergoing colectomy may benefit from specific advice about their food intake after surgery.
- Many patients with UC have iron deficiency anaemia and may require supplementation.
- Calcium intake and bone status should be monitored in those receiving corticosteroids for more severe disease.
- Patients with UC have ↑ risk of colon cancer and, in order to minimize this, those in remission should be advised to eat a healthy diet along the lines of the 'Balance of Good Health' (see 'Food-based dietary guidelines Chapter 2).

Coeliac disease

Coeliac disease is an immunomediated condition resulting in mucosal damage of the jejunum. It is caused by the ingestion of a protein, gluten, found in cereals such as wheat, rye and barley. Approximately 0.5–1.0% of the UK population have coeliac disease. Diagnosis is made by raised blood tissue transglutaminase levels and flat appearance of the jejunal mucosa.

Symptoms range from lethargy and tiredness, with or without anaemia, to diarrhoea bloating, abdominal discomfort, and weight loss. The range of gluten sensitivity is wide. The only treatment for the coeliac condition is the life-long exclusion of gluten from the diet. This is a major task for individuals to undertake and should always involve expert dietetic counselling with an annual dietetic review for all patients with coeliac disease.

The gluten-free (GF) diet

Foods can be categorized into three groups:
- foods that contain obvious sources of gluten derived from wheat and flour, e.g. bread, pasta, wheat-based breakfast cereals, cakes, biscuits;
- 'hidden' sources of gluten, where it is used as a thickener, filler, or carrier for flavours. These include many manufactured soups, sauces, sausages, cheese spreads, and ready meals.
- foods and ingredients that are naturally gluten-free include rice, maize, milk, eggs, fresh fruit and vegetables, fresh meats including poultry, fresh fish and seafood, butter, margarine, cooking oils. These can be safely used in the gluten free diet without limitation.

Prescribable products

GF products play an important role in the treatment of the coeliac condition. These are specifically manufactured without gluten and the range includes bread, biscuits, pasta, and flours. Some are made from carefully de-glutenized wheat while others are based on other sources, e.g. rice or potato. A limited assortment of GF products is prescribable to people with coeliac disease on the FP10 form. Further information can be found in the *British National Formulary*, Appendix 7, *Borderline substances* (see 'Prescription of nutritional products', Chapter 8). Others, including some more luxurious GF items like cakes and confectionery, can be purchased through some supermarkets and by mail order.

Food labelling

Food labels are an important factor when it comes to the GF diet as imprecise labelling may lead inadvertently to coeliac patients consuming gluten. New UK labelling regulations came into effect during 2005, which means that all ingredients present in a specific food will have to be listed, however small the quantity, and gluten will have to be identified as being present in the food item. In spite of this improvement, Coeliac UK recommends that food items are checked against their compiled list of manufactured products (www.coeliac.co.uk). GF manufactured products are often identified using the crossed grain symbol: ⊗

Contamination

A GF diet can become contaminated with gluten in a variety of ways. Naturally GF grains can become contaminated with wheat during the milling process, particularly when the same mills are used to process a number of different cereals. During manufacturing, contamination can also occur when the same production lines are used for GF and gluten-containing foods. Similarly, in the home, using the same toaster, bread board, or butter/margarine container for preparing GF and ordinary bread or sandwiches can lead to transfer of gluten via small breadcrumbs.

Other sources of gluten

- Medication and vitamin preparations may contain gluten; advice on specific products should be sought from a pharmacist.
- Wine, cider, liqueurs, and spirits (including whisky and malt whisky) are gluten-free but beer, lager, stout, and real ales should be avoided.
- Most communion wafers are made from wheat flour. GF wafers are available and permitted for use by the Roman Catholic church.

Oats

Traditionally, people with coeliac disease have been advised to avoid oats. Recent studies have suggested that this may not be necessary for everyone. Adults with coeliac disease who are well may be advised to take up to 50 g oats (one serving) per day. Children and adults who are particularly sensitive should continue to avoid oats and oat products. Oats are often stored, milled and processed with other cereals so only GF oats should be consumed (see Coeliac UK list described above).

Compliance

Strict dietary compliance is a problem with some coeliac patients. The non-compliance rates vary considerably from 45 to 94%. Those with poor compliance have ↑ risk of nutritional deficiency, reduced bone mineral density, and ↑ risk of malignancy. Following a strict GF diet for 5 years or more protects against malignancies. The reasons for non-compliance are numerous and varied but include:

- restrictions to everyday lifestyle;
- difficulties maintaining a strict diet when eating out, at school, whilst travelling or when on holiday;
- the diet being more expensive (although it should not be as many GF foods are prescribable);
- longer preparation and cooking;
- some patients can feel well and lack symptoms so perceive little benefit from following GF diet.

Intestinal failure and short bowel syndrome

Patients with intestinal failure (IF) require specialized nutritional support which is integral to their medical management. IF may result from either a loss of function or a reduction in gastrointestinal tract length (short bowel syndrome, SBS). Common causes include resection (often multiple) 2° to Crohn's disease, mesenteric infarction, radiation enteritis and traumatic injury.

Nutritional implications

- IF depends on the degree and site of intestinal disease or resection and whether there is continuity with the rest of the gut or a high output stoma.
- Parenteral support will usually be required in individuals with SBS with:
  - <100 cm of intestine + jejunostomy (fluid ± electrolytes only);
  - <75 cm of intestine + jejunostomy (parenteral nutrition);
  - <50 cm of intestine + colon intact (parenteral nutrition).
- The remnant gut may be able to adapt and increase absorptive capacity (depending on underlying condition) over a period of up to 3 years. Dietary modification and hormonal stimulation can help optimize this.
- Each patient must be individually assessed and advised by a registered dietitian with experience in IF/SBS. Most patients are treated at specialist centres where relevant expertise is available. Regular monitoring of nutritional status is an essential component of ongoing medical care.

Diet in SBS—Jejunum in continuity with colon

A high carbohydrate (60% energy), low fat (20% energy) diet is associated with reduced faecal weight and ↑ water absorption. Reducing fat intake is essential to help decrease steatorrhoea and thus maximize absorption of other nutrients although restrictions should be minimized to those needed to control symptoms because fat is a good source of energy. Medium chain triglycerides may be used to provide additional energy (see box in 'Steatorrhoea', this chapter). Fat soluble vitamins should be supplemented or status monitored. Oxalate intake should be minimized due to ↑ risk of calcium oxalate renal stones (ideally avoid rhubarb, spinach, beetroot, peanuts, and excessive tea).

Diet in SBS—Jejunostomy

By contrast, reducing fat intake is not necessary in patients with a jejunostomy as the proportion of fat absorbed remains constant as fat intake increases. Medium chain triglycerides do not increase overall energy absorption so confer no benefit. Hypotonic drinks should be avoided because fluids providing <90 mmol Na^+/l will result in sodium secretion into the lumen leading to ↑ fluid loss. A high salt intake is recommended due to jejunal losses of sodium, and patients will benefit from an oral rehydration solution containing 90 mmol Na^+/l.

Fistulae

GI fistulae are abnormal holes in the gut allowing the contents (partially digested food, secretions, water, and electrolytes) to escape either into another part of the thoracic or abdominal cavities or to the outside. Most (~80%) arise as a complication of surgery while some occur spontaneously in inflammatory bowel disease, diverticular disease, and radiation enteritis or as a result of trauma. The mortality, morbidity, and nutritional consequences are significant.

Nutritional implications

- Patients with fistulae are frequently undernourished because of their underlying disease and the consequences of nutrient loss via the fistula. Impaired nutritional status will adversely affect closure, whether surgical or spontaneous.
- Route of nutrient access must be considered if GI contents are leaking and absorption reduced:
  - In many cases parenteral nutrition is required (see 'Parenteral nutrition', Chapter 16). This should take account of the individual's losses via the fistula; depending on the site, additional fluid and electrolytes may be required to replace losses. Fistula output will also determine whether any oral intake should be permitted or whether solely parenteral nutrition should be provided. Currently there is no evidence on the difference in outcome of patients who are able to eat freely or remain nil by mouth while on parenteral nutrition.
  - Fistuloclysis, enteral feeding via the fistula, may be possible and desirable in some patients. This can be undertaken by accessing the GI tract distally to the fistula if high, e.g. oesophageal, gastric, jejunal. Again, an evaluation of fistula losses is required to facilitate adequate replacement of nutrients, fluid, and electrolytes and, in some patients, enteral feeding proximal to a fistula may increase output. Opinion is divided about whether high output fistulae (≥200 ml/d pancreatic, ≥500 ml/d intestinal) are less likely to spontaneously close. However, enteral feeding should not be automatically discounted in fistula patients due to its advantages associated with lower rates of infection and maintaining GI integrity.

Gastrointestinal stoma

Stoma differ from GI fistulae in that access to the GI tract is deliberate and aims to facilitate either:

- **Input** = nutrient intake into the stomach (feeding gastrostomy) or jejunum (feeding jejunostomy, (see 'Routes for enteral feeding'), Chapter 16).
- **Output** = effluent from the jejunum (jejunostomy), ileum (ileostomy), or colon (colostomy).

Jejunostomy See 'Intestinal failure and short bowel syndrome', this chapter.

Ileostomy

Usually formed after resection in inflammatory bowel disease. Although most patients eat a normal diet, depending on the length of remaining ileum, attention must be given to the fluid and electrolytes lost from the ileostomy effluent. Losses >1500 ml/d will require additional fluid and salt. Vitamin B_{12} is absorbed at the distal end of the ileum so patients with ileo-caecal resection will require supplementation, e.g. intramuscular injection 1 mg hydroxocobalamin every 3 months.

Some patients prefer to avoid specific foods if they experience unacceptable symptoms (see box). The identification of recognizable food remains, e.g. pips, skins, grain husks, in the effluent may concern some patients. Providing this is not associated with a high output or other symptoms, reassurance should be given and patients advised to chew their food well.

Reported effects

↑ Output: high fibre foods, beetroot, mushrooms, spicy foods, alcohol, fruit juice, milk

Flatus-producing: onions, peas, beans, carbonated drinks, spicy foods, beer, milk

Offensive odour: fish, onions, leeks, garlic, eggs

Colostomy

Like ileostomy, often formed after resection in inflammatory bowel disease although more common. As effluent leaves the GI tract distally to the ileum, there is less concern with fluid and electrolyte losses. Patients should ∴ eat as normally as possible but avoid specific foods that cause unacceptable symptoms (see box). Patients with a colostomy may experience constipation and should be encouraged to increase their intake of fruit and vegetables and wholegrain cereals (see 'Constipation' in 'Diseases of the colon', this chapter). Diarrhoea should be investigated if prolonged and exceeding 1000 g/d.

Intestinal transplantation

Transplantation of the intestine (small bowel) may be undertaken singly or in conjunction with other abdominal organs, including the liver and pancreas. Approximately 25 transplants have been undertaken in the UK (1989–2004), predominantly in children, with ~70 being undertaken annually in the USA.

Indications include intestinal failure where total parenteral nutrition is associated with cholestatic liver failure.

Long-term follow-up studies (up to 10 years) show that surviving patients can be sustained independently of parenteral nutrition and that growth velocity in children can be maintained although catch-up growth is rare. Post-operative transfer from parenteral to enteral nutrition should be managed on an individual basis, ensuring that nutritional status is maintained during the weaning process.

Disorders of the colon

Constipation

Constipation is a significant health problem in the UK and most high income countries and is associated with a high number of medical consultations and expenditure on laxatives, especially in older people.

Intractable and severe constipation requires investigation and treatment of any specific underlying pathology. However, in many cases, a regular and more frequent bowel habit can be achieved by simple dietary measures.

Nutritional management is compatible with the 'Balance of Good Health' (see 'Food-based dietary guidelines' Chapter 2) and is based on increasing dietary fibre (see 'Carbohydrate' Chapter 5) and taking an adequate fluid intake.

- Change to wholegrain bread and gradually increase daily intake to 200 g (6–7 average slices).
- Take a large bowlful (50 g) of wholegrain cereal daily.
- Increase fruit and vegetable intake to 400 g/d. This is equivalent to five portions per day.
- Try wholegrain rice and pasta as alternative to white varieties.
- Include nuts, beans, and pulses.

Other measures include the following.

- In order to be effective in increasing faecal bulk and promoting bowel activity, cereal fibre must be able to absorb fluid. In order to do this, there must be sufficient fluid in the colon. Fluid intake should be a minimum of 35 ml/kg/d (i.e. ~2½ litre for 70kg man) and should lead to passing of pale, straw-coloured urine.
- People with a very low fibre diet should be advised to increase their intake of fibre gradually to help the GI tract adapt and to avoid possible side-effects of abdominal distension and ↑ flatus. If these symptoms occur, they are often self-limiting and resolve spontaneously. If they do not, selective manipulation of fibre-containing foods may help identify ones that cause less difficulty but are still effective at promoting bowel evacuation.
- A high intake of cereal bran is not recommended as a first-line treatment in constipation because of the potential for sequestering micronutrients and thus reducing absorption. Its effects are variable—rapid in some people but less effective in others. In addition, bran has been associated with bowel impaction in elderly patients with a low fluid intake. If bran is used, it should be introduced slowly into the diet and limited quantities (<10 g/d) taken in conjunction with plenty of fluid and a well-balanced diet.
- Prunes and prune juice are frequently used to treat constipation and are probably effective through their content of sorbitol and phenolic compounds.

Diverticular disease

Diverticula are blind pouches found in the intestinal wall, particularly in older people, and probably arise in the colon from ↑ intraluminal pressure as a result of constipation and a low fibre diet. In themselves, diverticula are not considered pathological but, with a continued low fibre diet, may become inflamed and infected resulting in diverticulitis. This is manifest as colicky pain with diarrhoea and/or constipation; bleeding, abscesses, and perforation may complicate. An acute episode requires treatment with antibiotics and surgery in severe cases. On recovery, recurrence can be reduced by following a high fibre diet and an adequate fluid intake (see 'Constipation' above).

Haemorrhoids

Haemorrhoids (or piles) are swollen and inflamed blood vessels in the rectum and anus. They arise after prolonged constipation when pressure in the distended colon is combined with straining to evacuate the bowel and are most common in older adults and during/after pregnancy. Patients presenting with internal (non-prolapsing) haemorrhoids should be advised to increase their fibre and fluid intake. Others should be referred to a colorectal surgeon and will benefit from advice to ↑ fibre and fluid intake after treatment.

Increasing fibre intake is useful for softening faeces, relieving constipation, and thus reducing straining. Fibre supplementation reduces episodes of bleeding and discomfort in patients with internal haemorrhoids although this may take up to 6 weeks; it does not improve external (prolapsed) haemorrhoids. Cereal fibre is most effective in increasing stool weight (see 'Constipation' above) and bulk-forming laxative, ispaghula husk, may help.

Cancer of the colon and rectum

Approximately 37 500 cases are diagnosed in the UK annually, making this the third most common malignancy. It is more common in people aged >60 years. Nutritional factors may contribute to aetiology:
- obesity is strongly associated with ↑ risk;
- high intake of fruit and vegetables has a probable protective effect;
- low dietary fibre and high red meat intake is likely to increase risk but further studies are needed.

Treatment usually includes surgery (colectomy with or without formation of a temporary or permanent colostomy; see 'Gastrointestinal stoma', this chapter), and sometimes chemotherapy and/or radiotherapy (see 'Chemotherapy and radiotherapy', Chapter 20).

Nutritional management No specific dietary regime is required but maintaining an adequate and well-balanced intake may help to optimize the patient's nutritional status and his/her ability to withstand surgery or other treatment. Patients may seek dietary advice relating to a colostomy (see 'Gastrointestinal stoma', this chapter) or may benefit from guidance if the tumour or treatment is compromising nutritional intake. Depending on the stage of the tumour at diagnosis, long-term dietary advice compatible with the Balance of Good Health (see 'Food-based dietary guidelines', Chapter 2) may be appropriate whilst for others, nutrition support to counter weight loss (see 'Treatment of undernutrition', Chapter 16) or a more palliative approach to eating (see Chapter 29) should be considered.

Irritable bowel syndrome (IBS)

IBS is a functional gastrointestinal disorder that exhibits no known structural pathology. It accounts for 40–60% of referrals to gastroenterology outpatient clinics and affects all ages and races and ~ twice as many women as men.

Diagnosis of IBS*

IBS should be diagnosed if abdominal discomfort or pain has been present for ≥12 weeks (not necessarily consecutive) in the preceding 12 months which has ≥2 of the following features:
- pain relieved with defecation
- onset of pain associated with change in stool frequency
- onset of pain associated with change in stool form/appearance

The following additional features are considered supportive of the diagnosis:
1. <3 bowel movements per week
2. >3 bowel movements per day
3. hard or lumpy stools
4. loose (mushy) or watery stools
5. straining during a bowel movement
6. urgency (having to rush to have a bowel movement)
7. feeling of incomplete bowel movement
8. passing of mucus during a bowel movement
9. abdominal fullness, bloating, or swelling

Diarrhoea-predominant IBS includes one or more of features 2, 4, & 6 but none of 1, 3, or 5; constipation-predominant IBS includes one or more of features 1, 3, & 5 but none of 2, 4, or 6.

* Rome II criteria. See Thompson, W.G., et al. (1999). Functional bowel disorders and functional abdominal pain. *Gut* **45** (suppl.2), II 43–7.

Aetiology Possible causes include stress, post-infective dysfunction and diet. True food allergy is rare although intolerance to wheat, dairy products, and coffee is frequently reported. Lactose intolerance is found in 10% of IBS patients but low lactose diets rarely resolve the condition. Excessive caffeine intake may explain some symptoms.

Dietary management

- Standardized dietary advice is not appropriate for patients with IBS and should be individualized depending on symptoms.
- Self-imposed dietary restrictions are common but may be inappropriate. However, if they appear to benefit the patient without jeopardizing nutritional status, they need not be curtailed although the lack of scientific basis should be explained to the patient.
- Although food allergies are rare, evaluating 'offending' food items through a proper exclusion diet may provide reassurance. This should be managed with the assistance of a dietitian with experience in this area to ensure that the nutrient intake remains adequate.

- Strict elimination diets (avoiding all food except one meat and one fruit before gradual reintroduction of single items) may benefit up to 70% of those completing the regime; less stringent schemes yield benefits in ± 50% of patients.
- Patients with a high milk intake (>300 ml/d) may benefit from a low lactose diet (see 'Lactose intolerance', this chapter). If this does not relieve symptoms, the restriction should be curtailed.
- Keeping a 2-week food, stress, and symptom diary may help identify causal factors that can provide a basis for planning a healthy diet.
- Patients with constipation and diarrhoea may benefit from advice about increasing or decreasing dietary fibre respectively. Routinely prescribing bran is not appropriate.

Other treatment

Dietary management should be undertaken in conjunction with other therapies including listening to the patient, healthy lifestyle advice, relaxation approaches, and pharmacotherapy.

Further information

ones, J. et al. (2000). British Society of Gastroenterology guidelines for the management of irritable bowel syndrome:
http://www.bsg.org.uk/pdf_word_docs/man_ibd.pdf

Gall bladder disorders

Gallstones

Gallstones are relatively common in populations consuming a 'Western' diet and it is estimated that ~10% of adults in the UK have gallstones, two-thirds of whom are asymptomatic. The prevalence increases with age and is more common in women. Most gallstones (~80%) are composed of predominantly cholesterol while others have a higher proportion of bilirubin, calcium, and pigments. Cholesterol precipitates into stones when bile becomes (1) supersaturated and (2) gallbladder emptying is reduced.

Risk factors for cholesterol gallstones

- Age >40 years
- Female
- Genetic variation
- ↑ Fat, ↓ fibre diet
- Obesity
- Yo-yo dieting (repeated cycles of losing and re-gaining weight)
- Hyperlipidaemia
- Pregnancy
- Diabetes mellitus
- Cystic fibrosis
- Gall bladder dysmotility
- Bile salt loss (ileal disease ± resection)
- Nil enterally (fasting or parenteral nutrition)

Preventing gallstones

- A diet compatible with the 'Balance of Good Health' is optimal (see 'Food-based dietary guidelines' Chapter 2).
- Reduction of excess body weight using moderate energy restriction (very low calorie diet may exacerbate bile saturation).
- Eat regularly to minimize bile stasis, which accompanies fasting.
- Eat breakfast on rising (cholesterol concentrations are highest in bile produced overnight).

Cholecystitis

Approximately 1–4% of people with gallstones develop symptoms each year including pain (epigastric, upper or lower abdominal), nausea, and vomiting; generally these are non-specific. Acute cholecystitis features prolonged severe pain (right subcostal) and fever.

Dietary management of cholecystitis

Previously, a low fat diet was advocated on the basis that restricting fat intake reduced gall bladder contractions and reduced pain. However, the gallbladder is known to contract in response to the oral intake of most nutrients and also in anticipation of intake. Therefore, the restriction of dietary fat is unnecessary unless a stone obstructs the hepatic or common bile duct, precluding the delivery of bile to the gastrointestinal tract and thus provoking steatorrhoea (see 'Steatorrhoea', this chapter), jaundice, and nausea. This is relatively uncommon and requires medical intervention. If a patient is well enough to eat, s/he should be advised to follow the four points listed above under 'Preventing gallstones' and to only avoid specific foods if they are definitely associated with symptoms.

Pancreatic disease

Pancreatic disorders

Pancreatitis

Pancreatitis results from the auto-digestion of the pancreas by activated pancreatic enzymes with the following characteristics.

- Acute pancreatitis: severe pain, nausea, vomiting leading to pseudocysts, fistulae, shock, renal failure.
- Chronic pancreatitis: severe pain, weight loss, malabsorption secondary to lack of pancreatic enzymes.

The annual incidence in the UK is ~1 in 100 000 (chronic) and 1 in 10–20 million (acute). Risk factors include alcohol abuse, biliary tract disease, and abdominal trauma or surgery.

Nutritional management of pancreatitis

Patients are frequently very malnourished as a result of:

- poor intake due to lack of appetite and severe pain;
- malabsorption of nutrients consumed;
- frequent episodes of nil by mouth during treatment;
- ↑ requirements due to catabolic state.

Providing adequate nutritional support is ∴ paramount in supporting these patients and, because of the difficulties associated with achieving this, input from a registered dietitian with expertise in this area is required.

Key points for nutrition support:

- Patients with mild pancreatitis require no dietary restrictions and, if well enough to eat sufficient, will not benefit from enteral nutrition.
- Systematic review found inconclusive evidence of benefits of enteral versus parenteral feeding in acute pancreatitis. It is reasonable ∴ to recommend that feeding is attempted first via the enteral route because of its associated preservation of mucosal function, which is impaired in the inflammatory response, and its lower cost.
- Nasogastric feeding is feasible in ~80% of patients.
- Parenteral nutrition is preferable to no nutrient intake where enteral feeding cannot be undertaken, e.g. ileus >5 days.
- There is no evidence, at present, to support the use of specific formulae, e.g. standard, semi-elemental, elemental, or 'immune enhanced'.

Key points for dietary advice

- Patients with a poor appetite may benefit from practical advice about increasing oral intake (see 'Treatment of under nutrition', Chapter 16).
- If malabsorption is present, advice should be given about pancreatic enzyme replacement (see next section, this chapter).
- Low fat diets have little role to play in the treatment of pancreatitis as they will exacerbate energy depletion and steatorrhoea should be controlled by pancreatic enzyme replacement.
- Approximately one-third of patients with chronic pancreatitis will develop diabetes mellitus; a compromise should be reached between dietary advice to optimize blood sugar (see 'Goals and principle of dietary management', Chapter 18) and to enhance intake to maintain body weight or reverse weight loss.
- Abstaining from alcohol is advisable as continuing alcoholism is associated with ↑ morbidity and mortality.

Pancreatic cancer

Cancer of the pancreas is the 11th most common malignancy diagnosed in the UK (~7000 cases per year). It is equally common in men and women but more likely to occur in people aged >50 years. Smoking and a history of pancreatitis are risk factors.

Treatment may include surgery, chemotherapy, and radiotherapy (see 'Chemotherapy and radiotherapy', Chapter 20) depending on the stage of the tumour at diagnosis.

Nutritional management should include assessment of nutritional status and aim to provide an adequate energy and nutrient intake in a format that can be tolerated by the patient. Patients with pancreatic cancer are often undernourished on diagnosis as a result of poor intake and severe pain; depletion may be exacerbated by treatment. Appropriate nutritional support is ∴ essential but depends on the treatment given and overall prognosis.

- No dietary restrictions are needed.
- Nutritional support, preferably via the enteral route, may improve well-being.
- Pancreatic enzymes should be used to reduce steatorrhoea and to help control pain (even if steatorrhoea is absent).
- Supplementation with *n*-3 fatty acids (see box in 'Cardioprotective diet', Chapter 19) is associated with weight gain (including lean tissue) and improved quality of life.

Pancreatic enzyme replacement therapy (PERT)

Pancreatic enzymes include lipase, amylase, and proteases, e.g. trypsin, chymotrypsin, which contribute to the digestion of fat, carbohydrate, and protein, respectively. Their insufficiency can result in malabsorption but this can be treated effectively with PERT where combined enzymes are provided as capsules, granules, or tablets (Table 22.1). Patients require advice about the use of PERT in order to optimize the effects of therapy.

- The dose prescribed may need to be adjusted to resolve malabsorption and should be varied depending on what is eaten.
- Enzymes should be taken with all foods containing fat, protein, or starchy carbohydrate, e.g. meals and snacks. Sugary foods containing no fat and protein do not require PERT.
- Enzymes should be taken just before and/or with the meal or snack.
- Enzymes are deactivated by heat so should not be mixed with hot food or drinks.
- Enzymes are also deactivated by acidity (pH < 4). Capsules containing enterically coated microtablets should be swallowed whole or, if opened, swallowed without chewing the contents as this will expose the enzymes to the denaturing effects of gastric acid.
- H_2 antagonists may be prescribed to reduce gastric secretions and maximize the effects of PERT.
- Skin contact with enzymes taken as granules may cause irritation and should be avoided.
- High strength preparations are available; some have been associated with the development of large bowel strictures when taken by children <13 years. Total dose should not exceed 10 000 units lipase/kg body weight/day and adequate hydration should be ensured. New or changing abdominal symptoms should be investigated.

Table 22.1 Examples of pancreatic enzyme replacements available in the UK

Brand name (manufacturer)	Enzyme content (BP units/capsule*)		
	Lipase	Protease	Amylase
Pancrex (Paines & Byrne)	5 000	300	4 000
Pancrease (Janssen–Cilag)	5 000	330	2 900
Nutrizym 10 (Merck)	10 000	500	9 000
Creon 10 000 (Solvay)	10 000	600	8 000
Nutrizym 22 (Merck)	22 000	1100	19 800
Pancrease HL (Janssen-Cilag)	25 000	1250	22 500
Creon 40 000 (Solvay)	40 000	1600	25 000

* Except for Pancrex granules: enzyme content (BP units/g).

Liver disease

Introduction and nutritional assessment

Nutrition-related functions of the liver include:
- emulsification of dietary fat by bile prior to digestion;
- carbohydrate metabolism (maintain blood glucose, store glycogen);
- protein metabolism (synthesis and regulation of amino acids);
- lipid metabolism (production of triglycerides and lipoprotein);
- micronutrients (storage of vitamins A, B_2, B_3, B_6, B_{12}, K, folate).

Impairment of these functions, combined with poor nutrient intake, leads to many patients with liver disease being undernourished and requiring nutrition support.

Nutritional assessment

Assessment of nutritional status is difficult in patients with liver disorders because standard methods are confounded by the disease process, e.g. fluid retention distorts body weight (Table 23.1), impaired liver function precludes use of most biochemical markers. A global assessment can provide a reliable evaluation (see box).

> ### Key points for assessing global nutritional status in patients with liver disease*
>
> 1 Determine body mass index (derived from estimated dry weight) relative to 20 kg/m^2
> 2 Determine mid-arm muscle circumference (MAMC) relative to the 5th percentile of gender- and age-matched reference values (Bishop's standards; see Appendix 2)
> 3 Estimate adequacy of recent energy intake relative to estimated requirements (see 'Estimating requirements in disease', Chapter 16)
> 4 Follow algorithm (Fig. 23.1), using additional factors likely to impair nutritional status (e.g. ascites, malabsorption) if present to subjectively override final category of nutrition.
>
> * Madden, A.M. (1998) Nutritional status and body composition in patients with chronic liver disease. PhD Thesis, University of London.

Table 23.1 Guidelines for estimating fluid weight (kg) in patients with ascites and peripheral oedema*

	Ascites	Oedema
Minimal	2.2	1.0
Moderate	6.0	5.0
Severe	14.0	10.0

* Mendenhall (1992); Wicks, C. and Madden, A. (1994) *A practical guide to nutrition in Liver disease*, 2nd edn. BDA, Birmingham.

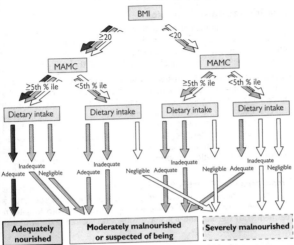

Subjectively override using additional factors likely to impair nutritional status.

Fig. 23.1 Algorithm for assessing nutritional status in patients with liver disease.

Hepatitis and cirrhosis

Hepatitis—acute and chronic

Hepatitis is an inflammation of the liver and can arise from a viral infection, e.g. hepatitis A, B, C, D, E, and G, an autoimmune response, or from other damage, e.g. alcoholic hepatitis. The nutritional implications vary depending on the severity of the condition and the time span.

Acute hepatitis In general, patients with acute hepatitis are very ill, have a poor appetite, and eat very little. No dietary restrictions should be imposed and patients should be encouraged to eat what they can. Small frequent snacks and nourishing drinks may be better tolerated than large meals. Fat restrictions used in the past are not evidence-based and dietary fat will not exacerbate the condition if the patient is able to eat it. Severe undernutrition may accompany acute alcoholic hepatitis and instigating early nutrition support, usually through enteral feeding, is recommended.

Chronic hepatitis Patients with chronic hepatitis may vary from those who are very undernourished following prolonged illness and poor intake to those who are obese, either incidentally or secondary to long-term treatment with steroids. Individual assessment is required and nutritional advice tailored accordingly.

Nutritional management

Appropriate nutritional management is important and influences prognosis.
- Undernourished patients who go on to liver transplantation have a greater risk of complications.
- Obesity is a risk factor for progression of chronic liver disease and associated with non-responsiveness to antiviral therapy.

Is it safe for women with viral hepatitis to breastfeed ?

- Hepatitis B. Small amounts of hepatitis B surface antigen have been detected in some samples of breast milk. However, the risk of transmission via breast milk is considered to be negligible compared to the risk of transmission at birth. It is advisable to abstain if nipples become cracked and bleed
- Hepatitis C. It is considered safe to breastfeed. It is advisable to abstain if nipples become cracked and bleed

Cirrhosis

Cirrhosis is irreversible damage of the hepatocytes. Most patients with cirrhosis have ↑ energy and protein requirements and are frequently undernourished (prevalence between 10 and 100% depending on population), ∴ requiring nutritional support. Dietary restrictions should not be routinely imposed. Complications arising from cirrhosis, including ascites, oedema, encephalopathy, and steatorrhoea, may benefit from dietary modification providing it is undertaken within a context of nutritional adequacy, i.e. feed first, restrict second.

Table 23.2 Energy and protein requirements in chronic liver disease recommended by the ESPEN* Consensus Group

	Non-protein energy (kcal/kg/d)	Protein (g/kg/d)
Compensated cirrhosis	25–35	1.0–1.2
Cirrhosis with malnutrition	35–40	1.5

* European Society for Parenteral and Enteral Nutrition. Plauth, M., et al. (1997). ESPEN guidelines for nutrition in liver disease and transplantation. *Clin. Nutr.* **16**, 43–55.

Ascites and oedema

Fluid retention is common in cirrhosis and end-stage liver disease and has relevance to nutrition.

- Abdominal distension can impair food intake leading to an inadequate nutritional status.
- Energy expenditure increases due to exertion of carrying additional weight.
- Negative nitrogen balance can be induced by repeated large volume paracentesis even if intravenous albumin infused.
- Restricting dietary sodium can help reduce or control the degree of fluid retention and thus improve symptoms.

Nutritional management of ascites and oedema

- Patients should be encouraged to eat as much as they are able and be tempted with tasty food.
- Small, frequent meals with snacks every 1–2 hours may optimize intake.
- The energy density of foods may be ↑ by the addition of extra sugar, honey, double cream, oil, and salt-free butter.
- Fat should not be restricted unless the patient finds it unpalatable or has clinically diagnosed steatorrhoea.
- Nutritional status should be monitored regularly. Body weight cannot be used; mid-arm muscle circumference and triceps skinfold thickness are most appropriate.
- Decisions about whether to restrict sodium intake must balance the potential benefits against the risk of reducing nutrient intake. Patients should be advised individually by a registered dietitian with experience in this area.

Low sodium diets for ascites and oedema

Patients are usually prescribed diuretics that ↑ urinary Na^+ output and ∴ induce negative Na^+ balance and fluid loss. Limiting dietary Na^+ intake will facilitate this and → a more rapid resolution, ↓ doses of diuretics being prescribed, and fewer associated complications. However, these advantages must be balanced against the negative effect that a low Na^+ diet may have on total nutrient intake. Two levels of restriction are generally advised.

1 No added salt diet (usually 80–100 mmol Na^+/day)

- Avoid salt at the table.
- Keep salt in cooking to minimum.
- Avoid high salt foods including most preserved or tinned items such as bacon, ham, sausages, tinned and packet soups, stock cubes, tinned vegetables, meats and fish, crisps and similar savoury snacks.
- Cheese (cheddar-type) should be limited to 100 g/week.
- Fast foods and ready-meals should be avoided unless they are known to provide <30 mmol Na^+ per portion.

2 Low sodium diet (40 mmol Na$^+$/day)

- Avoid all salt at the table and in cooking (prepare food separately).
- Avoid food prepared outside home unless specific arrangements have been made.
- Avoid high salt foods listed above under 'no added salt', including all cheese, fast food, and ready meals.
- Restrict bread intake to two slices per day.
- Use salt-free butter or margarine.
- Breakfast cereals should be salt-free, e.g. Puffed Wheat, Shredded Wheat.
- Restrict milk to half a pint (300 ml) per day.
- Use pepper, vinegar, spices, herbs, and lemon for flavouring.
- Fried food may be more appealing than boiled/grilled.

   Patients are rarely advised to restrict their intake to <40 mmol Na$^+$ although lower restrictions (~20 mmol/d) have been used in the past and these have required substituting ordinary bread and milk with unpalatable, low-sodium alternatives.

Other sources of sodium

- Antacids.
- Some antibiotics—check with pharmacist for suitable alternatives.
- Salt substitutes—most contain K$^+$ salts but some also contain Na$^+$.
- Sodium bicarbonate.

Portal systemic encephalopathy

Traditional treatment of portal systemic encephalopathy (PSE) included the restriction of dietary protein on the basis that nitrogenous compounds of dietary origin were implicated in the pathogenesis. Re-evaluation of the evidence has shown that dietary protein restriction is not an effective treatment[1] and can lead to rapid deterioration in nutritional status because protein requirements increase in chronic liver disease.

Nutritional management of PSE

- Sufficient protein to meet the estimated requirements should be provided (1.0–1.5 g/kg/d).
- Protein is best tolerated if spread out across the day. Eating several smaller meals and a bedtime snack is preferable to fewer large meals.
- Vegetable and dairy protein are better tolerated than protein from meat and fish.
- A high fibre diet, if acceptable to the patient, can contribute to a short gastrointestinal transit time, minimizing the opportunity for absorbing nitrogenous compounds of potential concern.

---

[1] See Soulsby CT and Morgan MY (1999) Dietary management of hepatic encephalopathy in cirrhotic patients. *Br. Med. J.* **318**,1391.

Steatorrhoea, fatty liver, and oesophageal varices

Steatorrhoea

Although ≥50% of patients with chronic liver disease have ↑ faecal fat excretion, relatively few have steatorrhoea. Those who do will benefit from restricting dietary fat to tolerance (see 'Low fat diet' in 'Steatorrhoea', Chapter 21).

Dietary fat contributes to the palatability of food and also provides:
- energy;
- fat-soluble vitamins;
- essential fatty acids.

A low fat diet is not recommended unless the symptoms of steatorrhoea are jeopardizing nutritional status or quality of life. Advice must be given to ensure that the diet remains adequate in all other nutrients, especially energy, fat-soluble vitamins, and essential fatty acids.

Steatorrhoea due to bile insufficiency cannot be treated with pancreatic enzyme replacement therapy although this may have a role if there is concomitant pancreatic disease.

Fatty liver

Lipid deposits in the liver are a common but reversible liver disorder associated with obesity and, in some patients, excessive alcohol intake. Usually fatty liver is asymptomatic but may progress to non-alcoholic steatohepatitis (NASH) and even cirrhosis. A moderate energy restriction that reduces excessive weight is associated with improvements in liver function tests and quality of life. There is debate over the optimum dietary composition to achieve this but in the absence of definitive evidence, patients should be advised to follow the 'Balance of Good Health' (see 'Food-based dietary guidelines', Chapter 2).

Oesophageal varices

Bleeding oesophageal or gastric varices are a life-threatening complication of chronic liver disease. Patients remain 'nil by mouth' during active bleeding and until their condition stabilizes. Nutritional implications arise if the patient's intake remains inadequate for prolonged periods, either because s/he is 'nil by mouth' or because of fear of eating.

There is no evidence that eating rough food, e.g. toast or crisps, increases the incidence of re-bleeding although some patients may prefer to take softer foods temporarily, particularly if they have undergone repeated endoscopic treatment. Nasogastric tubes can be used without increasing the incidence of re-bleeding or mortality or length of hospital stay.

Liver transplantation

Approximately 700 liver transplants are undertaken annually in the UK.

Pre-op Patients being worked up for transplantation should undergo a detailed nutritional assessment to establish their nutritional status and identify scope for nutritional support. Undernourished patients have a significantly greater risk of increased morbidity and mortality after surgery so implementing early pre-surgery nutritional support is vital.

Immediately post-op Post-operative nutrition support varies from centre to centre. Early feeding via a jejunally placed tube has been shown to be a safe and effective method of feeding post-transplant patients associated with reduced infections. Parenteral nutrition is only indicated if the gastrointestinal tract cannot be used for >5 days and, wherever possible, attempts should be made to feed via the gut.

Recovery in hospital When oral intake resumes, patients should be encouraged to eat an unrestricted diet; transient hyperglycaemia due to medication does not require dietary intervention. Attention to food hygiene is important because of immunosuppression, although no food restrictions are required.

Medium to long-term Following liver transplantation, most patients gain weight, especially in the first 6 months. This is appropriate if correcting pre-transplant undernutrition but >30% patients become obese at 3 years after surgery and up to 40% have hyperlipidaemia. Long-term cardiovascular risk is ∴ a concern. General dietary advice, e.g. the 'Balance of Good Health' (see 'Food-based dietary guidelines', Chapter 2) should be routinely made available to patients within the first 6 months and regular monitoring of body mass index and serum lipids used to identify those who need more specific guidance.

Renal disease

Introduction

Classification

- Acute renal failure (ARF): rapid deterioration of kidney function caused by injury or illness; often reversible.
- Chronic renal failure (CRF): abnormality of the structure or function of both kidneys, lasting >3 months; often progressive.
- End–stage renal failure (ESRF): chronic renal disease that has progressed so far that the patient's kidneys no longer function sufficiently to maintain life.

Prevalence

In the UK, it is estimated that ~5500 adults per million have CRF and ~400/million have ARF. Prevalence ↑ with age and co-morbidities, e.g. diabetes, cardiovascular disease, and in minority ethnic groups. ~7.5 children per million are referred annually to regional renal units.

Malnutrition

- 40–50% of all patients with ESRF are malnourished.
- Poor nutritional status prior to initiation of dialysis is also associated with poorer outcomes on dialysis, increasing the odds ratio of mortality × 2.5. Despite its limitations as an indicator of nutritional status, low serum albumin levels are independently associated with ↑ risk of death in haemodialysis (HD), peritoneal dialysis (PD), and transplanted patients.
- Malnutrition is caused by inadequate dietary intake or unmet increased nutritional requirements (see 'Contributing causes' in 'Undernutrition', Chapter 16).
- Body composition changes, especially muscle loss, occur during progressive renal failure. Metabolic responses to preserve protein balance are impaired when dietary protein is limited, resulting in degradation of essential amino acids, ↑ protein catabolism, and ↓ protein synthesis.

Contributing causes

Acute renal failure

- Hypovolaemia (shock)
- Cardiac failure
- Acute glomerulonephritis
- Toxic reaction, e.g. drugs, poison
- Obstruction of urinary output, e.g. tumour, renal stone disease

Chronic renal failure

- Diabetic nephropathy
- Hypertension
- Infection, e.g. chronic pyelonephritis or sepsis $2°$ to severe urinary tract infection
- Polycystic kidney disease
- Tumour, e.g. multiple myeloma, amyloidosis
- Familial, e.g. Alport's syndrome

Nutritional assessment

Nutritional status should be assessed in all ESRF patients using standard techniques (see Chapter 4). However, in the presence of renal impairment, biochemical markers require more specific interpretation.

- Serum albumin is a good predictor of mortality in ESRF. Patients with serum albumin <25 g/l have a risk ratio for dying 20 times higher than patients with serum albumin >40 g/l. Even those with levels in the normal range (35–40 g/l) have a twofold increase in mortality compared with those with serum albumin between 40 and 45 g/l. However, serum albumin requires careful interpretation: it can be influenced by fluid imbalance and an acute phase response as indicated by ↑ CRP levels (trauma, surgery, or infection). The large body pool and long half-life (14–20d) renders albumin relatively insensitive to immediate changes in nutritional status.
- Serum pre-albumin has a shorter half-life and smaller body pool than albumin, and is more influenced by the acute phase response and anaemia. Levels are elevated in CRF due to ↓ catabolism and excretion, volume changes, and interaction with ↑ retinol binding protein. Not a useful nutritional marker.
- Serum transferrin is not a good indicator of nutritional status in ESRF as serum levels ↑ in iron deficiency, and ↓ levels occur in uraemia *per se*, during an acute phase response, iron loading, and in patients with proteinuria.
- Haemoglobin (Hb) and iron stores should be monitored as anaemia, which is common in CRF, can reduce quality of life due to its effect on mental function, exercise tolerance, fatigue, appetite, and sleep patterns.
- Blood urea is derived from protein degradation, but influenced by diet, hydration, urine flow. Although ↑ blood urea is an indicator of impaired renal function, in ESRF a low level (<20 mmol/l) may indicate inadequate protein intake, and is predictive of a poor prognosis. However, type of protein consumed, degree of anabolism, residual renal function, and the amount of dialysis will also influence urea levels. Data from urea kinetic modelling can be used indirectly to estimate the protein intake.
- Protein catabolic rate (PCR) can be estimated from the calculated urea generation rate. In steady state, PCR correlates well with dietary protein intake. However, in catabolic patients, urea generated by muscle breakdown far exceeds that derived from dietary protein. Conversely, anabolism may produce falsely low PCR values. PCR is usually normalized for actual body weight (normalized PCR). However, extremes in body weight will influence the interpretation of nPCR, with obese or underweight patients showing inappropriately distorted values unless metabolically active fat-free mass is considered and the body weight adjusted accordingly.
- Serum potassium values < the normal range may indicate poor nutritional intake as potassium is found in a wide variety of foods. However, potassium excretion is influenced by the degree of residual

renal function. diarrhoea, anabolism, and the use of potassium-containing drugs, ACE inhibitors, or A2RBs.
* Serum phosphate. Low serum levels may indicate an overall poor food intake due to wide distribution of phosphate in foods. Low phosphate may also result as part of the metabolic imbalances associated with re-feeding syndrome.
* Lipid profile. Low total plasma cholesterol levels have been associated with ↑ mortality, possibly as an indicator of insufficient protein and energy intakes.

Dietetic treatment plan for pre-dialysis patients

Requires full dietary assessment from history and examination, nutritional support with advice tailored to the specific needs of the individual patient, and subsequent monitoring (Fig. 24.1).

Protein restriction will rarely be advised although patients with high intakes may need to modify these. Dietitians should be available in all low clearance or pre-dialysis clinics to give individual advice.

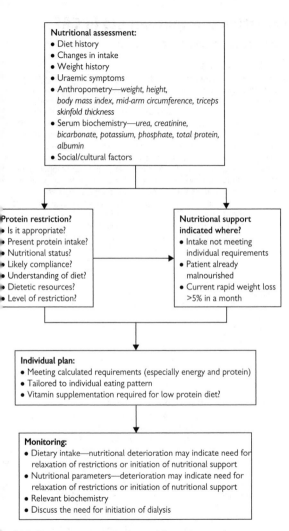

Nutritional assessment:
- Diet history
- Changes in intake
- Weight history
- Uraemic symptoms
- Anthropometry—*weight, height, body mass index, mid-arm circumference, triceps skinfold thickness*
- Serum biochemistry—*urea, creatinine, bicarbonate, potassium, phosphate, total protein, albumin*
- Social/cultural factors

Protein restriction?
- Is it appropriate?
- Present protein intake?
- Nutritional status?
- Likely compliance?
- Understanding of diet?
- Dietetic resources?
- Level of restriction?

Nutritional support indicated where?
- Intake not meeting individual requirements
- Patient already malnourished
- Current rapid weight loss >5% in a month

Individual plan:
- Meeting calculated requirements (especially energy and protein)
- Tailored to individual eating pattern
- Vitamin supplementation required for low protein diet?

Monitoring:
- Dietary intake—nutritional deterioration may indicate need for relaxation of restrictions or initiation of nutritional support
- Nutritional parameters—deterioration may indicate need for relaxation of restrictions or initiation of nutritional support
- Relevant biochemistry
- Discuss the need for initiation of dialysis

Fig. 24.1 Devising a treatment plan for pre-dialysis patients.

Nutritional requirements in CRF, ARF, and during dialysis

CRF (pre-dialysis)

- Energy requirements are normal, i.e. approx 35 kcal/kg/day. Some patients may be underweight and ∴ require additional calories.
- Protein intake should be maintained at 0.8–1.0 g/kg ideal body weight/day (a mild degree of restriction), especially in patients consuming excessive protein or in the short-term management of uraemic patients awaiting the start of dialysis. Protein restriction (0.6 g/kg/day or 0.3 g/kg/day + essential amino acid or ketoacid analogues) has been used to reduce uraemic symptoms and ↓ rate of decline in renal function. Benefits are marginal when compared with ↑ risk of malnutrition, even under close dietetic supervision. Compliance with low protein diets is often poor due to their unpalatability, monotony, and complexity. A ↓ protein intake may occur spontaneously as the glomerular filtration rate (GFR) falls below <25 ml/min. It is ∴ more likely that patients nearing ESRF will require nutrition support to achieve an adequate intake, rather than restrictions. Earlier initiation of dialysis should reduce the extent of malnutrition.
- Phosphate. Early restriction (i.e. if serum phosphate >1.6 mmol/l) may help prevent renal bone disease, secondary hyperparathyroidism, and may slow progression to ESRF.
- Fluid and potassium restriction are usually unnecessary in CRF unless:
  - urine output is markedly reduced (<1000 ml/day);
  - poorly controlled diabetic patients (relative insulin deficiency produces deficient glucose-potassium intracellular uptake; type IV renal tubular acidosis);
  - use of ACE inhibitors or A2RBs reduces renal potassium excretion
- Sodium intake. A mild restriction of 80–100 mmol (no added salt diet: see 'Ascites and oedema', Chapter 23) may be required if patients are hypertensive or oedematous.

Haemodialysis and peritoneal dialysis

In ESRF, appetite and food intake may gradually improve once dialysis has begun and uraemic symptoms have been alleviated. However, some patients may have ↑ malnutrition due to adverse effects of dialysis (HD or PD). Nutritional requirements for dialysis are shown in Table 24.1, although evidence from controlled trials is mostly lacking. When possible, general healthy eating guidelines are recommended, e.g. 50% total energy from complex CHO, high fibre (NSP) and 30–35% energy from fat (predominantly poly- and mono-unsaturated fatty acid source with low saturated fats). A high intake of soluble NSP is of particular importance in continuous ambulatory peritoneal dialysis (CAPD) when uptake of dialysate glucose may ↑ risk of hypertriglyceridaemia and poor glucose tolerance. If intake is poor, healthy eating guidelines may be relaxed to help achieve nutritional adequacy.

Table 24.1 Daily nutritional guidelines for patients on HD and PD

	HD	PD	Main food sources
Energy	30–35 kcal/kg	25–30kcal/kg [†]	Cereals, bread, rice, pasta, potato, sugar, fats
Protein	1–1.2 g/kg IBW	1.2–1.3 g/kg IBW	Meat, fish, eggs, pulses, milk (within allowance)
Potassium	0.8–1 mmol/kg	Restriction only necessary if hyperkalaemic: 1 mmol/kg	Fruit, vegetables, fruit juice, nuts, coffee, chocolate, crisps
Phosphate	<1000 mg	<1200 mg	Milk, yogurt, cheese, offal, shellfish, fish with bones
Sodium	80–100 mmol (no added salt)	80–100 mmol (no added salt)	Table salt, smoked/cured foods, tinned and packet foods, ready meals
Fluid	500 ml + previous day urine output	500 ml + previous day urine output + ultra filtration	Drinks, gravies, sauces, soups, jelly, yogurt

IBW, Ideal body weight.
[†] Adjusted for energy content of the dialysate fluid.

ARF

Nutritional status in ARF is usually influenced by the underlying aetiology of disease, pre-existing malnutrition, degree of catabolism, and prolonged hospitalization. Severely catabolic ARF patients usually require prompt nutritional support. The ↑ availability of dialysis and continuous filtration techniques means nutritional status no longer need be compromised in order to control electrolyte and fluid balance.

- Energy requirements in non-septic patients are similar to those of normal individuals. In sepsis, the BMR may be ↑ by up to 30%. Provision of adequate energy is essential to prevent the breakdown of endogenous and ingested protein for gluconeogenesis. Energy requirements are determined from energy expenditure, clinical circumstances, patient activity, and predicted BMR calculated from the Schofield equations (see Appendix 4). Indirect calorimetry can be used to assess directly the energy requirements of a patient with ARF (but is rarely used in clinical practice).

- Protein. Patients with ARF but no additional catabolic stress are usually able to maintain neutral or positive nitrogen balance. Catabolic patients may have a marked rise in blood urea nitrogen as nitrogen balance becomes negative. Urea nitrogen appearance can be measured to estimate total nitrogen balance. Protein requirements can be estimated using standard formulae, corrected for patient activity and underlying clinical condition (see 'Estimating requirements in disease states', Chapter 16). Dialysis-dependent patients require additional protein to replace losses during dialysis (Table 24.2).

- Electrolytes and minerals. Conservatively managed patients usually require dietary restriction of potassium, sodium, and phosphate. Patients undergoing continuous renal replacement therapy (CRRT) need a less restrictive diet, and many need full nutrition support. During CCRT many ARF patients develop hypokalaemia, hypophosphataemia, and hypomagnesaemia and require supplementation. These are important metabolic derangements, especially in ventilated patients, as electrolyte depletion can lead to increasing muscle weakness, alterations in acid–base balance, and to further nephrotoxicity (especially tubular damage). Daily monitoring is necessary. At different stages of ARF, supplementation or restriction can be necessary, often determined by the catabolic state of the patient and the modality of dialysis (e.g. intermittent or continuous).

Table 24.2 Amino acid (protein) losses during dialysis

	Estimated amino acid (protein) loss
HD	1–1.5 g (6–9 g)/session
CRRT	1.5–2.0 g (9–12.5 g)/24 h

Strategies for achieving nutritional aims

Energy

HD Patients generally have more difficulty achieving recommended energy intakes. This group more frequently needs advice aimed at increasing their energy intake, either using energy-rich foods or prescribed energy supplements.

PD Normal or overweight patients may require energy restriction to compensate for the additional calories absorbed from dialysate. Initial advice should concentrate on reducing excessive intake of fats and sugar (provide few nutrients other than energy). Excessive use of hypertonic dialysate to control fluid balance will increase energy intake. Fluid management and sodium restriction should then be emphasized.

Protein

HD Patients generally have sufficient intake of protein once energy requirements are attained. Combined energy and protein supplements or intradialytic parenteral nutrition may help.

PD The high protein requirements are often difficult to achieve by diet alone, particularly in those with poor appetite, or during and after peritonitis. Specific targets for protein-rich foods and snacks, and use of prescribed protein supplements may be required.

Potassium

HD Formal dietary K^+ restriction is usually required, but the level of restriction is partly dependent on residual renal function. Non-dietary causes of hyperkalaemia (Table 24.3) should be excluded.

Restriction of dietary K^+ intake is generally staged following review of the serum levels after each level of restriction.

- Limitation of K^+-rich food sources, including:
  - fruits: banana, rhubarb, avocado pear, dried fruit;
  - vegetables: spinach, mushroom, beetroot, jacket or instant potato, chips (if not parboiled), crisps;
  - drinks: fresh fruit juices, coffee, drinking chocolate, malted drinks, blackcurrant cordials;
  - other: chocolate, evaporated and condensed milk, yeast extract, liquorice, salt substitutes.
- Advice on suitable cooking methods (as K^+ is very water soluble):
  - use large volumes of water for boiling vegetables;
  - double boil method for cooking potatoes;
  - parboil vegetables before adding them to stews, soups, etc.;
  - avoid pressure cooker and microwave cooking (but re-heating is permitted);
  - limit portion size and quantities of fruit and vegetables;
  - review protein intake: as protein is also rich in K^+, ensure protein intake is not excessive by diet history (cross-check against serum biochemistry and nPCR).

Table 24.3 Non-dietary causes of hyperkalaemia

Metabolic factors	Hyperparathyroidism, acidosis, insulin insufficiency
Drugs	K^+-containing drugs, e.g. penicillin, senna.
	Drugs affecting K^+ excretion, e.g. ACE inhibitors, A2RBs, β-blockers, NSAIDs
	K^+-sparing diuretics, e.g. amiloride, spironolactone
Cellular trauma	Haemolysed blood sample, post-blood transfusion, infection, GI haemorrhage, crush injury, gangrene
Constipation	Reduced gut excretion
Dialysis	Inadequate dialysis

PD Dietary restriction is rarely needed in PD because of continuous clearance.

Phosphate

HD and PD Clearance of phosphate is not particularly effective with either PD or conventional HD. Daily dialysis and nocturnal dialysis achieve significantly better phosphate clearance, enabling some patients to relax their dietary restrictions and reduce their intake of phosphate binders. Management consists of dietary restriction of phosphate-rich foods, review of excessive protein portions and foods with added phosphate containing additives (polyphosphates). Review of compliance, dosage, and timing of phosphate binders and vitamin D analogues is essential.

Phosphate-rich foods include:
  milk;
  cereals;
  dairy products;
  cheese;
  chocolate;
  dried fruit;
  eggs;
  fish (bony);
  shellfish and seafood;
  beans and pulses;
  nuts;
  meat and poultry.

Vitamins

HD and PD Vitamin deficiency can occur in CRF due to dietary restriction, dialysate losses, and abnormal metabolism (see Table 24.4). Overt deficiency is rare. Most units prescribe a routine supplementary dose of the water-soluble vitamin B group, vitamin C, and folate, although good evidence for supplementation is lacking. Fat-soluble vitamins (A and E) are not routinely prescribed due to the risk of hypervitaminosis. However, vitamin E supplementation in ESRF may have antioxidant activity in relation to coronary heart disease prevention.

Table 24.4 Recommendations for vitamin requirements in CRF

Thiamin (B$_1$)	1.5 mg	Pantothenic acid	10 mg
Riboflavin (B$_2$)	1.7 mg	Biotin	300 µg
Pyridoxine (B$_6$)	10 mg	Folic acid	1000 µg
Cobalamin (B$_{12}$)	6 mg	Ascorbic acid (C)	60 mg
Nicotinamide	20 mg	Iron sulphate	150 mg

Iron

HD and PD Anaemia is common in CRF, due to a relative lack of erythropoietin, which develops when GFR falls to <35 ml/minute, and should be investigated if Hb <12 g/dl ($\male$ and post-menopausal $\female$) and <11 g/dl (pre-menopausal $\female$). Intravenous or oral iron can be given (see Table 24.4) so that ferritin levels are maintained between 400 and 800 ng/ml.

Minerals and trace elements

HD and PD Of the 14 essential minerals and trace elements (see 'Minerals and trace elements', Chapter 5), deficiencies in Zn, Cu, Mn, and Cr have been reported in CRF, mostly due to dietary restriction and drug interactions. Deficiency should be confirmed before starting supplementation.

Fluid and sodium

Fluid management in ESRF is influenced by the degree of residual renal function and mode of dialysis. Patients with substantial urine output (>1 l/day) do not usually require a strict fluid or Na$^+$ restriction. Patients with reduced urine output should restrict intake to the daily volume of urine plus 500 ml (insensible losses). Na$^+$ intake should be restricted to 'no-added-salt' (80–100 mmol/day) (see 'Ascites and oedema', Chapter 23). Hypertensive patients should have more aggressive Na$^+$ restriction. Patients should be educated about salt as the major drive to thirst, as restricting Na$^+$ intake **is likely** to lead to better fluid control than attempting to restrict fluid intake *per se*.

HD patients are usually anuric and often require severe fluid restriction (500 ml daily) and adjunctive Na$^+$ restriction. Interdialytic fluid gain should be kept to ~1 kg/day, or a maximum total increase of 3% dry body weight (adjusted for metabolically active tissue in obesity). See Table 24.5.

PD patients usually lose water by ultrafiltration dependent on the dextrose concentration of dialysate (up to 2 l/day). This is especially important to the anuric patient. The volume of ultrafiltrate may be added to the daily fluid intake. Long-term use of hypertonic solutions may cause damage to the peritoneal membrane, producing hyperpermeability and loss of peritoneal integrity, and weight gain. Use of higher dextrose concentration dialysate should be minimized especially in obese patients or those with diabetes or hypertriglyceridaemia. These patients need more stringent Na+ and fluid restrictions. Icodextrin dialysate may be especially beneficial.

Table 24.5 Strategies for achieving fluid restriction

Reduced fluid intake	Use small volume cup for drinks
	Suck ice cubes and ice lollies
	Take tablets with food (unless otherwise directed)
↑Awareness	Education about fluid content of certain foods, e.g. jelly, custard, soup, ice-cream, yogurt, dhal
	Measuring jug tally, e.g. fluid required throughout the day is extracted from a jug/bottle initially containing the desired daily volume
Thirst prevention	Reduce salt intake
Techniques	Take sugar-free sweets or chew gum
	Use of fruit (within K^+ restriction if applicable)
Regular mouth care	Use of mouth wash, lip salves, etc.

Nutrition support in renal patients

Renal patients who are malnourished or unable to achieve an inadequate intake from food should be advised and/or helped to supplement their oral intake using specific foods or proprietary products (see 'Treatment of undernutrition', Chapter 16) or provided with enteral or parenteral nutrition support (see 'Enteral nutrition' and 'parenteral nutrition', Chapter 16).

- Care must be taken to ensure that supplements are compatible with other dietary restrictions.
- Some patients may be unwilling to drink liquid supplements as they contribute to the daily fluid restriction. Where necessary, nutrient-dense supplements should be selected.
- If enteral feeding is required, attention must be given to the total fluid volume. Patients may need daily HD or more hypertonic PD exchanges.
- Gastrostomy feeding is increasingly being used in both HD and PD patients at home. In PD patients, a short period of peritoneal rest while the tube placement site heals is often instigated.
- Specifically formulated renal enteral feeds are available to provide fluid, electrolyte-restricted, nutrient-dense feeds (see Table 24.6).
- Parenteral nutrition may be preferred in patients with impaired gastro-intestinal function.
  - Energy requirements are best provided using a combination of both glucose and fat so as not to exceed the glucose oxidation rate 4–5 g glucose/kg/day (including glucose derived from dialysate during CRRT).
  - Excessive glucose is associated with ↑ risk of metabolic disturbances leading to ↑ CO_2 production and lipogenesis.
  - Provision of fat should not exceed 1 g/kg/day in ARF.
  - Routine use of low electrolyte parenteral nutrition regimens in patients with ARF receiving dialysis (especially CRRT) may cause electrolyte depletion, and necessitate administration of additional potassium, phosphate, or magnesium, or the use of standard parenteral nutrition formulae.
  - Close monitoring of serum biochemistry is paramount, especially at the onset of feeding.

Table 24.6 Nutritional products widely used in renal disease (also see 'Treatment of undernutrition', Chapter 16)

Type	Examples of prescribable brands
Energy supplements	
Glucose polymers	Caloreen (Nestlé Clinical), Polycal (Nutricia Clinical), Polycose (Abbott), Vitajoule (Vitaflo)
Fat	Calogen (SHS), Liquigen (SHS)
Combined	Duocal (SHS), Duobar (SHS)
Protein powders	Casilan 90 (Heinz), Maxipro Super Soluble (SHS), ProMod (Abbott), Renapro (KoRa)
Enteral feeds	
Nutrient dense	Ensure Plus (Abbott), Nutrison Energy (Nutricia Clinical)
Low fluid / electrolyte	Nepro (Abbott), Two CalHN* (Abbott)

*Not prescribable.

Intradialytic nutrition

- Intradialytic parenteral nutrition (IDPN) can be used to supplement energy and protein intakes during each HD session. It is expensive. It has the advantage of providing nutrients without additional fluid and ensuring patient compliance. Short-term evaluation of IDPN suggests it is of benefit in some patients, but few studies have evaluated the long-term benefits. Metabolic studies suggest that IDPN can switch a patient from a catabolic to an anabolic state, and can ↑ serum albumin, dry weight, muscle strength, and reduce mortality (no controlled trials). In principle it can provide up to 1000 kcal and 50 g protein per session. Metabolic side-effects of IDPN (including hyperglycaemia) and GI symptoms require close monitoring.
- Intraperitoneal amino acids have been used in CAPD patients. Studies using 1.1% amino acid dialysate solutions to replace 1–2 of the usual daily glucose exchanges may show some improvement in nutritional status, especially in those patients with moderate to severe pre-existing malnutrition. Expensive, only leads to a small improvement in nutrition, and the exchange must be done at the same time as a meal to enhance amino acid uptake.

Cardiovascular disease in renal patients

CVD accounts for 50% of deaths after renal replacement therapy has commenced and is also prevalent in patients in the early stages of renal disease. Renal patients present with raised cholesterol as well as raised triglycerides. In addition to hyperlipidaemia, patients exhibit many other risk factors associated with CVD, many of which can be improved with a combination of changes in diet, lifestyle, and physical activity (see 'Cardioprotective diet', Chapter 19).

The National Kidney Foundation - Kidney Disease Outcomes Quality Initiative (NKF-K/DOQI) Guidelines (2003) recommend that 'evaluation of dyslipidaemias should occur at presentation with chronic kidney disease'.[1] Renal patients with high cholesterol and /or high triglyceride levels have been advised to follow therapeutic lifestyle changes. For patients with very high triglycerides (>11.3 mmol/l), a very low fat diet (<15% energy) combined with fish oils may be beneficial (see box in 'Cardioprotective diet; Chapter 19).

---

[1] National Kidney Foundation (2003): Clinical practice guidelines for managing dyslipidemias in chronic kidney disease, *Am. J. Kidney Dis.* **41** (suppl. 3), 51–91. ▣ http://www.kidney.org/prof essionals/kdoqi/guidelines_lipids/jpegs/Table26L.jpg

Dietary issues specific to ethnic minority patients with renal disease

see 'Minority ethnic communities' in Chapter 13

- Vegetarian or vegan diets generally provide less protein and may be higher in potassium and phosphate. Protein supplementation may be required, especially in PD.
- Fasting. Energy and protein intakes are more difficult to achieve during fasting. For Hindus, pure foods, including fruit, nuts, yogurt, and milk, eaten during this time may be high in potassium and phosphate. Medications may be omitted inappropriately during a fast.
- Traditional cooking methods. Cooking methods for curries, stews, and stir-fries may conflict with potassium-lowering cooking techniques. Cooking utensils may contain iron, aluminium, or other trace elements, which can (rarely) accumulate.
- Traditional food items may be rich in the following:
  - potassium: spinach (sag, callaloo), karela, potato pakoras, plantain, yam, cassava, sweet potato, okra, banana, mango, paw-paw, nuts, coconut, sweetmeats, chevda;
  - phosphate: lassi, raita, Indian tea, nuts, sweetmeats;
  - sodium: chevda, pickles, salt fish and pork, soy sauce, monosodium glutamate.
- Toxicity. Rarely, some foods may be toxic in renal failure, for example, star fruit (*Averrhoa carambola*), which is eaten especially in Asia, causes severe intoxication in some renal patients leading to intractable hiccups, agitation, muscle weakness, confusion, fits, and can be fatal.

Nephrotic syndrome (NS)

Causes

- Focal segmental glomerulosclerosis (FSGS), 30%.
- Membranous nephropathy (MN), 25%.
- Diabetes, 20%.
- Minimal change nephropathy (MCN), 10%.
- Amyloidosis 4–10%.
- Others include systemic lupus erythmatosus, IgA nephropathy, toxic glomerulopathy, e.g. caused by gold or penicillamine.

Characteristics Proteinuria >3 g/day, hypoalbuminaemia, and generalized oedema. The following are also often observed: hyperlipidaemia, clotting problems, and hypertension.

Treatment

Aims to control oedema, reduce proteinuria, and treat complications that arise including infections, hyperlipidaemia, and clotting problems. Diet therapy has a role to play in several of these areas.

Oedema One of the main features of NS is oedema; this may present as swollen ankles, peri-orbital swelling, and pleural effusions. The oedema is due to Na^+ and water retention and patients benefit from a dietary Na^+ restriction: 80–100 mmol/day. Na^+ restriction can potentiate the antihypertensive and antiproteinuric effects of ACE inhibitors[1]. Fluid restriction may also be necessary, depending on the response to diuretics and other treatments such as albumin infusions.

❶ Note that oedema can mask the wasting signs of malnutrition.

Proteinuria/hypoalbuminaemia Treating the lesion that underlies the NS is possible in cases of MCN and, to a lesser extent, FSGS, which respond to steroids. However, MCN only accounts for 10% of cases and the proteinuria itself is now being targeted with ACE inhibitors, strict control of blood pressure, and good diabetes control. Historically, a high protein diet was advised with the aim of replacing protein losses. However, it is also known that a high protein intake causes ↑ permeability and hyperfiltration in the basement membrane of the kidney glomeruli which could exacerbate the proteinuria seen in NS. Studies comparing ↓ protein (0.7–0.8 g/kg) and normal /high protein (1.2 to 1.5 g/kg) diets showed that nitrogen balance could be achieved with the moderate protein restriction, proteinuria was also reduced, and some aspects of the disturbed protein metabolism ameliorated (fibrinogen levels were reduced), although not all studies showed a corresponding ↑ in plasma albumin levels. Other biochemical parameters such as phosphate, lipid, and renin levels also tended to improve on the lower protein diets. An intake of 0.8–1 g protein/kg ideal body weight/day is recommended.

[1] ACE (angiotensin converting enzyme) inhibitors can increase the serum potassium levels.

Hyperlipidaemia Both triglycerides and cholesterol are raised in NS due to ↑ liver synthesis of lipoproteins and ↑ metabolism of triglycerides. Incidence of myocardial infarction has been reported as 5–6 × greater in NS. Lipid lowering agents such as HMG-Co A reductase inhibitors and bile acid sequesters are used. Evidence exists for the cholesterol reducing effects of (↓ protein) vegetarian diets based on soy protein in conjunction with standard lipid lowering advice: 30% calories from fat including 10% calories from PUFA. Fish oils have been shown to ↓ triglyceride levels.

Thromboembolism 10–30% of adults with NS develop emboli, which may be in the lungs, legs, or renal vein. This is due to an imbalance between coagulation inhibitors and pro-coagulatory factors such as fibrinogen. A ↓ protein diet has been shown to improve fibrinogen levels.

Infections NS patients are prone to infections possibly because of loss of protective immunoglobulins. Iron, copper, zinc, and vitamin D are also lost as a result of the proteinuria. Vitamin D losses can result in derangements of calcium metabolism and supplementation may be necessary. A balanced, nutritious diet will help maintain micronutrient levels.

Summary

- Protein: 0.8–1 g/kg ideal body weight per day
- Calories: 'normal requirements': 30–35 kcal/kg IBW/day
- Fat: <30% total kcal, low saturated fat, encourage MUFA, PUFA
- Micronutrients: ensure adequate intake, monitor for signs vitamin D deficiency
- Sodium: 80–100 mmol/d
- Potassium: Monitor as may ↑ with ACE inhibitors

Renal transplantation

Renal transplantation is considered to offer the patient with ESRF the best chance of rehabilitation and good quality of life. A patient may have spent several years on dialysis and possibly a couple of years in the pre-dialysis stage before receiving a transplant. Even with careful management, they will be showing signs of the long-term metabolic effects of chronic renal failure, including:

- anaemia;
- bone disease;
- muscle wasting;
- cardiovascular disease.

Immunosuppressive therapy, which is used to prolong the life of the transplanted kidney, can exacerbate all of the above conditions as well as creating additional problems (see box).

> **Immunosuppressive treatment is associated with many side-effects**
>
> - Protein hypercatabolism
> - ↑ Appetite leading to obesity
> - Hyperlipidaemia
> - Glucose intolerance/↑ risk of diabetes (~20% of patients)
> - Hypertension
> - Hyperkalaemia
> - Interference with vitamin D metabolism
> - ↑ Cancer risk
> - ↑ Infection risk (opportunistic viral and bacterial infections that may ↓ appetite and ↑ nutrient requirements)
> - Gum hypertrophy

The positive effects of transplantation are to relieve the patient from dietary and other lifestyle restrictions imposed by dialysis. Patients experience a general improvement in well-being; waste products that were the cause of uraemic symptoms are removed more efficiently, and they no longer have to undertake the exhausting process of dialysis.

Immediately post-transplant

Nutritional care should be the same as for any other post-surgical patient: monitoring biochemistry and urine output, ensuring the return of normal gut function and appetite, and meeting requirements with supplements if necessary. The rate at which biochemistry and urine output return to normal can vary (sometimes within a couple of days after surgery, or it can take several weeks) and needs to be monitored closely. Treatment varies accordingly from fluid and electrolyte (Na^+ and K^+) restrictions to intravenous support, if urine output is excessive and serum electrolyte levels drop below normal. Dehydration at this stage can damage the new kidney.

Once kidney function has improved and stabilized

The main aims of dietary therapy are to encourage a healthy balanced diet and reduce the risk factors for cardiovascular disease, which is the cause of ~60% of deaths in transplant patients. The incidence of obesity (BMI >25 kg/m^2) can ↑ dramatically post-transplantation and dietary advice should be given to the patient prior to hospital discharge with regular follow up in outpatient clinics in order to prevent excessive weight gain. This advice should include healthy eating, exercise, and other lifestyle improvements: stress management and avoidance of smoking and of exposure to too much sun. As the patient is more susceptible to infections, some advice on food hygiene and safe handling of food is also useful. Barriers to eating a healthy diet may be due to the habits formed whilst adhering to the previous dietary restrictions. Patients who have been on a K$^+$ restriction may be reluctant at first to ↑ intake of fruit and vegetables, and other 'cardioprotective' foods such as oily fish may have been restricted on the dialysis diet. Conversely, there may be a temptation to overconsume some of the previously restricted foods such as alcohol, chips, crisps, dairy products, fruit juices, nuts, and chocolates, etc., contributing to a rapid ↑ in body fat. Additionally, there can be reluctance, partly due to loss of confidence, to exercise because of years of inactivity and fear of damaging the new kidney.

Longer-term

Weight management and improvement in lipid levels have been achieved with diet and exercise interventions. These interventions will help reduce the risk of metabolic syndrome and diabetes, although many patients also need medication to control blood lipids. Improved lean body mass (muscle) and bone strength may also result from diet and exercise advice. Alendronate, vitamin D, and calcium supplements may be required to improve bone strength. Ideally, in addition to the renal physician, a team of specialists should be available to help with the rehabilitation of the transplant patient including a dietitian, nurse, physiotherapist, and social worker or counsellor.

Summary

- Monitor biochemistry, especially blood cholesterol, triglycerides, glucose, K$^+$, bone minerals, PTH, haemoglobin
- Monitor blood pressure control
- Aim for acceptable body mass index
- 'Balance of Good Health' is an appropriate food model to use
- Emphasize eating a good variety of fruit and vegetables
- Encourage high fibre foods
- Encourage fish particularly oily fish, lean meats, and pulses
- Foods high in sugar, saturated fat, and salt should be used sparingly
- Encourage ↓ fat dairy products
- Ensure Ca requirements are met
- Advise alcohol within usual recommendations
- Be aware of good food hygiene practices
- Encourage physical activity and regular exercise
- Avoid smoking and too much sun exposure

Renal stone disease (Nephrolithiasis/renal calculi)

Incidence

Stone formation is $2-4 \times$ more frequent in men than women, usually appearing after the age of 30, with a recurrence rate of 50% within 10 years. 10% of men and 5% of women may suffer from kidney stones in their lifetime. There are significant differences in incidence in different populations, which suggests genetic and/or environmental influences such as diet and climate. The populations of the developed world are more at risk with greater incidences seen in Whites > Asian and Hispanic > Black. Water hardness is not thought to be a predisposing factor.

Stone formation

- Renal stone formation can occur anywhere in the kidney, ureter, or bladder.
- The size of stone can vary from microscopic to the large 'staghorn' calculi and can lead to kidney failure if the kidney or urinary tract becomes obstructed.
- The stones vary in composition and analysis is useful in order to help determine the cause (see Table 24.7).
- Biochemical risk factors include ↑ urinary concentration of promoter substances and ↓ concentration of inhibitor substances (see Table 24.8).
- Stone formation can also be linked to congenital abnormalities as seen in polycystic kidneys, horseshoe kidneys, and medullary sponge kidney or to short bowel syndromes such as Crohn's disease or to recurrent infections with urease-positive organisms.
- About 50% of stone formers excrete ↑ urinary calcium, >7.5 mmol/day in men or >6.2 mmol/day in women. Hypercalcuria may be due to ↑ absorption of calcium from the gut, calcium resorption from the bone, or ↓ ability of the kidney tubules to reabsorb calcium. Vitamin D and PTH levels may be normal or elevated. Only 5% of patients have an elevated PTH level but in 95% of cases it is due to 1° hyperparathyroidism.
- Stone formation is exacerbated by ↓ urine output volume. This may result from a low fluid intake or ↑ losses via other routes including sweat, e.g. in tropical areas, and GI tract, e.g. intestinal failure.

Dietary treatment of renal stone disease

A number of dietary factors can contribute to the management of stone disease, specifically those that influence the appearance in the urine of any of the promoters or inhibitors or factors that alter the urine acidity or volume (and thus dilute the concentration of stone forming salts). The diet of the affluent world has been scrutinized with respect to intake of animal protein, sodium, calcium, oxalate, and purine. It appears that even with identical dietary intakes stone formers will form larger crystals than non-stone formers. The number of long-term, randomized controlled trials to pinpoint individual dietary factors is low.

Table 24.7 Composition, incidence, and causes of the main types of stone

Composition	Incidence (%)	Possible causes
Calcium oxalate: up to 50% may contain calcium hydroxyl phosphate	75	Idiopathic hypercalciuria 1° Hyperparathyroidism ↓ Urine citrate Hyperoxaluria Hyperuricosuria
Magnesium ammonium phosphate (struvite or triple phosphate)	10–20	Bacterial infection
Uric acid	5	Low urine pH Hyperuricosuria
Cystine	1–2	Cysteinuria

Table 24.8 Promotors and inhibitors of stone formation

Promoters	Inhibitors
↓ Urine volume, particularly <1000 ml/d	Urine output >2000 ml/d
↑ Urinary concentrations of: calcium, sodium, oxalate, urate, cystine	↑ Urinary concentrations of: magnesium, pyrophosphate, citrate
Bacterial products	Nephrocalcin
↓ Urine acidity	

Fluid An adequate fluid intake of 2–3 l/d is encouraged to ensure a urine output >2 l/d. Specifically, patients are told to drink 250 ml every 4 waking hours + 250 ml at meals. New stone formation within 5 years may be prevented in up to 60% of patients with idiopathic calcium urolithiasis and the average interval for recurrences can be ↑ from 2–3 years. A hot climate and activities such as heavy exercise and long distance travel can result in concentrated urine.

Calcium There are a number of dietary factors that can cause hypercalciuria.

- Calcium intake or absorption. Restriction is not advisable and the aim is to meet the recommended nutrient intake for calcium of 700–800 mg/d (preferably from diet rather than supplements). Paradoxically ↓ calcium intake will ↑ intestinal absorption of oxalate and hence lead to hyperoxaluria (another risk factor for stone formation). Patients may also be at risk of osteoporosis on a ↓ calcium diet.
- Sodium intake. Sodium causes precipitation and crystal formation. Additionally, ↑ dietary sodium of 100 mmol/d increases calcium excretion by 0.6 mmol/d. A moderate intake of 2–3 g/d (90–100 mmol) sodium is recommended. This will, however, affect the perceived palatability and convenience of foods eaten.
- Protein intake. ↑ Animal protein intake can promote stone formation in a number of ways: ↑ acidity of the urine due to breakdown of sulphur-containing amino acids, calcium, uric acid, and also ↑ cystine excretion. The acidifying effects of an ↑ protein intake also results in ↓ urinary citrate. An intake of 1 g protein/kg body weight is thought to be appropriate. Factors that reduce hypercalciuria are ↑ alkali load (from fruit and vegetables), dietary fibre, potassium, and phosphate.

Oxalate is mostly formed endogenously (from vitamin C and glycine metabolism). Approximately 10–15% of urinary oxalate is derived from dietary intake. Oxalate absorption from the gut increases with ↓ calcium intake (perhaps through ↓ precipitation in the gut) or if competition for absorption decreases, e.g. fatty acid malabsorption. Nonetheless, a high intake of foods with highly bio-available oxalate, such as rhubarb or spinach, can ↑ urinary oxalate excretion to near or above the normal limits, resulting in the urinary calcium oxalate concentration reaching saturation point. High doses of vitamin C, e.g. >1 g/day, can ↑ oxalate production, although the metabolic pathway is usually saturated. Pyridoxine is involved in conversion of glyoxalate to glycine and epidemiological studies have shown an inverse relationship between B_6 intake and stone formation. Pyridoxine (100–300 mg/day) is used to ↓ oxaluria.

Oxalate-rich foods—bio-availability varies

Drinks	Beer, cocoa, Ovaltine, black tea, juices from high oxalate fruits, instant coffee powder
Fruit	Gooseberries, strawberries, raspberries, blackberries, blueberries, rhubarb, kiwi, tangerines
Vegetables	Beets, celery, green beans, leeks, runner beans, okra, parsley, spinach, sweet potato, watercress, yam
Legumes	Baked beans, soy products, e.g. tofu
Grains	Wheat germ, bran
Nuts & seeds	Pecans, peanuts, almonds, cashews, sesame seeds, sunflower seeds
Other	Plain chocolate, soy sauce

Uric acid is an end product of purine metabolism (largely from DNA) and dietary restriction of purines and animal protein will ↓ urinary excretion. Acidic urine will precipitate uric acid salts and alkalinization has been achieved with citrate salts. Orange juice is high in citrate without containing too much oxalate.

Purine-rich foods

Meat	Liver, kidney, brain, heart, goose, partridge
Fish	Anchovies, crab, herring, mackerel, mussels, roe, sardines, scallops, shrimps, sprats, whitebait
Other	Yeast, meat extract, e.g. Bovril, Oxo

Summary of dietary treatment in renal stone disease

- Fluid: >2 litres of fluid a day (take particular care if exercising or in a hot climate)
- Protein: 1 g protein/kg ideal body weight
- Calcium: 700–800 mg/d
- Sodium: ~100 mmol/d
- Oxalates: if 24 hour urinary oxalate is >440 mmol check for ↑oxalate containing foods and megadoses of vitamin C. Pyridoxine supplements may ↑ stone formation
- Purines: if 24 hour urinary uric acid is >4 mmol check for ↑ purine containing foods. If uric acid stones are identified, drinking orange juice may help prevent formation of stones
- Other: Potassium, magnesium, fibre, fruit, and vegetables are associated with ↓ risk; ↓ refined carbohydrate may ↑ risk

Useful websites

▯ DH (2004) National Service Framework for Renal Services.
http://www.dh.gov.uk/PolicyAndGuidance/HealthAndSocialCare
Topics/Renal/fs/en
▯ European Guidelines for the Nutritional Care of Adult Renal Patients.
http://www.edtna-erca.org
▯ National Kidney Foundation—Kidney Disease Outcomes Quality
Initiative. http://www.kidney.org/professionals/kdoqi/guidelines/

Respiratory disease and cystic fibrosis

Respiratory disease

Asthma

Pathogenesis Evidence suggests that a sub-optimum intake of an[ti] oxidant micronutrients contributes to the development of asthma. This [is] supported by studies showing that people consuming a diet rich in fru[it] and vegetables have better respiratory health. A diet compatible with th[e] 'Balance of Good Health' (see 'Food-based dietary guidelines', Chapter [?]) may ∴ help reduce risk. Obesity is also associated with ↑ risk of asthm[a] and weight loss has been shown to improve respiratory symptoms [in] overweight patients. An ↑ sodium intake is associated with airway reactivi[ty] and ↑ symptoms in patients with asthma; an excessive salt intake shou[ld] ∴ be avoided.

Food allergy Cow's milk has anecdotally been linked to asthma b[ut] objective testing suggests that diet and food allergy is only important in [a] minority of individuals; in these, food avoidance can improve symptom[s] and reduce drug therapy and hospital admission (see 'Food hypersensit[iv]ity', Chapter 32). There is no evidence that feeding infants soya-base[d] rather than cow's milk formula reduces the risk of having asthma; brea[st] milk remains the feed of choice for all babies for at least the first 6 mont[hs] of life (see 'Breast versus bottle feeding', Chapter 10).

Chronic obstructive pulmonary disease (COPD)

Patients with COPD are frequently malnourished (prevalence 25–60%[).] This is of concern because undernutrition is associated with poor respir[a]tory function and ↑ susceptibility to infection and, in COPD, is associate[d] with poor prognosis. Instinctively, providing nutritional support seems a[n] appropriate mode of treatment, although one recent systematic revie[w] concluded that nutritional support had no significant effect on anthr[o]pometric measurements, lung function, or exercise capacity in patien[ts] with stable COPD. However, a wider review of evidence in hospital an[d] community-based COPD patients shows that oral nutrition support c[an] have beneficial effects on respiratory and skeletal muscle strengt[h,] walking distance, and well-being in underweight patients who gain >2 [kg] and, importantly, is not associated with any detrimental effects.

Lung cancer

Lung cancer is the second most common malignancy in the UK with a[n] annual incidence of ~37 000. Smoking contributes to 90% of cases. [A] higher intake of fruit and vegetables has a slightly protective effect. Th[is] had been attributed to their antioxidant content but trials have show[n] that antioxidant β-carotene supplements do not yield the same benefi[t] and are, in fact, associated with ↑ risk of lung cancer. Eating fruit an[d] vegetables rather than taking supplements is thus recommended.

Patients with lung cancer are frequently undernourished, especially [in] the more advanced stages. Nutrition support should be considered in th[e] context of their treatment and prognosis (see 'Nutrition goals in anticanc[er] treatment', Chapter 20).

Lung transplantation

Approximately 120 lung transplants are undertaken in the UK each year. Patients with end-stage lung disease are frequently malnourished. Those with a BMI <17 or >27 kg/m^2 have a greater chance of dying at 90 d after transplant compared to those with BMI between 17 and 25 kg/m^2. Pre-surgical nutritional support has been shown to be effective in increasing body weight in underweight patients; nutritional assessment and advice before transplant may help improve outcome.

Tuberculosis (TB)

Worldwide, ~9 million new cases of active TB are diagnosed each year. The prevalence of TB has been increasing in the UK since 1990 after decades of decline (2003: ~7000 individuals diagnosed in England and Wales, 40% in London, 60% pulmonary TB, 90% born outside UK; <10% also HIV +ve). Undernutrition is a risk factor for developing TB and patients who are malnourished are at greater risk of dying than those who are not; vitamin D deficiency has been implicated. Patients with TB and those at risk do not require a special diet but would benefit from a well-balanced diet providing an adequate intake of all macro- and micronutrients.

Cystic fibrosis (CF)

Approximately 7500 people in the UK have CF, an autosomal recessive inherited disorder that affects the exocrine glands leading to pancreatic insufficiency and chronic lung disease. Weight loss and undernutrition are associated with a worse clinical outcome.

Causes of weight loss and undernutrition in CF

Impaired nutrient absorption Inadequate secretion of pancreatic enzymes should be treated by replacement therapy (see 'Pancreatic enzyme replacement therapy', Chapter 22). If adequate pancreatic enzymes are taken, there is no need to limit dietary fat in almost all patients. Fat restriction may have detrimental consequences because of the associated restriction in energy intake. However, in a very small minority of cases where steatorrhoea cannot be controlled adequately in spite of appropriately taken high dose pancreatic supplements, a modest fat restriction should be tried; energy intake must be maintained.

Increased requirements Energy needs increase due to the ↑ costs of respiration. It is estimated that energy requirements are 120–150% of normal. Protein requirements are also likely to be ↑ as a result of ↑ nitrogen losses via the gut and sputum; an intake of 120% of the reference nutrient intake is recommended (see Appendix 6).

Poor food intake Appetite may be poor due to tiredness and repeated chest infections. ↑ respiratory tract secretions may discourage the intake of some supplement drinks. The nutrient density of the diet should be considered to ensure that requirements are met within the limited quantity of foods consumed.

Nutritional management

This should include the following.
- Regular review by a registered dietitian with experience in this area; nutrient intake is significantly greater in CF patients when they are reviewed at least annually by a dietitian.
- Consideration of oral supplements. While some patients may be able to consume sufficient ordinary food to meet their needs, others will benefit from home-made or commercial supplements (see 'Treatment of undernutrition Chapter 16).
- Consideration of overnight tube feeding. This may be useful for patients who are unable to maintain an adequate oral intake in the long term or for shorter periods following an exacerbation of respiratory problems. It is particularly beneficial in children where overnight feeding for 6 months is associated with improved nutritional status and catch-up growth.
  - Nasogastric tubes can be passed nightly or a gastrostomy inserted, preferable by endoscopy (see 'Routes for enteral feeding', Chapter 16).

- Feeding regimes should take account of the higher requirements in CF and aim to provide 30–50% of energy needs (assuming that oral intake will provide the rest).
- Energy-dense feeds may be useful, but otherwise general feeding guidelines relevant to the age of the patient should be followed.
- Pancreatic enzyme replacement may be given before feeding commences but fat content is often tolerated better because the feed is delivered slowly over several hours.

Infants with CF

Ideally CF babies should be breastfed. They require pancreatic enzymes with each feed.

Alternatively, regular infant formulae can be given, again with pancreatic enzymes.

Pancreatic enzymes should be mixed with a little breast milk or formula and given to the infant on a spoon. They should not be given with formula milk in a bottle or feeder.

Some infants with higher energy requirements may need additional supplementation. This should be undertaken with the advice of a registered dietitian with paediatric experience.

Complicating factors

CF and diabetes mellitus Due to ↑ survival, up to 30% of CF patients develop diabetes and the dietary advice for the two conditions needs to be reconciled. It is imperative to maintain an adequate energy intake so it should not be restricted but some saturated fat can be replaced by monounsaturates. As a bulky, ↑ carbohydrate diet may not be practical, foods contributing refined carbohydrate should not be restricted but eaten in conjunction with other items to dissipate the glycaemic effect.

CF and liver disease occur in up to 25% of CF patients. Additional problems with malabsorption may occur if bile composition is altered or output is ↓ and this may not be remedied by increasing pancreatic enzyme supplementation. If it is ∴ necessary to ↓ fat intake (and this should be avoided if possible), then an adequate energy intake must be maintained using carbohydrate and protein sources. Liver transplantation may be necessary and usually leads to an improvement in pulmonary function as well as restoration of liver function.

Human immunodeficiency virus (HIV) infection

Introduction

Infection with HIV leads to progressive suppression of immune function eventually rendering the body susceptible to opportunistic infections and tumours. While there is no cure, antiretroviral drugs to suppress HIV replication have been developed. Combining ≥3 of these agents to form highly active antiretroviral therapy (HAART) has greatly improved clinical outcome. Nutritional issues are diverse, reflecting the complexity of the disease and its pharmacological management.

Nutritional goals

Avoidance of nutritional deficiencies Nutrition and immunity are cohesively linked and optimal intake of energy, protein, and micronutrients may help augment immune function.

Prevention/treatment of unintentional weight loss Wasting, a feature of symptomatic disease, is associated with ↑ morbidity and mortality.

Management of complications associated with HAART Metabolic side effects include hyperlipidaemia, insulin resistance, and hyperglycaemia.

Nutritional assessment should be undertaken regularly including diet history, height, weight, and BMI. In addition, skinfold measurements and circumferences (see 'Anthropometry', Chapter 4) may help monitor body composition/shape changes (see below).

Avoidance of nutritional deficiencies

Diet advice should follow the guidelines of the 'Balance of Good Health' (see 'Food-based dietary guidelines', Chapter 2). The exact micronutrient requirements in HIV infection are unknown but may be higher than in the general population. A complete daily vitamin and mineral supplement around the level of reference nutrient intake (see Appendix 6) may be appropriate and is clearly indicated if diet is compromised.

Unintentional weight and lean tissue loss

Although the incidence and severity of wasting has reduced since the introduction of HAART, it remains a significant clinical problem. The aetiology is multifactorial, the main precipitating factors being:
- ↓ nutritional intake;
- altered metabolic requirements;
- malabsorption;
- testosterone deficiency.

Management of weight loss
- Treatment of underlying opportunistic infections and optimization of antiretroviral therapy are a priority.
- Nutritional status and requirements should be assessed using standard methods.
- Aim to ↑ energy and protein intake.
  - Small, frequent nutritious meals, snacks, and drinks.
  - Appropriate use of proprietary energy and protein supplements.
  - Symptoms such as nausea, vomiting, diarrhoea, taste changes, and anorexia must be taken into account (see 'Chemotherapy and radiotherapy' in Chapter 20).
  - Resistance exercise may help aid accretion of lean body mass.
- Artificial nutrition support should be considered if nutritional needs are not met orally despite intervention.
  - Nasogastric for short-term support.
  - Percutaneous endoscopic gastrostomy (PEG) for longer term intervention (see 'Routes for enteral feeding', Chapter 16).
- Pharmacotherapy.
  - Testosterone replacement may aid lean tissue accretion in hypogonadal men with wasting.
  - Anabolic steroids can ↑ weight and lean tissue in men with wasting. However, they are associated with hyperlipidaemia, body fat loss, and possible liver disturbances and may be best avoided in those at risk of HAART-related metabolic complications.
  - The progesterone derivative, megestrol acetate, is an effective appetite stimulant. However, weight gain tends to be fat rather than lean and it is associated with adrenal insufficiency and hyperglycaemia.

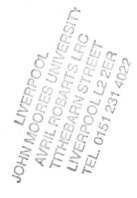

Lipodystrophy associated with HAART

Lipodystrophy includes a number of morphologic and metabolic complications that can be observed individually or in combination.

• Visceral, breast, and dorso-cervical fat accumulation.
• Lipoatrophy: loss of subcutaneous fat from limbs, buttocks, and face.
• Dyslipidaemia: elevated total and LDL cholesterol and triglycerides. Low HDL cholesterol.
• Insulin resistance and hyperglycaemia.

Aetiology

• Unclear.
• Thought to relate to the interaction between HIV, immune reconstitution, and antiretroviral therapy.
• Various protease inhibitors (P I) and the nucleoside analogues D4T and possibly AZT have been implicated.

Clinical significance

• Body shape changes may have an adverse psychological impact and potentially affect adherence to HAART.
• Dyslipidaemia, insulin resistance, and hyperglycaemia may ↑ risk of CVD. Risk may further ↑ by the pro-inflammatory nature of HIV.

Management

• Awareness, monitoring, careful choice of HAART, and dietary advice may help prevent lipodystrophy.
• Patients commencing HAART should undergo cardiovascular risk assessment.
• Advice based on the 'Balance of Good Health' (see 'Food-based dietary guidelines', Chapter 2) and Mediterranean diet principles is recommended. Those with hyperlipidaemia or elevated CVD risk should receive more intensive dietary advice. Mediterranean/cardioprotective diet includes:
  • ↑ omega 3 fatty acids (oily fish, rapeseed oil, olive oil), fruit, vegetables, beans, and pulses;
  • reduced saturated and trans fatty acids and replacement with monounsaturated fatty acids.
• Exercise should be encouraged as it may benefit metabolic parameters and abdominal shape.
• Additional modifiable risk factors to address include smoking, hypertension, and obesity.
• Dietary treatment of diabetes should follow Diabetes UK guidelines (see 'Goals and principles of dietary management', Chapter 18).
• Morphological changes may be more difficult to manage than metabolic aberrations. Weight reducing advice may help reduce visceral adiposity

Additional dietary issues

Food and drug interactions
- HAART regimens can be complex and involve food restrictions.
- Presence or absence of food in the gut may affect drug absorption or modify risk of side-effects. Drugs prescribed change over time, hence the importance of referring to up to date manufacturers information.

Food and water safety
- Food and water borne infection is more common in the immuno compromised host. Good food hygiene and avoidance of high-risk foods (e.g. raw/undercooked eggs, unpasteurized milk products, raw/undercooked meat and fish) are advisable.
- *Cryptosporidium* may occasionally be found in tap-water supplies. Immunosuppressed patients, particularly those with CD4 counts <200 cells/mm^3, should be advised to boil water to destroy this protozoan.

Further information
1. Grinspoon, S. and Mulligan, K. (2003). Weight loss and wasting in patients infected with human immunodeficiency virus. *Clin. Infect. Dis.* **36** (Suppl. 2), 569–78.
2. British HIV Association (2005). BHIVA guidelines for the treatment of HIV infected adults with antiretroviral therapy 2005. www.bhiva.org.

Nutrition in mental health

Introduction, pharmacotherapy, and care in the community

Introduction

It is estimated that 3 out of every 10 people in the UK will experience problems with their mental well-being every year. Only ~1 in 10 will be diagnosed with a mental health problem but this still means that a large proportion of the population is affected. The interrelationship between mental health and nutrition includes a diverse range of topics ranging from those close to 'normal' healthy behaviour to the 'extremes' of mental ill health (see Table 27.1).

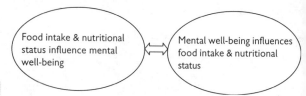

Food intake & nutritional status influence mental well-being ⟷ Mental well-being influences food intake & nutritional status

Table 27.1 Relationship between mood and eating*

Mood disorder and symptoms	Potential nutrition consequences
Depression	
Loss of appetite	Inadequate/inappropriate intake
Apathy & disinterest in food	Compromised nutritional status
Tiredness—unable to cook	Weight loss/gain
Loss of thirst sensation	Tiredness/lack of concentration
Food craving/erratic eating habits	Dehydration
	Constipation
Anxiety	
Restlessness/hyperactivity	↑ Energy expenditure
Dry mouth	Inadequate/excessive intake
Nausea, vomiting, diarrhoea	Difficulty chewing and swallowing
Loss of appetite	Compromised nutritional status
Food refusal	Weight loss/gain
Comfort eating	Tiredness/lack of concentration

*Note. Many of the nutritional consequences will contribute to the symptoms and potentially exacerbate them, e.g. tiredness in depression is associated with poor food intake → inadequate ingestion of energy and nutrients → further tiredness.

Pharmacotherapy

Drugs used in treating mental health problems may influence food intake and/or nutritional status. It should not be assumed that every patient taking medication will experience any or all of the side-effects associated with specific drugs. When side-effects arise, they are sometimes managed by adjusting the dose or changing prescription to a similar preparation that may be better tolerated. However, as some pharmacotherapy is long-term, e.g. taken for many years, there may be nutritional implications that require intervention (see box).

Examples of possible nutrition-related side-effects associated with selected drugs used to treat mental illness

Antidepressants
- Tricyclic, e.g. dosulepin, → dry mouth, sour metallic taste, constipation
- 5-Hydroxytryptamine re-uptake inhibitors, e.g. fluoxetine, → anorexia, nausea, & vomiting (usually mild) may occur in first 10 days but tend to resolve
- Monoamine oxidase (MAO) inhibitors, e.g. phenelzine, → patients taking these drugs should avoid foods containing high levels of tyramine, e.g. mature cheese, yeast extracts, soya bean products, pickled herring, and certain wine (see 'Drug–nutrient interactions', Chapter 8)

Antipsychotics
- Atypical antipsychotics, e.g. clozapine, olanzapine, → ↑ appetite, weight gain, diabetogenic
- Thioxanthenes, e.g. flupentixol decanoate (used as depot injection), → ↑ appetite, weight gain

Mood stabilizers
- Lithium salts, e.g. lithium carbonate → nausea, metallic taste (~ mild, controlled by adjusting dose), serum electrolytes must be checked (see 'Drug–nutrient interactions', Chapter 8).

Anticonvulsants
- Barbiturates, e.g. phenobarbital*, → ↓ vitamin D levels, ↓ folate levels; e.g. phenytoin* → ↓ vitamin D absorption, ↑ turnover, & ↓ absorption of folate

*No longer 1st choice of treatment but many patients continue to take it

---

Nutritional care in the community

The vast majority of people with mental health problems live in the community, some autonomously and others requiring considerable support. Obtaining, preparing, and eating a well-balanced diet can be a challenge and poor diet can exacerbate both short-term symptoms and the risk of chronic health problems associated with mental illness. The community mental health team should be aware of this and facilitate support. Specialist training in nutrition is rarely required and dietitians are well-placed to guide support workers in how to optimize their clients' nutritional status. In addition to considering the nutrients supplied by food, the pleasure of eating and the empowerment associated with preparing an edible meal can also make a valuable contribution.

Eating disorders

- Defined as persistent disturbance of eating (± behaviour) that impairs physical health or psychosocial functioning or both and that is not 2° to any other medical or psychiatric disorder.
- Include anorexia nervosa, bulimia nervosa, and binge eating disorder.
- Individuals who do not fall within strict diagnostic criteria are describe as having an atypical eating disorder or disordered eating.

Anorexia nervosa

- Diagnosed on basis of key features (ICD-10 and DSM-IV):
  - active maintenance of very low body weight, e.g. 15% less than idea or BMI <17.5 kg/m^2;
  - cognitive disturbance including 'relentless pursuit of thinness' and 'morbid fear of fatness';
  - amenorrhoea.
- Prevalence: 0.5–2.5/1000 in UK; predominantly ♀ aged 10–30 yrs; ~10% are ♂.
- Predisposing and maintaining factors include dieting, family history of eating disorder and depression, and personal history of depression, perfectionism, low self-esteem.

Management

- Patients may be reluctant to seek treatment so forming a 'collaborative therapeutic relationship' is important. May also involve family.
- Establish healthy eating habits and normal weight (see below).
- Address issues that are likely to cause relapse. Usually includes cognitive behavioural and family therapy.

Nutritional aspects

- Depends on severity of weight loss and setting (in- or outpatients).
- If severe, aim to introduce regular meals and snacks that provide 1000–1500 kcal /d within first few days of admission. Care may be needed, especially in extreme emaciation, to avoid re-feeding syndrome (see 'Re-feeding syndrome', Chapter 16).
- ↑ Intake to 'normal' meals and snacks that provide ~2000 kcal/d within 2 weeks.
- Aim towards intake that will achieve target weight gain of 1.0–1.5 kg/week. This may require an intake >3000 kcal. Supplement drinks may be helpful if the quantity of food is otherwise unacceptable.
- Body weight should be monitored daily initially, then weekly.
- Target weight should be agreed with patient, encompass a 3 kg band (to facilitate natural fluctuation), and be achievable without dieting.
- Phase out supplement drinks on reaching target.
- Education about healthy/normal eating with gradual transfer of control to the patient.

Bulimia nervosa

- Diagnosed on basis of key features (ICD-10 and DSM-IV):
  - frequent bulimic episodes, e.g. 'binges' of very large quantities of food, average 3000 kcal, with feeling of loss of control;
  - extreme measures to control body weight including vomiting and use of laxatives and diuretics;
  - cognitive disturbance including 'relentless pursuit of thinness' and 'morbid fear of fatness'.
- Prevalence: 10–20/1000 in UK and USA; predominantly ♀ aged 16–40 y; rare in ♂.
- Clinical features: restrained eating between binges; often follow complex food rules; breaking rules may trigger binge; not overtly thin; dental erosion may be visible on palatal surface of front teeth (from vomiting gastric acid); callus may be visible on dorsal surface of dominant hand from inducing vomiting; electrolyte disturbances following vomiting or purging with laxatives or diuretics.

Management

- Patients may be reluctant to seek treatment and most regard behaviour with great shame. Medical help often sought for other conditions.
- Usually managed in outpatient setting.
- Specialized cognitive behavioural therapy (CBT), e.g. 20 sessions over ± 5 months, can result in substantial improvements.
- Establish healthy eating habits and normal weight (see below).

Nutritional aspects

- Monitor weight by weekly weighing.
- Introduce a meal plan to establish 'normal' (non-dieting) eating behaviour.
- Educate *re* healthy balanced diet/normal weight and fluctuation.
- Use self-monitoring diary (see Table 27.2) to support CBT.

Table 27.2 Example of a self-monitoring diary*

Time of intake
Food eaten
Quantity consumed
Where eaten
With whom
How did you feel ?
Were you hungry ?

* Reproduced from Thomas B (2001), *Manual of Dietetic Practice*, Table 2.18, p191. Permission requested from Blackwell Publishing.

Binge eating disorder

Diagnostic criteria are not defined by ICD-10 or DSM-IV but research diagnostic criteria describe binge eating episodes on 2 days per week. It is estimated that as many as 20–30% of individuals seeking help for obesity have a binge eating disorder, characterized by binge eating without the extreme weight-control measures of starving, vomiting, purging, or excessive exercise.

• Potentially, this means that more patients will need nutritional management than the combined number with anorexia nervosa and bulimia nervosa.
• Patients with binge eating disorder have a higher rate of anxiety, mood and personality disorders, and depression than those with bulimia nervosa.

Nutritional management

Although a less-pronounced condition with fewer serious health implications than bulimia nervosa, nutritional management should follow similar guidelines.

Dementia

Dementia is 'the development of multiple cognitive deficits that are sufficiently severe to cause impairment in occupational or social functioning and represent a decline from a previously higher level of functioning'.[1] It affects:
- ~700 000 people in the UK;
- ~2% of people aged between 65 and 75 years;
- ~20% of those >80 years.

Causes of dementia
- Alzheimer's disease;
- Vascular disease;
- Lewy body disease;
- Huntington's disease;
- AIDS;
- Acquired head injury;
- Prion disease (e.g. CJD);
- Multiple sclerosis;
- Wernicke–Korsakoff syndrome;
- Syphilis.

Factors influencing eating & drinking in dementia

- Poor memory: forgetting to eat or that they have eaten, forgetting to shop or the names of foods to buy
- Poor coordination: inability to put food on to cutlery, move food into the mouth, peel or unwrap food
- Inability to sequence activities needed to prepare meals
- Drug side-effects: dry mouth, drowsiness, constipation, dysphagia
- Poor concentration: easily distracted from meals by noise and other activity
- Tremor: spilling drinks, food
- Eating slowly: food becomes unappetizing or removed by carer
- Poor vision/confusion: food not recognized
- Agitation and restlessness: increases energy requirements while reducing opportunities to eat and drink
- Hallucinations: reluctance or refusal to eat food that appears to contain, foreign bodies
- Tooth/mouth problems: pain or discomfort, altered taste
- Choking/swallowing problems: reluctance to eat and drink, food may be hoarded in the mouth, spat out, or may lead to aspiration and repeated chest infections
- 'Sun-downing': cognitive function often reduced in the late afternoon/evening so later meals often not eaten
- Depression: a very common additional diagnosis, leading to reduced appetite and reluctance to eat

---

[1] American Psychiatric Association (1994). *Diagnostic and statistical manual of mental disorders IV*, APA, Washington DC.

Improving nutrition in dementia

- Routine, regular screening for nutritional risk.
- Monitor weight; people with dementia are often thin because they do not eat enough, not because it is part of the illness.
- Help older people maintain an active lifestyle; this helps maintain appetite and energy intake.
- Keep support flexible: help with shopping, cooking, company for meals, verbal prompts.
- Maintain independence by offering help rather than interference.
- Offer snacks; some older people adopt 'grazing' eating patterns, with snacks between meals. Ensure snacks are nutritious so that total intake is not compromised.
- Try to provide choice by allowing people to select from plates of food so that they can eat immediately.
- Avoid patterned crockery, tablecloths, etc. as these may confuse people with dementia and reduce their attention given to food.
- Try coloured drinks in clear glasses as they are easier to see than drinks in cups, beakers, or cartons.
- Allow enough time for eating; hurried meals cause agitation, distress, and reluctance to eat.
- Limit noise and other distractions while people are eating.
- Ensure adequate light so that food can be seen properly.
- Keep the dining room just for meals rather than other activities so that entering the room acts as a cue for eating and drinking.
- Talk about food and encourage eating by chatting about the meal.
- Ensure adequate resources allocated to catering in institutional settings.

Increasing nutrient intake using ordinary food

- Ensuring an adequate energy intake will help increase the intake of other nutrients.
- Use whole milk (not skimmed or semi-skimmed) in all cooking and for drinks. Channel Island or 'gold top' milk contains more energy.
- Use sugar or honey in puddings and not artificial sweeteners.
- If people like sugar in drinks or on cereals, try adding glucose as well. It has the same calories as sugar but is only half as sweet.
- Try honey or syrup on porridge or hot instant cereals. They don't add more calories than ordinary sugar, but can encourage people to eat more if they like the flavour.
- Alcohol can stimulate the appetite. Try adding small amounts to milky coffee, hot chocolate, fruit drinks, or prescribed supplements.
- Include some fried food on the menu, and provide 'proper' puddings and cakes every day.
- Make a cooked breakfast available as people often eat better earlier in the day.
- Add butter, margarine, or grated cheese to mashed potato and other vegetables.
- Tinned and packet soups and gravy have almost no food value. Home-made soups are usually better but ideally should contain meat, milk, peas, beans, or lentils.

- If food needs to be moistened to puree or mash it, add butter, margarine, or white sauce rather than gravy or water.
- Make fruit mousses or fruit fools with custard and add some cream.
- Offer high-energy between-meal snacks with drinks, e.g. cake, biscuits, ice cream, fruit and cream, instant desserts, trifles, sandwiches, chocolate.
- Make food and drink available at night if people sleep poorly.

Finger foods

Using finger foods (Table 27.3) may help people who cannot remember how to use cutlery, or those who have lost the use of one hand, e.g. after a stroke. They can allow people to feed themselves and help to maintain independence and dignity whilst the greater interaction with food often results in a better food intake. As with all institutional catering, finger food menus need full nutritional analysis and audit.

Table 27.3 Examples of finger foods

Starchy & cereal	Protein-rich	Dairy	Fruit & vegetables	Energy dense
Buttered rolls	Chicken nuggets	Cheese cubes	Apple slices	Biscuits
Chips	Fish cakes	Sliced cheese	Banana pieces	Chocolate
Crumpets	Fish fingers	Yogurt-covered raisins	Carrot sticks	Crisps
Potato cakes	Hard-boiled egg		Celery sticks	Ice cream cones
Roast potatoes	Meatballs		Cherry tomatoes	Jam tarts
Tea cakes	Samosas		Grapes	Slices of cake
Toast fingers	Sandwiches		Orange segments	
	Sausages			

Soft diets

If a person is unable to chew, care should be taken to ensure that food provided supplies an adequate energy, protein, and micronutrient intake (see 'Dysphagia' in 'Cerebrovascular accident/stroke', Chapter 19). Simply liquidizing ordinary food is rarely adequate and oral nutrition supplements should be considered (see Table 16.4 in 'Treatment of under nutrition', Chapter 16).

Nutrition in neurological conditions

Multiple sclerosis (MS)

MS is an autoimmune disorder of the central nervous system with a UK prevalence of ~1.2 in 1000. Damage is caused to the myelin sheath surrounding nerves, thus impairing the conduction of impulses. The condition varies from a relapsing/remitting pattern (~80% patients) to a progressive form that may be fatal within a few years. Nutritional implications relate to (1) the cause of the condition, (2) its progression, and (3) the management of neurological symptoms that arise.

Pathogenesis

Genetic susceptibility and environmental factors have been implicated. Dietary factors include:
- an association between a high prevalence of MS and ↑ saturated fat and ↓ polyunsaturated fatty acids intakes;
- a possible link with vitamin D status.

The fatty acid hypothesis is interesting because myelin is composed of ~70% fatty acids, including ~ a third of polyunsaturates. However, at present, the evidence is considered non-conclusive and further studies are needed.

Disease progression

The potential role for diet to ameliorate disease progression is uncertain. Evidence suggests that a ↓ fat diet (<20 g/d) and supplements of *n*–3 and *n*–6 fatty acids may reduce the progression of disability. On the basis of this, a dose of 17–23 g/d of *n*–6 linoleic acid is recommended. This intake is ~6–10 times the minimum individual dietary reference value and could be taken by consuming a variety of different food sources (see box).

Good sources of linoleic acid (quantity providing 4 g linoleic acid)

- Safflower oil: 5 g (~1 teaspoonful)
- Corn or sunflower seed oil: 8 g (~1½ teaspoonful)
- Polyunsaturated margarine: 9 g (~2 level teaspoonful)
- Walnuts: 13 g (~5 halves)
- Brazil nuts: 16 g (~4 medium nuts)

It is recommended that ↑ linoleic acid intake should not be taken in isolation but should be consumed within the context of a well-balanced and varied diet (see 'Balance of Good Health' in 'Food-based dietary guidelines', Chapter 2). This will ensure that total fat intake is not excessive and that sufficient antioxidant micronutrients are taken to accompany ↑ linoleic acid intake. The median survival of MS patients is 40 years after diagnosis and ∴ concern about long-term nutritional health is important.

Management of neurological symptoms

Fatigue, loss of balance, weakness, numbness, tingling, and bladder problems are among the most common symptoms experienced by MS patients. Difficulty in swallowing is relatively uncommon except in the very late stages but may have a profound impact on food intake and nutritional status.

- Routine nutritional assessment will help to identify patients whose nutritional intake is suboptimum before depletion results in clinical impairment.
- Practical support, e.g. help with shopping or meal preparation, may be sufficient to help some patients 'normalize' their intake.
- Nutritional supplements may help to increase nutrient intake where sufficient food cannot be consumed (see 'Treatment of undernutrition', Chapter 16).
- Overweight is common, ~40% of patients diagnosed 10–13 years, and related to reduced mobility and ↑ fatigue. A moderate energy-restricted diet that provides all other nutrient requirements is advisable (see Appendix 6).
- Constipation, reported in ~40%, may be alleviated by a ↑ fibre intake and drinking sufficient fluid, >2 litre/d (see 'Constipation' in Disorders of the colon', Chapter 21).
- Swallowing difficulties should be evaluated by a speech and language therapist and dietitian with expertise in this area (see 'Dysphagia' in 'Cerebrovascular accident/stroke', Chapter 19).
- If an adequate nutritional intake cannot be maintained orally, feeding via a PEG may help improve quality of life (see 'Routes for enteral feeding', Chapter 16).

Alternative diets and MS

- Patients with MS may be offered a variety of allegedly therapeutic diets through the popular press and other media.
- Some include specific dietary restrictions that may compromise the adequacy of their nutrient intake.
- Other regimes involve the purchase of specific food items or supplements that are not prescribable and often expensive.
- At present, there is little evidence to support dietary manipulation other than that described above.
- Patients may need advice about the potential harms and benefits associated with some alternative diets.

Motor neurone disease (MND)

MND (or amyotrophic lateral sclerosis) is a group of related progressive disorders involving the degeneration of the motor neurones and leading to muscle weakness and wasting. Sensory neurones, e.g. taste, are not affected but difficulty chewing and swallowing may arise. The prevalence in the UK is ~5 in 100 000 and most patients have a life expectancy of <5 years at diagnosis.

Undernutrition

Inadequate nutrient intake often leads to poor nutritional status (~20%). This may further impair muscle function and is associated with ↓ survival.

Causes

- Dysphagia: lip and tongue dysfunction, palatal incompetence, impaired swallow reflex, pharyngeal weakness, and reduced laryngeal elevation.
- Arm weakness: dependence on others to be fed.
- Social consequences: difficulty in eating and excessive salivation may inhibit eating with other people.

Treatment

- Assessment of nutritional status by a dietitian (see Chapter 4).
- Evaluation of swallow and appropriately textured diet by speech and language therapist and dietitian—good coordination is essential (see 'Dysphagia' in 'Cerebrovascular accident/stroke', Chapter 19).
- Gastrostomy insertion (endoscopically or radiologically) if:
  - >10% loss of body weight despite supplementation;
  - unsafe swallow;
  - bulbar symptoms;
  - life expectancy >3 m;
  - able to provide consent and manage feeds (or carer who can).

Overweight

A small number of patients, particularly those whose mobility is compromised by leg muscle weakness, are overweight. A modest energy restriction that does not compromise other nutrient intakes should be advised.

Antioxidants

The role of antioxidants in treating MND, i.e. to combat the oxidative stress contributing to disease progression, has been examined in a number of studies but a recent systematic review revealed no significant benefits or contraindications. Whilst there is no specific evidence to support the use of supplements, diets of altered texture that are provided to patients with swallowing difficulties are often relatively ↓ in antioxidants and this could be addressed by the inclusion of suitably prepared fruit and vegetables.

Parkinson's disease (PDis)

PDis is a chronic progressive neurological condition with a UK prevalence of 150–200 per 100 000. Although it is associated with older people, the mean age at onset is 55 years with 1 in 10 people aged >80 years affected. Symptoms including hypokinesis (reduced movement and fatigue), rigidity, tremor, and depression can contribute to a poor food intake and impair nutritional status, particularly in the later stages.

• *Constipation* may arise from a poor overall food intake, a ↓ fibre diet as a result of texture modification, or as a side-effect of anti-parkinsonian medication. Increasing dietary fibre and an adequate fluid intake (>2 litre/d) is advisable. Fibre can be provided for patients requiring a soft/puree diet as oat porridge, pureed or mashed fruits including bananas, prunes, and dates, and thickened lentil-type soups.

• *Weight loss* will result from an inadequate intake possibly as a result of declining ability to shop or prepare food, increasing tremor that makes self-feeding difficult, or swallowing difficulties (see below). An evaluation of the patient's physical status and nutritional needs will help identify how to best address undernutrition (see Chapter 4).

• *Swallowing difficulties* are common and occur in up to 84% of patients, although in most they are relatively mild and do not impair food intake until a later stage. The patient's ability to swallow should be evaluated by a speech and language therapist and dietitian with expertise in this area to coordinate advice and an appropriately textured diet (see 'Texture modification' in Cerebrovascular accident/stroke' in Chapter 19).

• *Dry mouth* may arise as a side-effect of medication. Moist meals served with appropriate sauce may help. Sharp flavour, e.g. lemon and grapefruit, may stimulate saliva.

Other nutritional management

Protein restriction   The potential competition between circulating amino acids and PDis medication, L-dopa, led to investigation of diets providing ↓ protein diets (<10 g/d) during the day. Although pre-1993 studies looked promising, the long-term nutritional effects have not been examined. There is insufficient evidence to recommend restricting dietary protein as a means of treating PDis. However, patients experiencing fluctuating symptoms may benefit from manipulating the timing of their protein intake by (1) avoiding taking their medication with high protein meals and (2) eating a greater proportion of their dietary protein in the evening.

Antioxidants   Free radicals are implicated in the neurological damage of PDis. Studies have investigated the potential therapeutic effects of countering these with dietary antioxidants including vitamin E. No convincing evidence has emerged that can be translated into dietary recommendations. However, a well-balanced diet including 5 portions of fruit and vegetables per day will help provide a good baseline intake of antioxidants.

Palliative care

Palliative care

Most of this book is concerned with using nutritional strategies to improve health through promoting good health, reducing risk associated with poor nutrition, and treating or managing disease or illness (for cancer see chapter 20). These issues are no longer relevant for many people approaching the end of their life but nutritional care can play a role in maximizing their quality of life and well-being. In order to do this, nutritional care must be seen within the context of the patient's total management and objectives established and agreed with the patient, as appropriate, their carers, and all health-care staff. Points to consider include the following.

• First, do no harm. The potential benefit of nutritional support should be evaluated against the potential side-effects, e.g. nausea, diarrhoea.

• Palliative care may last for a few days or even years. Each individual will have different physical, emotional, and spiritual requirements and ∴ the contribution made by food and nutrition will also vary

• Abruptly stopping nutritional support, even if some side-effects occur, may be interpreted as a withdrawal of care. Tailoring-down support or leaving it as an option for the patient may be more acceptable.

• Pain-relieving medication may have side-effects that impact on food intake, e.g. constipation and drowsiness. Expertise within the palliative care team may facilitate drug manipulation to optimize pain relief and minimize side-effects. Communication is important.

• Eating and/or drinking may remain one of a limited number of enjoyable experiences and relaxing dietary restrictions to take account of this may be appropriate. The potential consequences of doing so must be considered in the context of the patient's likely prognosis.

• Nutrition does not need to be medicalized and regular meals may be one of the more 'normal' activities during a time that can otherwise be very stressful. Eating can be a social pleasure, so spending meal times with others may be enjoyable even if little is consumed. Conversely, eating together may become stressful if the patient fails to meet others' expectations of what s/he should eat. A balance is needed.

• Encouraging carers to provide favourite foods or special dishes may help them to demonstrate their love for the patient and feel actively involved in their care, even when there is no prospect of recovery. The patient's changing desires or reducing ability to accept such gifts can cause feelings of guilt or rejection and may need sensitive support.

• If eating is no longer possible and nutrition support is inappropriate, hydration can be maintained through drinks using a straw, spoon, or moistened sponge.

• For some patients, not eating or drinking may be part of the natural dying process.

Formal decisions to continue or withdraw feeding or hydration from patients who are terminally ill are sometimes made in the court if agreement between patients, carers and staff cannot be reached. The position changes in response to case law and the latest ruling (July 2004) which reflects the European Convention on Human Rights is available from the General Medical Council's web page on ethical guidance:

🖥 http://www.gmc-uk.org/guidance/witholding_lifeprolonging.asp

A court ruling is required before artificial nutrition and hydration is withdrawn from a patient in a persistent vegetative state in England, Wales, and Northern Ireland. This is not specified as required in Scotland but it is advisable to seek a legal opinion in each individual case.

Inherited metabolic disorders

Definitions and management

Definitions
- Metabolism: cellular biochemical reactions that occur within the body. This involves the breakdown (catabolism) and formation (anabolism) of chemical compounds.
- Metabolic pathways: sequence of chemical reactions of metabolism.
- Enzymes: proteins that control the chemical reactions (or steps) in a metabolic pathway.

Inherited metabolic diseases (IMD) are due to deficient activity of an enzyme (or occasionally multiple enzymes) in a metabolic pathway. The deficiency 'blocks' the metabolic pathway and the clinical consequences of this arise because:
- substrates prior to the 'block' accumulate and can be toxic;
- essential products beyond the 'block' are not formed;
- other compounds may be formed via alternative pathways which may be toxic.

Patients can present at any age: as neonates, throughout childhood, and in adulthood. The severity of the disorder may vary widely depending upon the degree of enzyme deficiency. IMD occur in many pathways of amino acid, carbohydrate, lipid, and vitamin metabolism.

Treatment is based upon an understanding of the biochemistry. The mainstays of therapy are the following.
- Therapeutic diet (see Table 30.1) to:
  - limit the intake of substrate that cannot be catabolized;
  - provide the product that cannot be formed.
- Large doses of precursor vitamins.
- Medicines that conjugate with toxic metabolites and the product is excreted in urine.

IMDs are rare and complex so it is essential patients are managed in a specialist metabolic centre by a multidisciplinary team including specialist consultants, dietitians, nurses, with supporting specialized laboratory services. For detailed information on presentation, medical and dietary management and outcome of IMD see:

📖 Fernandes, J., et al. (2000). Inborn metabolic diseases: diagnosis and treatment, 3rd edn. Springer-Verlag, Berlin.

📖 Dixon, M., et al. (2001). Inborn errors of metabolism. In Clinical paediatric dietetics, 2nd edn, (ed. V. Shaw and M. Lawson), pp. 233–316. Blackwell Science, Oxford.

Table 30.1 Summary of dietary management of some inherited metabolic diseases

Disorder	Dietary management
Amino acid disorders	
Classical phenylketonuria	Low phenylalanine diet + phenylalanine-free, tyrosine enriched amino acid supplement
Maple syrup urine disease*	Low leucine, isoleucine, valine diet + leucine, isoleucine, valine-free amino acid supplement. Amino acid supplement given during illness
Tyrosinaemia type I and II	Low protein diet (to limit tyrosine intake) + tyrosine, phenylalanine-free amino acid supplement
Classical homocystinuria	Low methionine diet + methionine-free, cystine enriched amino acid supplement
Organic acidaemias*	
Methylmalonic acidaemia*	Low protein diet (to limit methionine, threonine, valine, isoleucine intake) + methion-
Propionic acidaemia*	ine, threonine, valine, isoleucine-free amino acid supplement sometimes recommended
Isovaleric acidaemia*	Low protein diet (to limit isoleucine intake)
Urea cycle disorders*	
Ornithine carbamoyl transferase deficiency*	Low protein diet (to limit waste nitrogen for excretion) + l-arginine supplements. Essential
Citrullinaemia*	amino acid supplements may be needed
Argininosuccinic aciduria*	
Carbohydrate disorders	
Classical galactosaemia	Minimal galactose and lactose diet. Infant soya milk substitute
Glycogen storage disease type I* and type III*	Frequent supply of exogenous glucose provided as:
	Continuous overnight tube feeds and either 2 hourly daytime feeds or uncooked cornstarch
	Type III—milder disorders require less intensive dietary treatment
Fatty acid oxidation*/lipid disorders	
Very long chain acyl-CoA dehydrogenase deficiency*	Minimal long chain fat, ↑ CHO diet and medium chain triglyceride supplements. Frequent
Long chain 3-hydroxyacyl CoA dehydrogenase deficiency*	daytime feeding and continuous overnight tube feeds or uncooked cornstarch
Medium chain acyl-CoA dehydrogenase deficiency*	Emergency regimen during illness
Familial hypercholesterolaemia	Healthy eating—restricted saturated fat, replace with poly- and monounsaturated fats

* Disorders requiring emergency regimen during metabolic stress such as intercurrent illnesses, e.g. colds, ear infections, etc.

Emergency regimens for IMD

Metabolic stress, e.g. intercurrent infections, combined with a poor oral intake and fasting, anaesthesia, or surgery can precipitate severe metabolic decompensation in some IMD. Decompensation is due to catabolism with concomitant ↑ production of toxic metabolites. An emergency regimen (ER) is given to provide energy and help minimize the effects of catabolism. The basic ER is similar for all disorders.

- Glucose polymer drinks are given 2 to 3 hourly day and night.
- Carbohydrate concentration of these and volume given depend on age and weight (see Table 30.2).
- Glucose polymers can be flavoured to improve palatability.
- If an oral rehydration solution is prescribed for treatment of gastroenteritis, additional glucose polymer needs to be added to provide a final concentration of 10 to 12% carbohydrate. Too concentrated a solution may exacerbate diarrhoea.
- For some disorders, additional specific therapy is given such as drugs to promote excretion of toxic metabolites or amino acids to promote anabolism.
- If the ER is not tolerated an admission to the local hospital for stabilization with IV fluids (10% dextrose) is often necessary.
- Parents ∴ need to have explicit, hand-held, written ER instructions that explain the disorder, hospital management, and provide contact details for the specialist metabolic centre.
- ERs are not nutritionally complete and prolonged use can result in protein malnutrition. The child's usual diet should at least start to be reintroduced after 24–48 hours of ER.

Table 30.2 *Emergency regimens—composition and fluid volume for age*

Age	Glucose polymer concentration (% CHO)	Energy (kcal/100 ml)	Suggested daily fluid volume
0–6 m	10	40	150 ml/kg
7–12 m	10	40	120 ml/kg (up to 1200 ml/day maximum)
1–2 y	15	60	11–20 kg: 100ml/kg for 1st 10 kg + 50ml/kg for next 10kg
2–10 y	20	80	≥20kg: 100ml/kg for 1st 10kg + 50ml/kg for next 10kg + 25ml/kg thereafter (up to 2500 ml/day maximum)
>10 y	25	100	

Phenylketonuria (PKU)

PKU is due to a deficiency of the enzyme phenylalanine hydroxylase that converts the essential amino acid phenylalanine to tyrosine. Phenylalanine (phe) accumulates in plasma and is neurotoxic. Tyrosine, which is essential for the synthesis of protein and the catecholamine neurotransmitters, becomes deficient. Untreated, patients will develop severe mental retardation. Newborn screening for PKU was established in the UK in 1968. Patients are treated with a low phe diet that is continued throughout childhood; some adults also remain on diet. During pregnancy, a low phe diet is crucial to prevent damage to the unborn baby.

Low phe diet—main principles

- Restrict intake of dietary protein to maintain plasma phe concentrations within recommended reference range for age (Table 30.3).
- Provide daily phe allowance. Daily phe intake varies between patients and depends upon the level of enzyme activity:
  - phe prescribed is based on plasma phe concentrations;
  - phe intake is measured using a system of 50 mg phe exchanges or 1 g protein exchanges if phe content of food is unknown;
  - phe is provided in breast milk/infant formula for babies or low protein foods, e.g. potato, pasta, for older infants and children;
  - phe intake is divided evenly across the day.
- Give a phe-free amino acid supplement (protein substitute) with added tyrosine (essential because phe restriction limits natural protein intake to below that needed for normal growth).
  - Generous intakes of phe-free amino acids are recommended: 0–2 years = 3.0 g/kg body weight/day; 3–10 years = 2.0 g/kg/day.
  - Amino acid supplement is given 3–4 × throughout the day combined with some of the measured phe foods.
  - A range of age-dependent prescribable amino acid supplement is available. These vary in nutrient composition and presentation, e.g. infant formula, gels, and juice or milk-type drinks which need reconstitution, Tetrapak ready-made drinks, tablets, bars, capsules (see *British National Formulary* and 'Prescription of nutritional products', Chapter 8).
  - Flavourings need to be added to improve palatability/acceptability of some of these products, particularly the older formulations.
- Give a vitamin and mineral supplement to meet normal dietary requirements. Some amino acid supplements provide adequate amounts of vitamins and minerals; if not, a separate supplement will be needed.
- Provide adequate energy intake for growth from a combination of:
  - naturally very ↓ protein foods (e.g. pure fats, sugar, fruit, some vegetables);
  - special ↓ protein, prescribable manufactured foods, e.g. bread and flour mixes, pasta and rice, biscuits, crackers, chocolate, snack pots, cereals.

Low phe diet—monitoring

Low phe diet is monitored by regular measurement of plasma phe concentrations. See Table 30.3 for frequency of monitoring and aims for plasma phe concentrations at different ages. Parents collect blood samples for phe analysis (usually on to a Guthrie card and send by 1st class post to the biochemistry laboratory). Ideally, blood should be taken at the same time, in the morning before the amino acid supplement. Parents need to be promptly advised of any necessary dietary changes depending on plasma phe results.

Reasons for high plasma phe concentrations:
- intercurrent illnesses;
- too much dietary protein/phe;
- insufficient amino acid supplement;
- unintentional use of non-PKU amino acid supplement or gluten-free rather than low protein manufactured foods.

Reasons for low plasma phe concentrations:
- inadequate intake of protein/phe;
- growth spurt;
- ↑ requirement post-illness.

Table 30.3 Recommended reference range for blood phe concentrations and frequency of phe monitoring in PKU

Age (years)	Plasma phe (µmol/l)	Frequency of monitoring
0 to 4	120–360	Weekly
5–10	120–480	Fortnightly
>11	120–700	Monthly

Epilepsy and ketogenic diets

The ketogenic diet (KD) is a high fat, restricted carbohydrate regime that has been used as a treatment for epilepsy since the 1920s. It has been shown to reduce seizure frequency by half in at least 50% of children using it, many of whom will become seizure-free

KD is designed to induce a similar metabolic response to starvation, with ketone bodies, acetoacetate, and β-hydroxybutyrate becoming the primary energy source for the brain in the absence of adequate glucose supply. Although the precise mechanism of action is unclear, initiation and maintenance of this state of ketosis is important for optimal seizure control.

Types of KD

- Classical KD. Used since the 1920s. Based on a ratio of fat to carbohydrate and protein, usually 4:1 (90% dietary energy from fat). Fat is mainly from foods, such as cream, butter, oil, and mayonnaise. Carbohydrate is usually limited to small servings of vegetables and/or fruits. Protein is based on minimum requirements for growth.
- Medium chain triglyceride (MCT) KD. Developed in the 1970s, the addition of MCT increases ketosis, thus allowing more carbohydrate and protein, and a more 'normal' diet. The traditional MCT diet provides 60% energy from MCT; a modified version uses 30% energy MCT and an extra 30% from fat in foods. MCT is given as an oil or emulsion (e.g. Liquigen, SHS International Ltd, Liverpool), both available on prescription.

Both types of KD require the calculation of an individual dietary prescription by an experienced dietitian; this is then used to plan meal recipes. Food exchange lists can also be used, especially on MCT diet. All food needs to be weighed to ensure dietary accuracy. Full vitamin, mineral, and trace element supplementation is necessary to avoid nutritional deficiencies.

Indications for KD use

- Age. Mainly used to treat childhood epilepsy; current UK NICE guidelines do not recommend KD use in adults. Can be successful in infants, although requires a more cautious approach to initiation and monitoring.
- Seizure type. Traditionally used to treat generalized seizures, but no current evidence to show special benefits on any one type of seizure or syndrome.
- Medications. Generally not used until at least two anti-epileptic medications have failed. Can be used alongside other anti-epileptic medications, although initiation should done with caution in patients taking topiramate due to ↑ risk of acidosis and excess ketosis.
- Dietary restriction. Can be used for both oral and tube (NG/gastrostomy) fed patients. Can be used in dairy-free, gluten-free, and vegetarian diets. A vegan KD would be difficult to implement without the use of a prescribable source of protein, due to the necessary carbohydrate restrictions.

Contraindications for KD use

- Inborn errors of fat metabolism (β-oxidation defects), and disorders that require a high dietary carbohydrate content as treatment.
- History of hyperlipidaemia or renal stones.
- Use with caution if also taking diuretics or medications that increase risk of acidosis. Concomitant steroid use may limit ketosis.
- KD has limited success if pre-existing behavioural feeding problems

Initiating the KD

Can be started at home, without a fast, if carefully monitored by hospital team. Adverse effects on initiation could include excess ketosis, acidosis, hypoglycaemia, vomiting, diarrhoea, and food refusal. Tolerance to KD should be built up gradually, by starting at a lower ratio (classical diet), or reduced amount of MCT (MCT diet); full diet achieved within 1–2 weeks.

Monitoring the KD

- Dipsticks used to measure urine ketone (acetoacetate) levels twice daily. Aiming for high readings (8–16 mmol/l). Finger-prick blood ketone (β-hydroxybutyrate) monitors have recently been developed and may improve accuracy of ketone monitoring. Some centres monitor blood glucose levels during dietary initiation and fine-tuning.
- Routine serum biochemistry every 3–6 months, including plasma lipids, nutritional indices, and carnitine.
- Urine tested for haematuria every 3 months, also calcium–creatinine ratio. Renal ultrasound may be needed if stones suspected.
- Regular measures of weight and height to ensure adequate growth.

Complications of the KD

- Gastrointestinal symptoms (commonly constipation; occasionally vomiting, diarrhoea, and abdominal pain).
- Hyperlipidaemia—common, although long-term effects on cardiovascular system undetermined.
- Renal stones—reported in 5–8% of cases.
- Growth problems—risk of compromised linear growth in younger children; may be related to lower protein intakes.
- ↑ Infections—reported in 2–4% of cases, although no specific immunodeficiency determined.
- Other—literature reports include bleeding abnormalities and bruising, cardiac complications, pancreatitis, hypoproteinaemia, and potentiation of valproate toxicity.

Food hypersensitivity

Classification and diagnosis

Classification

Food hypersensitivity reactions can be categorized as immune-mediated (food allergies) and non-immune-mediated (food intolerances). Immune-mediated (food allergy) can be subdivided into:

- IgE-mediated food hypersensitivity:
  - characterized by immediate symptoms;
  - prevalence of 4–8% in childhood and 1.3–4% in adults;
  - causes 33 to 61% of all cases of anaphylaxis.
- Non-IgE mediated and non immune mediated food hypersensitivity:
  - onset of symptoms usually delayed;
  - the perceived prevalence high; actual prevalence hard to measure although thought to be 0.23% for food additives.

Diagnosis

- Clinical history—the cornerstone of diagnosis: speed of onset of reaction, type of symptoms, foods suspected, and other factors such as exercise, other allergies, family history, occupation, pets, and seasonal factors.
- Skin prick test (SPT)—good first-line test for all food hypersensitivity: inexpensive, immediate, 95% negative predictive value, good sensitivity; wheal over certain size highly positively predictive for some foods; poor specificity and positive predictive value; using fresh foods can improve this; not suitable if patient has taken antihistamines or if anaphylaxis is reported symptom.
- Serum IgE—good for validating SPT or if SPT not possible; good negative predictive value and sensitivity with cut off levels that are highly positively predictive for some foods; first choice of test if patient has taken antihistamines or experienced an anaphylactic reaction; expensive, no immediate result, not a good predictor for wheat, soy, fruits, and vegetables.
- Diagnostic diets—essential if no suitable tests are available: 4-week avoidance of a food group, food additive or naturally occurring substance in food followed by open or blind challenge if symptoms improve; useful if discordance between tests and clinical history or if no tests available; total exclusion, elimination, or 'few foods' diets rarely used for IgE-mediated allergy but may be useful for other food hypersensitivities; diagnostic diets should be supervised by a dietitian to ensure dietary adequacy; no need for diagnostic avoidance diet if test result is concordant with clinical history.
- Food challenge—the gold standard of diagnosis; used to establish a diagnosis for IgE-mediated food allergy if discordance between history, test results, and diagnostic diet; definitive diagnostic test for most non-IgE-mediated food allergy or non-immune-mediated food hyper-sensitivity; can also be used to check whether children have outgrown their food allergy; speed of onset and symptom severity normally dictates whether changes should be carried out in hospital or at home, and whether they should be open or blinded.

• There are many non-validated diagnostic tests available, e.g. the laboratory analysis of hair samples, that claim to diagnose food allergies. Patients should be discouraged from using the results from these services as a basis for implementing dietary change.

Management

The main management for any food hypersensitivity reaction will be avoidance of the food(s) concerned. EU directive (2003/89/EC) requires that cereals containing gluten, crustaceans, eggs, fish, peanuts, soybeans, milk, nuts, celery, mustard, sesame seed, and sulphur dioxide and sulphites at >10 mg/litre/kg to be declared on the label of all packaged food. For most foods the avoidance advice will be similar but degree may vary depending on the severity of symptoms and type of reaction.

Cow's milk

- Allergy outgrown before 5th birthday in 90% of cases.
- Diet excludes all cow milk, milk solids, lactose, casein, whey, goat and sheep's milk and foods containing milk, e.g. flavoured crisps, baked beans, vegetarian cheese, and breakfast cereals.
- Infants 0–6 months: breast milk or extensively hydrolysed formula milk only.
- Commence weaning 6 months; can include infant formula soy milk and soy foods.
- Milk substitutes fortified with energy, calcium, and B vitamins can be used in >5 years.
- Calcium supplements may be needed by both children and adults.
- Nutritional adequacy of milk-free diets that do not include a milk replacement may be compromised.
- Milk can cause other food hypersensitivities, e.g. lactose intolerance, and has been anecdotally linked to asthma and gastrointestinal symptoms.

Eggs

- Common cause of allergy in children aged 6 months to 3 years.
- In adults, the allergy is a cross-reaction associated with bird allergy.
- There is cross-reactivity between hen, duck, and goose eggs.
- Cooking reduces allergenicity but raw or semi-cooked eggs may still be present in foods, e.g. royal icing, marzipan, meringue (pavlova), marshmallows, mayonnaise, and bun wash.

Fish and seafood

- Affects children and adults and is usually life-long and often severe.
- There is high cross-reactivity between different fish species, and also between fish and crustaceans (prawns, lobster, crab) and molluscs (mussels, oysters).
- It is prudent for people with fish allergy to avoid all seafood due to cross-contamination.
- Allergens in fish are affected by heat; canned fish may be tolerated.
- Decomposing fish can cause scombroid poisoning, sometimes mistaken for an allergy. It is advisable to eat only very fresh fish.

Wheat and other grains

- This allergy is more common in children than adults. Wheat implicated in a rare form of food allergy that does affect adults, exercise-induced anaphylaxis, where the reaction only occurs when eating wheat is combined with exercise.
- SPT and serum IgE are poor predictors of wheat allergy.
- There is high degree of cross-reactivity between wheat and grass pollen so that 80% positive SPT to wheat has no clinical significance in people with grass pollen allergy.
- Wheat also involved in other food hypersensitivity reactions such as coeliac disease (see 'Coeliac disease', Chapter 21) and linked to gastrointestinal symptoms.
- Corn/maize, barley, and malt have all been reported to cause food allergy.

Fruit and vegetables

- Can be primary allergy with sensitization through ingestion but more commonly caused by a cross-reaction between tree pollen and foods known as oral allergy syndrome (OAS).
- OAS affects 6–47% of pollen-sensitive individuals with symptoms usually triggered by apples, stone fruits and tree nuts.
- Allergens from other pollens and from latex also cross-react to plant foods.

Peanuts and tree nuts

- Can develop at any age; most likely to be life-long, although 20% could outgrow peanut allergy.
- Peanuts most commonly reported food to provoke anaphylaxis.
- Recent changes in the labelling; declaration of ingredients and nut trace warnings may help decrease accidental exposure.
- Up to 60% of peanut allergic individuals sensitized to other nuts, but this may not be manifest clinically.
- Prevalence of allergy to some nuts increasing, e.g. cashew nut allergy.
- Usual dietary advice is to avoid all nuts and foods containing nuts, e.g. pastries, biscuits, cereals, ice cream, pesto (which may contain cashew nut), oriental and Asian cuisine.
- Refined oils usually allowed but unrefined nut oils should be avoided.
- Even if only peanuts or a tree nut are causing problem, advice is still to avoid all nuts due to risk of contamination rather than cross-reactivity.
- Most common seed allergy is sesame—botanically unrelated to peanuts but cross-reacts with them.
- Mustard seed is also a highly potent allergen.

Food additives

These are often implicated in food hypersensitivity but evidence is variable. They Include:
- natural food colourings—carmine (cochineal), annatto, turmeric, carotenoids, both synthetic and naturally occurring, and saffron;
- azo dyes, e.g. tartrazine (E102), sunset yellow (E110), found in foods and drugs;

- benzoates (E210–219)—beer, jam, fruit products, pickled foods, yogurt, salad cream, cinnamon, cloves, tea, prunes, raspberries, and cranberries;
- monosodium glutamate (MSG)—sauces, soups, gravy, pre-cooked meals, dried foods, Chinese food;
- sulphites (E220–E227)—white wine, dried onions, apricots, and potato products, lemon/lime juice, grape juice, wine vinegar, and fruit cordial or 'squash'.

Naturally occurring food intolerance triggers

- Salicylates—oil of wintergreen, bilberries, blackcurrants, grapes, peaches, strawberries, tomatoes, toothpastes, chewing gum, and tea.
- Histamine—parmesan, blue and roquefort cheese, red wine (chianti and burgundy), spinach, aubergines, yeast extract, tuna, mackerel. Some foods, such as egg white, chocolate, strawberries, ethanol, tomatoes, and citrus fruits, do not contain histamine but can trigger the degranulation of mast cells.

Food labels

Food labelling law from November 2005 requires pre-packed food sold in the EU to show if it contains the following ingredients:

- Celery
- Cereals containing gluten (including wheat, rye, barley, oats)
- Crustaceans (including prawns, crabs, lobsters)
- Eggs
- Fish
- Milk
- Mustard
- Nuts (almonds, hazelnuts, walnuts, brazils, cashews, peanuts, pecans, pistachios, macadamia)
- Sesame seeds
- Soya
- Sulphites & SO_2 >10 mg/kg

Rheumatology and bone health

Osteoarthritis (OA)

It is estimated that >2 million people visit their doctor about OA and >50 000 hip replacements are undertaken in the UK each year. These numbers are likely to increase as the population ages as this condition primarily affects people aged over 40 years. The hands, knees, hips, and feet are most commonly affected.

Nutritional risk factors

- Obesity is the most important, potentially modifiable risk factor for developing OA in weight-bearing joints, e.g. ↑ BMI by 2 kg/m^2 increases relative risk of knee OA by 1.36.
- People with ↓ serum vitamin C and D have ↑ risk of OA; antioxidant vitamin C plays a role in collagen synthesis.

Nutritional advice

- No special diet is indicated in OA and a varied intake compatible with the 'Balance of Good Health' (see 'Food-based dietary guidelines', Chapter 2) is advisable.
- Weight loss is recommended for those with a BMI ≥25 kg/m^2. Ideally, dietary advice (see 'Obesity', Chapter 17) should be combined with exercise, which is considered the single most important intervention.
- Glucosamine (glucose with an amino group) is a shell-fish derived compound described as a 'nutritional supplement'. A recent meta-analysis concluded that glucosamine reduced pain (standardized mean difference −0.61, 95% CI −0.28 to −0.95). It is not prescribable and is considered safe in the dose tested (~500 mg orally × 3 daily).
- No clinical trials have reported on the potential anti-inflammatory effects of n-3 fatty acids (eicosapentaenoic and decosahexaenoic) in osteoarthritis. *In vitro* studies using osteoarthritic models have demonstrated benefit from both n-3 and n-6 fatty acids but results are not consistent. Further studies are needed before recommendations can be made.
- There is no evidence of benefit from selenium or vitamin E supplements. Anecdotal reports of improvements with cider vinegar and/or honey have not been tested.
- Patients with advanced OA may have difficulty in shopping or preparing food and as a result their intake and nutritional status may fall. Appropriate support is required.

Rheumatoid arthritis (RA)

This chronic, autoimmune condition affects ~10 people in 1000. Joint inflammation causes swelling, pain, muscle weakness, and functional impairment with ~10% of sufferers experiencing severe disability <5 years after diagnosis. RA is associated with a greater risk of cardiovascular disease and an estimated reduction in life expectancy of 3–10 years.

Nutritional risk factors

- Systematic review has shown that diet may play a role in the aetiology of RA. A diet providing olive oil, oil-rich fish, fruit, and vegetables may be protective while people with low serum antioxidant levels have ↑ risk.
- There is no evidence that high coffee intake increases risk of RA but drinking coffee is frequently associated with cigarette smoking, which is an independent risk factor.

Nutritional issues

- Some patients with RA have poor nutritional intake with a low intake of energy, micronutrients, and fibre but relatively high levels of saturated fat. Poor intake may arise 2° to loss of appetite and difficulty in preparing food, especially during periods of inflammatory exacerbation.
- Total energy expenditure in RA is lower than in matched controls, mainly because of a reduction in energy expended through physical activity. Basal metabolic rate may increase during inflammatory exacerbations but only if expressed per kg lean body mass.

Nutritional advice

- Patients with RA do not need a restricted diet but should aim to eat a nutritionally adequate intake, e.g. based on the 'Balance of Good Health' (see 'Food-based dietary guidelines', Chapter 2).
- Attempts should be made to gently reduce overweight or, conversely, to address undernutrition.
- Fatty acids—the anti-inflammatory effects of *n*–3 and *n*–6 fatty acids have been investigated extensively in RA. Evidence shows that *n*–3 fatty acids (α-linolenic, eicosapentaenoic, and decosahexaenoic) are beneficial although the optimum dose has not been determined. The best dietary sources of *n*-3 fatty acids are oil-rich fish including mackerel, salmon, and sardines (see box in 'Cardioprotective diet', Chapter 19).
- Antioxidants—although ↑ intake is protective against developing RA, the treatment effects of vitamin C, E, and selenium supplementation have been disappointing. Dietary sources have not been evaluated but it seems reasonable to recommend a diet that provides good food sources of antioxidant micronutrients, not least because of their benefits in relation to cardiovascular disease. Five portions of fruit and vegetables daily will provide this.
- Folic acid supplementation (<5 mg/week) is beneficial in patients treated with folate antagonist, methotrexate. Vitamin B_{12} status should be checked before starting.

- Exclusion/allergy diets are frequently followed by RA patients. These may include eliminating meat, dairy products, or 'acidic' foods or periods of fasting. Evaluative studies, mostly of limited quality, have reported mixed results but provide inconclusive evidence. Patients should be advised to eat a well-balanced diet that provides good sources of the micronutrients described above and only restrict their intake if there is evidence of benefit. Review by a registered dietitian will help ensure that nutritional adequacy is maintained.
- Calcium and vitamin D status. Corticosteroids are an effective treatment for RA but patients are susceptible to steroid-induced bone disease (vertebral bone density 85–95% of control values). There is no evidence of benefit from Ca or vitamin D supplementation but it seems reasonable to advise that adequate amounts should be consumed from food in the diet.
- Difficulties in obtaining, preparing, and eating food should not be underestimated in patients whose hands or jaws are particularly affected. Advice and practical support from an occupational therapist and dietitian may help overcome this.

Gout

Gout is a metabolic disorder manifest as acute joint disease. It is caused by the deposition of urate crystals in the joints, tendons, and tissues leading to inflammation and severe pain.

Pathogenesis and nutritional issues

- High serum urate levels are associated with ↑ deposition, but do not always lead to gout. They may arise from: (1) metabolism from endogenous purines; (2) metabolism from dietary purines, e.g. from offal meat, fish, yeast extract, beer, and some vegetables; (3) reduced urinary excretion.
- Obesity and excessive alcohol intake (acute and chronic) is associated with ↑ endogenous urate production and ↓ urinary excretion.
- 95% of patients with gout also have hyperinsulinaemia.
- 25–60% of patients with gout also have hyperlipidaemia.
- Raised serum urate levels are considered a marker of insulin resistance.

Nutritional advice

- Losing excess body weight is the first priority. This should be undertaken by a modest ↓ dietary energy and ↑ exercise. Crash dieting may worsen hyperuricaemia and precipitate an attack so sudden weight loss should be avoided. Aim for a reduction of 0.5–1.0 kg / week.
- Saturated fat should be replaced by mono- or polyunsaturates, especially if hyperlipidaemia is present.
- An energy-restricted diet with ↓ fat (~30% energy), ↓ carbohydrate (~40% energy), and ↑ protein (~30% energy) has been shown to be compatible with weight loss and improvement in gout symptoms. However, further studies are required before it can be recommended as the optimum diet.
- Restricting dietary purines has a limited effect on reducing urate levels; avoiding excessive amounts seems reasonable but is less important than previously thought and than other dietary advice.
- There is no evidence that *n*-3 or *n*-6 fatty acids supplements yield any benefit in gout.
- There is no evidence that antioxidant supplements are beneficial.

Systemic lupus erythematosus (SLE)

SLE is a chronic autoimmune condition where antibodies attack the connective tissues. People of all ages can be affected but it is most common in women of child-bearing age and has a higher incidence in Black and Asian than White women.

Nutritional issues and advice

- There is no good evidence that nutrition is implicated in the pathogenesis of SLE.
- SLE is associated with ↑ risk of cardiovascular disease. A cardioprotective diet of low saturated fat, ↑ fruit and vegetables and oily fish is recommended to patients who are well and have a good appetite.
- The anti-inflammatory effects of n–3 fatty acids may be beneficial. Dietary supplementation with ≡ 500 mg eicosapentaenoic acid and 350 mg decosahexaenoic acid is associated with a significant ↓ in systemic lupus activity measure[1]. This is equivalent to eating oily fish twice per week, e.g. 2 × 170 g (6 oz) fresh salmon/mackerel.
- Corticosteroids may be used in long-term treatment and SLE patients taking them have ↑ risk of osteoporosis. They should be advised to consume an adequate intake of dietary calcium and vitamin D and increase weight-bearing exercise. One pint (600 ml) of semi-skimmed/whole milk provides the reference nutrient intake for women aged 19–50 years, e.g. 700 mg Ca.
- Some patients with SLE may develop renal failure and may need specific dietary modification. Individual advice should be given by a renal dietitian.
- The health of patients with SLE can vary from relatively well to an acutely ill, hypercatabolic state. Nutritional support may be required if food intake is compromised and should be instigated promptly because poor nutritional status is associated with a worse outcome (↑ in systemic lupus activity measure).

---

[1] Duffy EM et al (2004). The clinical effect of dietary supplementation with omega-3 fish oils and/or copper in systematic lupus erthematosus. *J Rheumatol.* **31**, 1551–1556.

Osteoporosis

Osteoporosis, thinning of the bones, affects ~3 million people in the UK, predominantly those >50 years, and is associated with ~230 000 bone fractures annually.

Nutritional risk factors

- Generally poor diet, including inadequate calcium and vitamin D intake.
- High alcohol intake.
- Malabsorption, e.g. coeliac disease, Crohn's disease.

However, most risk factors are not nutrition-related: early menopause, family history, treatment with corticosteroids, immobility.

Prevention through an optimum diet

- Peak bone mass is reached in adolescence and young adulthood, i.e. decades before most people are concerned about osteoporosis. It cannot be ↑ in later life so good early bone health is essential.
- Calcium intake should meet reference nutrient intakes (mg/d) given in Table 33.1. It is estimated that ~10% of boys and ~20% of girls fail to meet these recommendations (thus reducing their chance of achieving peak bone mass—see 'Nutritional problems of children and adolescents', Chapter 11) and that up to 16% of women have a Ca intake <400 mg/d. An inadequate dietary intake will accelerate age-related bone loss and contribute to osteoporosis. See Table 33.2 for good dietary sources.
- Vitamin D is required in Ca metabolism. It is obtained from:
  - adequate exposure to sunlight, e.g. face and arms, 30 min/day in direct sunlight between April and October. There is recent concern that many people in Europe do not achieve this and as a result have a poor vitamin D status;
  - dietary sources. There are no reference nutrient intake values for the ages of 1–65 years in the UK (see Appendix 6). Most European countries recommend 5–10 μg/d. For good food sources, see Table 33.3.
- Excessive alcohol intake should be avoided. Safe limits are ≤21 units/ week for men; ≤14 units/week for women.
- Weight-bearing exercise including brisk walking, is recommended: at least 3 × 20 minutes weekly.
- Recent studies have suggested that a low vitamin K intake and high salt, protein, and vitamin A intakes are detrimental to bone health. These issues are complex and at present there is insufficient information on which to base recommendations. A varied diet based on the 'Balance of Good Health' (see 'Food-based dietary guidelines', Chapter 2) is likely to be safe and contribute to good bone health.

Table 33.1 Reference nutrient intakes (mg/day) of calcium*

Age	Male	Female
7–10 years	550	550
11–18 years	1000	800
>18 years	700	700

* For younger children see Appendix 6.

Table 33.2 Sources of calcium

Providing ~200 mg Ca		Providing ~50 mg Ca	
Source	Weight (g)	Source	Weight (g)
Milk*, cupful	170	White bread	30
Yogurt, small carton	130	Wholemeal bread	50
Cheese, e.g. cheddar	30	Baked beans	100
Cottage spread	40	Muesli, Swiss	50
Sardines, canned with bones	40	Spinach	30
Sesame seeds	30	Orange	100

* Whole, semi-skimmed, or skimmed.

Table 33.3 Sources of vitamin D

Providing ~5 µg vitamin D		Providing ~5 µg vitamin D*	
Source	Weight (g)	Source	Weight (g)
Cod liver oil	2	Ghee	260
Herring, grilled	30	Pork chop, grilled	450
Salmon, tinned/steamed	50	Butter	550
Pilchards, tinned	60	Whole egg	600
Margarine (all types)	60	Lamb, roasted	650
Egg yolk	100	Beef, roasted	700

*The right-hand column shows quantities >> normal portions and are not recommended because of the high quantity of associated saturated fat.

Nutritional management

- When osteoporosis is diagnosed, management should include review of dietary adequacy.
- All postmenopausal women should aim for a dietary intake of calcium of 1000 mg/d.
- Housebound, frail elderly women should receive 1000–1200 mg calcium and 20 μg vitamin D daily.
- Men with a history of low bone mineral density and/or fracture should receive 500 mg calcium and 10 μg vitamin D daily.
- Antiresorptive medication is less effective when calcium and vitamin D levels are low. It is recommended that most patients should receive all three together.
- Calcium supplements are available as tablets, effervescent tablets, chewable tablets, granules, and syrup. As the required dose is large, the tablets are usually of considerable size. Major side-effects are rare but some gastrointestinal symptoms may occur. Splitting the daily does into smaller quantities and altering the time of dosing, e.g. before or after food, may help.
- Combined calcium and vitamin D preparations are available.

Hospital catering

In the UK, NHS hospital catering provides ~1 million meals each day. These are consumed by individuals who vary from those who are in good health to those who are very sick and may have highly specialized nutritional requirements. Food may be provided in the form of a single meal or as an individual's exclusive intake over a long period of time (>3 months) or even indefinitely. The nutritional needs of such individuals vary considerably and yet the importance of providing optimum nutrition is imperative to promote healing and recovery, to minimize complications associated with poor nutrition, and to maintain and optimize health and quality of life. Meeting all these aims, providing food people want to eat, and achieving a balance between and under- and overnutrition in an environment of financial constraint and where food is often regarded as being of little significance is a major challenge. Provision of food is one important factor amongst many that influence the nutritional status of hospital patients (see 'Contributing causes' in 'Undernutrition', Chapter 16).

Better hospital food (BHF)

The BHF project was launched in 2001 with four initial aims:
- to produce a range of tasty and nutritious recipes that every NHS hospital could use;
- to redesign printed menus to make them easier to read and understand;
- to introduce 24-hour catering services so that food is available day and night;
- to ensure that hot food is available both at midday and early evening mealtimes.

Whilst the popular media have derided some features of the initiative, e.g. the so-called celebrity menus, other aspects have the capacity to improve nutritional intake and ∴ positively influence patient well-being (see box). An evaluation of the impact of BHF is required to support further development.

🖳 www.betterhospitalfood.com

Council of Europe (CoE)

The CoE report (2003) makes 117 recommendations, which include topics covered elsewhere, e.g. nutritional screening (see 'Nutritional Screening', Chapter 16), nutritional support (see 'Treatment of undernutrition Chapter 16), as well as aspects of ordinary food, the distribution of responsibility for nutritional care, communication, nutrition education, organization of food service (including contract food services), eating environments, food hygiene and economic cost.[1] The implementation of these recommendations requires agreement at national and local level. Within the UK, this is being led by the Hospital Caterers Association and British Dietetic Association.

---

[1] Council of Europe (2003). *Food and Nutritional care in hospitals: how to prevent undernutrition.* Council of Europe Publishing, Strasbourg.

Possible ward scenario

- Patient X admitted for investigations prior to major surgery
- Weight loss ±12 kg in last 3 months, now BMI = 18.1 kg/m^2 (see 'Anthropometry', Chapter 4)
- Misses breakfast for three consecutive mornings as nil by mouth prior to investigative procedures
- Misses lunch on two of these days as off ward at meal time and on third day as asleep following sedation
- Early evening ward round followed by student teaching curtails time available to eat supper
- Eats small amount of supper but unable to achieve adequate nutrient intake for whole day at one meal

BHF

- *Ward kitchen services* means tea, toast, fruit juice available 24 hours so that an early breakfast can be provided before nil by mouth restrictions start
- *Snack box* can be ordered so that patient missing lunch due to visits to X-ray, physiotherapy, etc. can eat on his/her return, e.g. sandwiches, cheese and biscuits, fruit, and drink
- *Protected meal times* mean that non-urgent clinical activity stops so that patients can eat without interruptions and that ward staff can provide food-related assistance, e.g. feeding, when it is required. This includes ward rounds, teaching, and visiting times

Red tray project

Some UK hospitals have adopted a system where patients who are at nutritional risk are given their food on an easily identifiable tray (e.g. coloured red) so that their intake can be monitored and appropriate eating/nutritional support given at meal times. Concurrent staff training has been undertaken and limited audit to date has shown a positive response.

Red Tray Project education at Milton Keynes General* Hospital NHS Trust

Remember the vulnerable patient in need of extra help at mealtimes
Encourage and assist patients where necessary
Dietary intake may be improved by extra attention at mealtimes

Tell patients and relatives about the benefits of the Red Tray Project
Remove red tray only after recording food consumption
Assess and weigh patients regularly
You can improve the patients' mealtime experience!

* Reproduced with permission from Milton Keynes General Hospital NHS Trust. Concept initiated at West Wing, Cardiff Royal Infirmary by Lindsey Bradley and Colin Rees, co-authors of the original work and article in the Nursing Standard/March 12/Vol 17/no 26/2003.

Types of hospital food production

Cook–serve   Food is prepared within the hospital site and served immediately to patients and staff.

Cook–chill   Food is prepared either within the hospital site or at another venue and rapidly chilled to ~0–4°C and stored for up to 5 days before regeneration (reheating) either in the hospital kitchen or at ward level.

Cook–freeze   Food is prepared either within the hospital site or at another venue and rapidly frozen to approximately −18°C and stored for up to 3 months before regeneration (reheating) usually in the hospital kitchen.

Types of hospital food service

Plated meal service   Individual trays are served out for each patient in the main hospital kitchen and transported to the ward either in insulated trolleys (if hot and cold food) or chilled trolleys (if regeneration takes place at ward level).

Bulk service   Large containers of food are sent from the kitchen to each ward/dining area where staff, e.g. nursing, care or catering assistants, or ward hostesses, serve out the meals for each patient. Food sent in bulk containers may be already hot or still be chilled and regenerated at ward level.

Popular diets

This section is included to help orientate health-care professionals to diets that their patients may initiate or possibly seek advice about. It does not validate their efficacy. For many, evidence of benefit in the form of a randomized controlled trial is not available. However, the concerns, described below, about potential harm resulting from some diets are based on scientific principles.

- **Atkins Diet.** A low carbohydrate, high protein diet for weight reduction (see 'Treatment: introduction and dietary management', Chapter 17).
- **Beverley Hills Diet** is based on the belief that enzymes are required to break-down specific foods and that certain foods provide these enzymes while undigested food in the gastrointestinal tract leads to the gain of fat. There is no scientific evidence to support this hypothesis.
- **Blood Group Diet or Eat Right For Your Type.** This diet is based on the idea that blood groups evolved at different times during evolution and that a diet that reflects this period is optimum for health and weight control. There is no evidence that different types of blood group relate to different historical eating patterns or that modifying current dietary intake on the basis of blood groups influences energy balance and thus weight loss.
- **Bristol Diet.** The nutritional guidelines recommended by the Bristol Cancer Help Centre for people with cancer (see 'Other dietary approaches to cancer', Chapter 20).
- **Cabbage Soup Diet.** Advocates weight loss through consuming large quantities of home-made cabbage soup plus very limited other food. The soup recipe provides little energy but also few other nutrients. Whilst this regime may lead to rapid weight loss through a very low energy intake, nutrient intake is very likely to be inadequate and following the diet is incompatible with established nutritional principles.
- **Detox diets.** Recommend strict avoidance of all potential dietary 'toxins', e.g. alcohol, caffeine, food colouring, and preservatives, as a means of reducing body weight. Perceived 'natural' foods, e.g. organic produce including fruit, vegetables, and nuts, are usually allowed, although short-term fasting is also recommended on some regimes. No formal studies have been undertaken to evaluate efficacy but it is likely that weight loss associated with this type of diet is due to a reduction in energy intake as a result of the limited foods permitted. The total nutrient intake is likely to be inadequate overall, especially as foods providing protein and calcium are often restricted.
- **Food combining diets.** The rationale is based on the theory that overweight occurs as a result of defective digestion caused by eating the wrong types of food at the same time, e.g. eating protein-rich food and carbohydrate at the same meal. The diet ∴ advises careful separation of these foods so that they are not consumed together. There is no scientific basis for this theory and no evidence that a food combining diet is effective in reducing excess body weight. If weight loss occurs while following the regime, it will be because total energy intake falls below energy expenditure and this is likely to happen on this diet because the complexity of the rules discourages food intake.

Although the diet could be potentially adequate and nutritious, it is complex and time-consuming to follow and does not address long-term changes in eating habits.

- *Gerson diet.* A regime used in treating cancer (see 'Other dietary approaches to cancer', Chapter 20).
- *Glycaemic index (GI) diet* uses the sound scientific principle that foods with a low GI index, e.g. apples, lentils, yogurt, are more satiating and have other health benefits compared to high GI foods, e.g. white bread, cornflakes, sugar, and that the former will help followers to limit their total energy intake and thus reduce overweight. Weight loss will only occur if total energy intake is < total energy expenditure rather than by eating low GI foods *per se*, but these can help and are compatible with a well-balanced and varied diet.
- *Hay diet.* See 'Food-combining ducts above.
- *Macrobiotics.* Describes a philosophical approach to life that includes balancing yin and yang elements. The dietary element is based on predominantly vegetarian, high carbohydrate, low fat food with regular consumption of soya and sea vegetables. Although some aspects of the diet follow healthy eating principles, more extreme versions are nutritionally inadequate and cannot be recommended for health reasons; the low energy and protein density is a particular concern in patients with a poor appetite.
- *Plant diet.* A regime used in treating cancer (see 'Other dietary approaches to cancer', Chapter 20).
- *Sugar Busters.* Advocates a sugar-free diet for weight loss. Although avoiding all refined carbohydrate is compatible with a healthy, weight-reducing diet, avoiding sugar on its own is insufficient to ensure long-term successful weight loss.
- *Zone diet* is based on the theory that an optimum diet should comprise a fixed proportion of macronutrients at each meal: carbohydrate 40%, fat 30%, and protein 30%. These values differ from values currently recommended for healthy adults (50%, 35%, and 15%, respectively) and there is no evidence that weight loss is optimized by the proposed quantities.

Appendices

Weights and measures

Volume

1 fl oz = 28.41 ml
1 pint = 568.3 ml
1 litre = 1.76 pint

Table A1.1 Approximate volume conversion

fl oz/pint	ml/l	ml/l	fl oz/pt
1 fl oz	28 ml	50 ml	1.75 fl oz
¼ pint (5 fl oz)	142 ml	100 ml	3.5 fl oz
$^1/_2$ pint	284 ml	200 ml	7 fl oz
1 pint	568 ml	500 ml	8.8 fl oz
2 pints	1.1 l	1 l	1.76 pints
3 pints	1.7 l		
4 pints	2.3 l		
5 pints	2.8 l		

Mass/weight

1 ounce = 28.35 g
1 pound (16 oz) = 454 g (0.45 kg)
1 stone (14 lb) = 6.35 kg
1 g = 0.0352 ounces
1 kg = 2.2 pounds

Table A1.2 Approximate weight conversion

g to oz		oz to g	
g	oz	oz	g
1	0.04	1	28
10	0.35	2	57
15	0.53	3	85
20	0.71	4	113
30	1.06	5	142
40	1.41	6	170
50	1.76	7	198
60	2.12	8	227
70	2.47	9	255
80	2.82	10	284
90	3.17	11	312
100	3.53	12	340
		13	368
		14	397
		15	425
		16	454

Anthropometrics

Length/height conversions

1 inch = 2.54 cm
1 foot (12 in) = 30.48 cm
1 yard (36 in) = 91.44 cm
1 cm = 0.394 inch
1 m = 39.37 inches

Table A2.1 Approximate length conversions

Inches to centimeters		Centimetres to inches	
Iin	cm	cm	in
1	2.54	1	0.39
2	5.08	2	0.79
3	7.62	3	1.18
4	10.16	4	1.57
5	12.70	5	1.97
6	15.25	6	2.36
7	17.78	7	2.76
8	20.32	8	3.15
9	22.86	9	3.54
10	25.40	10	3.94
20	50.80	20	7.87
30	76.20	30	11.81
40	101.60	40	15.75
50	127.00	50	19.69
60	152.40	60	23.62
70	177.80	70	27.56
80	203.20	80	31.50
90	228.60	90	35.43
100	254.0	100	39.37

Table A2.2 Approximate height conversions

m	ft and in	m	ft and in
1.22	4'0"	1.6	5'3"
1.23	4'½"	1.61	5'3½"
1.24	4'1"	1.63	5'4"
1.26	4'1½"	1.64	5'4½"
1.27	4'2"	1.65	5'5"
1.28	4'2½"	1.66	5'5½"
1.29	4'3"	1.68	5'6"
1.31	4'3½."	1.69	5'6½"
1.32	4'4"	1.7	5'7"
1.33	4'4½"	1.71	5'7½"
1.35	4'5"	1.73	5'8"
1.36	4'5½"	1.74	5'8½"
1.37	4'6"	1.75	5'9"
1.38	4'6½"	1.76	5'9½"
1.4	4'7"	1.78	5'10"
1.41	4'7½"	1.79	5'10½"
1.42	4'8"	1.8	5'11"
1.43	4'8½"	1.82	5'11½"
1.45	4'9"		
1.46	4'9½"	1.83	6'0"
1.47	4'10"	1.84	6'0½"
1.49	4'10½"	1.85	6'1"
1.5	4'11"	1.87	6'1½"
1.51	4'11½"	1.88	6'2"
		1.89	6'2½"
1.52	5'0"	1.9	6'3"
1.54	5'0½"	1.92	6'3½"
1.55	5'1"	1.93	6'4"
1.56	5'1½"	1.94	6'4½"
1.57	5'2"	1.96	6'5"
1.59	5'2½"	1.97	6'5½"
		1.98	6'6"

Mass/weight conversions

1 ounce = 28.35 g
1 pound = 454 g or 0.45 kg
1 g = 0.0352 ounces
1 kg = 2.2 pounds

Table A2.3 Approximate weight conversions

kg	st	lb	kg	st	lb	kg	st	lb	kg	st	lb
0.5		1	44	6	13	83	13	1	122	19	3
1		2	45	7	1	84	13	3	123	19	6
1.5		3	46	7	3	85	13	6	124	19	7
2		4	47	7	6	86	13	7	125	19	10
2.5		6	48	7	8	87	13	10	126	19	11
3		7	49	7	10	88	13	11	127	20	0
3.5		8	50	7	13	89	14	0	128	20	1
4		9	51	8	0	90	14	3	129	20	5
4.5		10	52	8	3	91	14	4	130	20	7
5		11	53	8	4	92	14	7	131	20	8
5.5		12	54	8	7	93	14	8	132	20	11
6		13	55	8	10	94	14	11	133	20	13
			56	8	11	95	14	13	134	21	1
10	1	8	57	9	0	96	15	1	135	21	3
15	2	6	58	9	1	97	15	4	136	21	6
20	3	1	59	9	4	98	15	6	137	21	8
21	3	4	60	9	6	99	15	8	138	21	10
22	3	7	61	9	8	100	15	10	139	21	13
23	3	8	62	9	11	101	15	13	140	22	0
24	3	11	63	9	13	102	16	1	141	22	3
25	3	13	64	10	1	103	16	3	142	22	5
26	4	1	65	10	3	104	16	6	143	22	7
27	4	3	66	10	6	105	16	7	144	22	10
28	4	6	67	10	7	106	16	10	145	22	11
29	4	8	68	10	10	107	16	11	146	23	0
30	4	10	69	10	13	108	17	0	147	23	1
31	4	13	70	11	0	109	17	3	148	23	5
32	5	0	71	11	3	110	17	5	149	23	6
33	5	3	72	11	4	111	17	7	150	23	8
34	5	6	73	11	7	112	17	8	151	23	11
35	5	7	74	11	8	113	17	11	152	23	13
36	5	10	75	11	11	114	17	13	153	24	1
37	5	11	76	12	0	115	18	1	154	24	3
38	6	0	77	12	1	116	18	5	155	24	6
39	6	1	78	12	5	117	18	6	156	24	7
40	6	3	79	12	6	118	18	8	157	24	10
41	6	7	80	12	8	119	18	10	158	24	13
42	6	8	81	12	10	120	18	13	159	25	0
43	6	11	82	12	13	121	19	0	160	25	3

Body mass index (BMI)

Height (m)

Weight (kg)	1.36	1.40	1.44	1.48	1.52	1.56	1.60	1.64	1.68	1.72	1.76	1.80	1.84	1.88	1.92	1.96	2.00
125	68	64	60	57	54	51	49	46	44	42	40	39	37	35	34	33	31
123	67	63	59	56	53	51	48	46	44	42	40	38	36	35	33	32	31
121	65	62	58	55	52	50	47	45	43	41	39	37	36	34	33	31	30
119	64	61	57	55	52	49	46	44	42	40	38	37	35	34	32	31	30
117	63	60	56	53	51	48	46	44	41	40	38	36	35	33	32	30	29
115	62	59	55	53	50	47	45	43	41	39	37	35	34	33	31	30	29
113	61	58	54	52	49	46	44	42	40	38	36	35	33	32	31	29	28
111	60	57	54	51	48	46	43	41	39	38	36	34	33	31	30	29	28
109	59	56	53	50	47	45	43	41	39	37	35	34	32	31	30	28	27
107	58	55	52	49	46	44	42	40	38	36	35	33	32	30	29	28	27
105	57	54	51	48	45	43	41	39	37	35	34	32	31	30	28	27	26
103	56	53	50	47	45	42	40	38	36	35	33	32	30	29	28	27	26
101	55	52	49	46	44	42	39	38	36	34	33	31	30	29	27	26	25
99	54	51	48	45	43	41	39	37	35	33	32	31	29	28	27	26	25
97	52	49	47	44	42	40	38	36	34	33	31	30	28	27	26	25	24
95	51	48	46	43	41	39	37	35	34	32	31	29	28	27	26	25	24
93	50	47	45	42	40	38	36	35	33	31	30	29	27	26	25	24	23
91	49	46	44	42	39	37	36	34	32	31	29	28	27	26	25	24	23
89	48	45	43	41	39	37	35	33	32	30	29	27	26	25	24	23	22
87	47	44	42	40	38	36	34	32	31	29	28	27	26	25	24	23	22
85	46	43	41	39	37	35	33	32	30	29	27	26	25	24	23	22	21
83	45	42	40	38	36	34	32	31	29	28	27	26	25	23	23	22	21
81	44	41	39	37	35	33	32	30	29	27	26	25	24	23	22	21	20
79	43	40	38	36	34	32	31	29	28	27	26	24	23	22	21	21	20
77	42	39	37	35	33	32	30	29	27	26	25	24	23	22	21	20	19
75	41	38	36	34	32	31	29	28	27	25	24	23	22	21	20	20	19
73	39	37	35	33	32	30	29	27	26	25	24	23	22	21	20	19	18
71	38	36	34	32	31	29	28	26	25	24	23	22	21	20	19	18	18
69	37	35	33	32	30	28	27	26	24	23	22	21	20	19	18	18	17
67	36	34	32	31	29	28	26	25	24	23	22	21	20	19	18	17	17
65	35	33	31	30	28	27	25	24	23	22	21	20	19	18	18	17	16
63	34	32	30	29	27	26	25	23	22	21	20	19	19	18	17	16	16
61	33	31	29	28	26	25	24	23	22	21	20	19	18	17	17	16	15
59	32	30	28	27	26	24	23	22	21	20	19	18	17	17	16	15	15
57	31	29	27	26	25	23	22	21	20	19	18	17	16	16	15	15	14
55	30	28	27	25	24	23	21	20	19	19	18	17	16	16	15	14	14
53	29	27	26	24	23	22	21	20	19	18	17	16	16	15	14	14	13
51	28	26	25	23	22	21	20	19	18	17	16	15	15	14	14	13	13
49	26	25	24	22	21	20	19	18	17	17	16	15	14	14	13	13	12
47	25	24	23	21	20	19	18	17	17	16	15	14	14	13	12	12	11
45	24	23	22	21	19	18	18	17	16	15	15	14	13	13	12	12	11
43	23	22	21	20	19	18	17	16	15	15	14	13	13	12	12	11	11

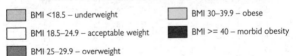

BMI <18.5 – underweight

BMI 18.5–24.9 – acceptable weight

BMI 25–29.9 – overweight

BMI 30–39.9 – obese

BMI >= 40 – morbid obesity

Fig. A2.1 Adult BMI ready reckoner.

Table A2.4 WHO cut-offs for BMI in adults

BMI	Weight status	Risk of co-morbidities
Below 18.5	Underweight	Low
18.5–24.9	Normal	Average
25.0–29.9	Overweight	Increased
30.0–39.9	Obese	Moderate–severe
Above 40	Very obese	Severe

Table A2.5 International cut-off points for body mass index for overweight and obesity between 2 and 18 y*

Age (years)	Body mass index 25 kg/m²		Body mass index 30 kg/m²	
	Males	Females	Males	Females
2	18.41	18.02	20.09	19.81
2.5	18.13	17.76	19.80	19.55
3	17.89	17.56	19.57	19.36
3.5	17.69	17.40	19.39	19.23
4	17.55	17.28	19.29	19.15
4.5	17.47	17.19	19.26	19.12
5	17.42	17.15	19.30	19.17
5.5	17.45	17.20	19.47	19.34
6	17.55	17.34	19.78	19.65
6.5	17.71	17.53	20.23	20.08
7	17.92	17.75	20.63	20.51
7.5	18.16	18.03	21.09	21.01
8	18.44	18.35	21.60	21.57
8.5	18.76	18.69	22.17	22.18
9	19.10	19.07	22.77	22.81
9.5	19.46	19.45	23.39	23.46
10	19.84	19.86	24.00	24.11
10.5	20.20	20.29	24.57	24.77
11	20.55	20.74	25.10	25.42
11.5	20.89	21.20	25.58	26.05
12	21.22	21.68	26.02	26.67
12.5	21.56	22.14	26.43	27.24
13	21.91	22.58	26.84	27.76
13.5	22.27	22.98	27.25	28.20
14	22.62	23.34	27.63	28.57
14.5	22.96	23.66	27.98	28.87
15	23.29	23.94	28.30	29.11
15.5	23.60	24.17	28.60	29.29
16	23.90	24.37	28.88	29.43
16.5	24.19	24.54	29.14	29.56
17	24.46	24.70	29.41	29.69
17.5	24.73	24.85	29.70	29.84
18	25	25	30	30

*From Cole et al. (2000). Br. Med. J. 320 (7244), 1240, Table 4. 6th May 2000 edition. Amended with permission from the BMJ publishing group.

Waist circumference cut-offs for risk of metabolic complications and mindex and demiquet measures of adiposity

Table A2.6 WHO waist circumference cut offs and risk of associated metabolic complications

	Increased risk	Substantially increased risk
♂	≥94 cm	≥102 cm
♀	≥80 cm	≥88 cm

Mindex and demiquet

Measures of adiposity >64 y using demispan as proxy for height:

$$\text{Mindex } (♀) = \frac{\text{wt (kg)}}{\text{demispan (m)}}$$

$$\text{Demiquet } (♂) = \frac{\text{wt (kg)}}{\text{demispan (m}^2)}$$

Table A2.7 Deciles for mindex (♀)*

	10	20	30	40	50	60	70	80	90
64–74 y	68.3	73.3	77.8	82.2	84.8	88.4	92.3	99.9	110.6
75+ y	63.1	68.4	73.6	78.1	81.7	85.3	88.4	94.6	102.2

*Reprinted from *Clinical Nutrition*, 1: 18–23, Lehman Copyright (1991) with permission from Elsevier.

Table A2.8 Deciles for demiquet (♂)*

	10	20	30	40	50	60	70	80	90
64–74 y	87.6	96.1	99.6	102.4	106.7	111.6	117.1	123.7	130.7
75+y	84.5	92.8	98.9	103.1	106.3	109.1	113.4	119.3	125.3

*Reprinted from *Clinical Nutrition*, 1: 18–23, Lehman Copyright (1991) with permission from Elsevier.

Upper arm anthropometry

Table A2.9 Midarm circumference (MAC) (cm)[*]

Age group (y)	Percentile						
	5th	10th	25th	50th	75th	90th	95th
♂							
18–74	26.4	27.6	29.6	31.7	33.9	36.0	37.3
18–24	25.7	27.1	28.7	30.7	32.9	35.5	37.4
25–34	27.0	28.2	30.0	32.0	34.4	36.5	37.6
35–44	27.8	28.7	30.7	32.7	34.8	36.3	37.1
45–54	26.7	27.8	30.0	32.0	34.2	36.2	37.6
55–64	25.6	27.3	29.6	31.7	33.4	35.2	36.6
65–74	25.3	26.5	28.5	30.7	32.4	34.4	35.5
♀							
18–74	23.2	24.3	26.2	28.7	31.9	35.2	37.8
18–24	22.1	23.0	24.5	26.4	28.8	31.7	34.3
25–34	23.3	24.2	25.7	27.8	30.4	34.1	37.2
35–44	24.1	25.2	26.8	29.2	32.2	36.2	38.5
45–54	24.3	25.7	27.5	30.3	32.9	36.8	39.3
55–64	23.9	25.1	27.7	30.2	33.3	36.3	38.2
65–74	23.8	25.2	27.4	29.9	32.5	35.3	37.2

[*]Bishop, C.W., Bowen, P.E., and Ritchley, S.L. (1981). Norms for nutritional assessment of *Am. J. Clin. Dietet.* **34** 2530–9.

Table A2.10 Mid-arm muscle circumference (MAMC) (cm)*

Age group (y)	Percentile						
	5th	10th	25th	50th	75th	90th	95th
♂							
18–74	23.8	24.8	26.3	27.9	29.6	31.4	32.5
18–24	23.5	24.4	25.8	27.2	28.9	30.8	32.3
25–34	24.2	25.3	26.5	28.0	30.0	31.7	32.9
35–44	25.0	25.6	27.1	28.7	30.3	32.1	33.0
45–54	24.0	24.9	26.5	28.1	29.8	31.5	32.6
55–64	22.0	24.4	26.2	27.9	29.6	31.0	31.8
65–74	22.5	23.7	25.4	26.9	28.5	29.9	30.7
♀							
18–74	18.4	19.0	20.2	21.8	23.6	25.8	27.4
18–24	17.7	18.5	19.4	20.6	22.1	23.6	24.9
25–34	18.3	18.9	20.0	21.4	22.9	24.9	26.6
35–44	18.5	19.2	20.6	22.0	24.0	26.1	27.4
45–54	18.8	19.5	20.7	22.2	24.3	26.6	27.8
55–64	18.6	19.5	20.8	22.6	24.4	26.3	28.1
65–74	18.6	19.5	20.8	22.5	24.4	26.5	28.1

*Bishop, C.W., Bowen, P.E., and Ritchley, S.L. (1981). Norms for nutritional assessment of American adults by upper arm anthropometry. *Am. J. Clin. Dietet.* **34**, 2530–9.

Table A2.11 Triceps skinfold thickness (cm)*

Age group (y)	Percentile						
	5th	10th	25th	50th	75th	90th	95th
♂							
18–74	4.5	6.0	8.0	11.0	15.0	20.0	23.0
18–24	4.0	5.0	7.0	9.5	14.0	20.0	23.0
25–34	4.5	5.5	8.0	12.0	16.0	21.5	24.0
35–44	5.0	6.0	8.5	12.0	15.5	20.0	23.0
45–54	5.0	6.0	8.o	11.0	15.0	20.0	25.5
55–64	5.0	6.0	8.0	11.0	14.0	18.0	21.5
65–74	4.5	5.5	8.0	11.0	15.0	19.0	22.0
♀							
18–74	11.0	13.0	17.0	22.0	28.0	24.0	37.0
18–24	9.4	11.0	14.0	18.0	24.0	30.0	34.0
25–34	10.5	12.0	16.0	21.0	26.5	33.5	37.0
35–44	12.0	14.0	18.0	23.0	29.5	35.5	39.0
45–54	13.0	15.0	20.0	25.0	30.0	36.0	40.0
55–64	11.0	14.0	19.0	25.0	30.5	35.0	39.0
65–74	11.5	14.0	18.0	23.0	28.0	33.0	36.0

*Bishop, C.W., Bowen, P.E., and Ritchley, S.L. (1981). Norms for nutritional assessment of American adults by upper arm anthropometry. *Am. J. Clin. Dietet.* **34**, 2530–9.

Child growth foundation charts

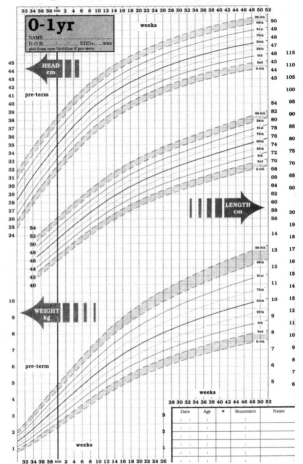

Fig. A2.2 Child Growth Foundation 9-centile growth chart for boys, 0–1 years. Permission requested from the Royal College of Paediatrics and Child Health (www.rcpch.ac.uk).

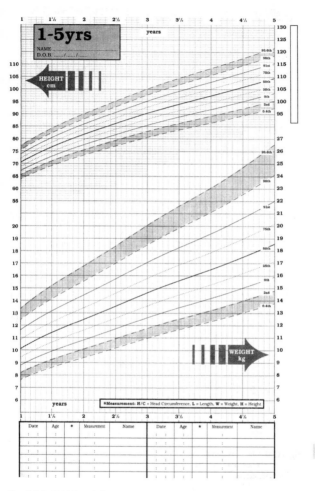

Fig. A2.3 Child Growth Foundation 9-centile growth chart for boys 1–5 years. Permission requested from the Royal College of Paediatrics and Child Health (www.rcpch.ac.uk).

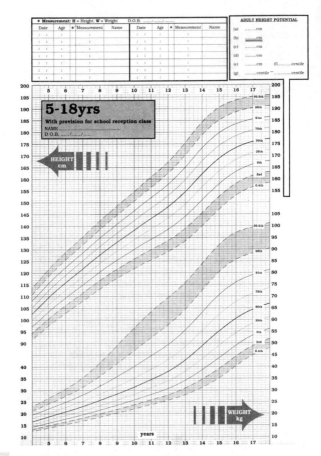

Fig. A2.4 Child Growth Foundation 9-centile growth chart for boys 5–18 years. Permission requested from the Royal College of Paediatrics and Child Health (www.rcpch.ac.uk).

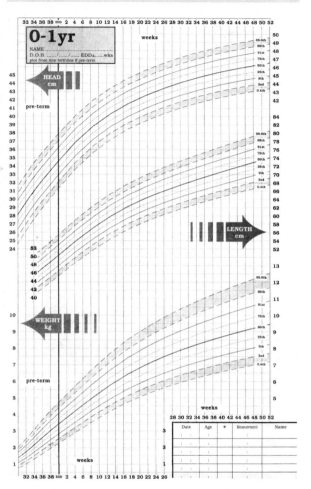

Fig. A 2.5 Child Growth Foundation 9-centile growth chart for girls 0–1 year. Permission requested from the Royal College of Paediatrics and Child Health (www.rcpch.ac.uk).

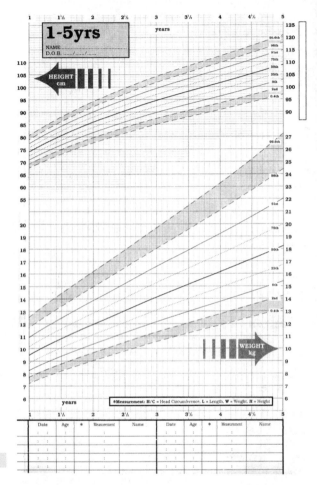

Fig. A 2.6 Child Growth Foundation 9-centile growth chart for girls 1–5 years. Permission requested from the Royal College of Paediatrics and Child Health (www.rcpch.ac.uk).

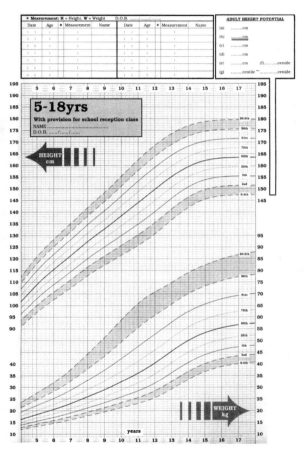

Fig. A 2.7 Child Growth Foundation 9-centile growth chart for girls 5–18 years. Permission requested from the Royal College of Paediatrics and Child Health (www.rcpch.ac.uk).

Conversion factors

Dietary energy

Units used in energy balance

1000 joules = 1 kJ
1000 kJ =1 MJ
1 kcal = 4.184 kj (The Royal Society (London) recommended conversion factor)
1 kJ = 0.239 kcal
1 W = 1 joule per second
0.06 W = 1 kJ per min
86.4 W = 1 kJ per 24 h

Table A3.1 Nutrient energy yields

Nutrient	Energy yield per gram	
	kcal	kJ
Protein	4	17
Carbohydrate	3.75	16
Fat	9	37
Alcohol	7	29
Medium chain triglyceride (MCT)	8.4	35

Protein/nitrogen

Dietary protein/dietary nitrogen

Dietary protein (g)= dietary nitrogen (g) x 6.25.[1]
Dietary nitrogen (g)= dietary protein (g) ÷ 6.25.[1]

[1] This conversion factor is only appropriate for a mixture of foods. For milk or cereals alone, the factors 6.4 or 5.7 should be used.

Vitamin A

The active vitamin A content of a diet is usually expressed in retinol equivalents.

1 µg retinol equivalent = 1 µg retinol or 6 µg β carotene

1 IU vitamin A = 0.3 µg retinol or 0.6 µg β carotene

Vitamin D

1 µg vitamin D = 40 IU
1 IU = 0.025µg vitamin D

Nicotinic acid/tryptophan

1 mg nicotinic acid = 60 mg tryptophan

Nicotinic acid content mg equivalents = Nicotinic acid (mg) + (tryptophan (mg)/60

Mineral content of compounds and solutions

Table A3.2 Mineral content of compounds and solutions

Solution/compound	Mineral content	
1 g sodium chloride	393 mg Na	17 mmol Na
1 g sodium bicarbonate	273 mg Na	12 mmol Na
1 g potassium bicarbonate	524 mg K	13.4 mmol K
1 g calcium chloride (hydrated)	273 mg Ca	7 mmol Ca
1 g calcium carbonate	400 mg Ca	10 mmol Ca
1 g calcium gluconate	93 mg Ca	2.3 mmol Ca
1 litre normal saline	3450 mg Na	150 mmol Na

Energy expenditure prediction equations

The following equations are used as a basis for calculating energy expenditure (DRVs)[1]: They have been derived from a large number of studies,[2] including the classic work of Harris and Benedict[3] (1919), which measured energy expenditure in healthy subjects. In clinical practice, these are often referred to as the Schofield equations.

Table A4.1 Equations for estimating basal metabolic rate from weight (MJ/24 h)[*]

Age range (y)	♂	♀
10–18	0.074W + 2.754	0.056W + 2.898
18–30	0.063W + 2.896	0.062W + 2.036
30–60	0.048W + 3.653	0.034W + 3.538
>60	0.049W + 2.459	0.038W + 2.755

[*] W = body weight in kg.

Table A4.2 Equations for estimating basal metabolic rate from weight (kcal/24 h)[*]

Age range (y)	♂	♀
10–18	17.69W + 659	13.39W + 693
18–30	15.06W + 692	14.83W + 487
30–60	11.48W + 874	8.13W + 846
>60	11.72W + 588	9.09W + 659

[*] W = body weight in kg.

Notes on tables

- The equations in Table A4.2 were derived from those in Table A4.1 using a conversion factor of 1 kcal = 0.004182 MJ.
- The equations published for children aged 10–18 years are rarely used for those aged less than 15 years.
- The equations published for men and women aged >60 years are derived from data from only 50 and 38 individuals, respectively, so are least robust. All other equations are derived from data from between 300 and 2900 individuals.

[1] Department of Health (1991). *Dietary reference values for food and nutrients for the united Kingdom*. HMSO, London.
[2] Schofield, W.N. (1985). Predicting basal metabolic rate, new standards and review of previous work. *Hum. Nutr. Clin. Nutr.* **39C** (suppl.1), 5–41.
[3] Harris, J.A. and Benedict, F.G. (1919). *A biometric study of basal metabolism in man*. Carnegie Institution of Washington, Washington DC.

Table A4.3 Calculated physical activity level (PAL) values for light, moderate, and heavy activity (occupational and non-occupational)[*]

| Non occupational activity level | Occupational activity level | | | | | |
| | Light | | Moderate | | Heavy | |
	♂	♀	♂	♀	♂	♀
Sedentary	1.4	1.4	1.6	1.5	1.7	1.5
Moderately active	1.5	1.5	1.7	1.6	1.8	1.6
Very active	1.6	1.6	1.8	1.7	1.9	1.7

[*] Department of Health (1991). *Dietary reference values for food and nutrients for the united Kingdom*. HMSO, London.

Clinical chemistry reference ranges

❶ The values given are for guidance purposes only. Values will vary between laboratories. Check normal ranges in use at applicable setting before making clinical decisions.

Table A5.1 Adult normal values*

Substance	Value	Substance	Value
Albumin	32–50 g/l	Red Cell Count	
Bicarbonate	20–29 mmol/l	Males	$4.5–6.5\times10^{12}$/l
Bilirubin	<17 µmol/l	Females	$3.8–5.8\times10^{12}$/l
Calcium	2.15–2.55 mmol/l	Mean cell haemoglobin (MCH)	27–32 pg
Chloride	97–107 mmol/l	Mean cell volume (MCV)	77–95 fl
Total cholesterol	<5 mmol/l	Mean cell haemoglobin conc	32–36 g/dl
Creatinine	60–125 mmol/l	White blood count (WBC)	$4.0–11.0\times10^{9}$/l
Glucose (fasting)	<6.1 mmol/l	Neutrophils	$2.0–7.5\times10^{9}$/l
Phosphate	0.7–1.5 mmol/l	Eosinophils	$0.04–0.4\times10^{9}$/l
Magnesium	0.7–1.0 mmol/l	Monocytes	$0.2–0.8\times10^{9}$/l
Osmolality	278–305 mosmol/kg	Basophils	$0.0–0.1\times10^{9}$/l
Potassium	3.5–5.0 mmol/l	Lymphocytes	$1.5–4.5\times10^{9}$/l
Sodium	135–150 mmol/l	Platelets	$150–400\times10^{9}$/l
Total protein	63–80 g/l	Erythrocyte sedimentation rate	2–12 mm/1st hour
Triglycerides	0.55–1.90 mmol/l	Ferritin (varies with age)	14–200 µg/l
Urate	0.14–0.46 mmol/l	Pre-menopausal women	14–148 µg/l
Urea	3.0–6.5 mmol/	Serum B_{12}	150–700 ng/l
Haemoglobin		Serum folate	2.0–11.0 µg/l
Male	13.0–18.0 g/dl	Red cell folate	150–700 µg/l
Female	11.5–16.5 g/dl	Prothrombin time (PT)	12–14 s
Newborn male	16.0–21.0 g/dl	Activated partial thromboplastin time (APTT)	26.0 33.5 s
2–6 month female	10.5–12.5 g/dl		
Haematocrit (PCV)		Thrombin time (TT)	± 3s of control
Male	0.40–0.52		
Female	0.36 0.47		

* Adapted from Provan J. (2005) *Oxford Handbook of Clinical and laboratory investigation*, 2nd edn. By permission of Oxford University Press, Oxford.

Table A5.2 Adult normal urine levels

Substance	Value
Albumin	< 20 mg/24 h
Calcium	<7.5 mmol/24 h
Creatinine	9–15 mmol/24 h
Phosphate	15–50 mmol/24 h
Osmolality	50–1500 mosmol/24 h
Potassium	14–120 mmol/24 h
Protein	< 150 mg/24 h
Sodium	100–250 mmol/24 h
Urate	<3.0 mmol/24 h
Urea	250–600 mmol/24 h

Table A5.3 Adult normal faecal values

Substance	Value
Faecal fat	<18 mmol/24 h
Nitrogen	70–140 mmol/24 h

Dietary reference values (DRVs)

Estimated average requirements (EARs)

Table A6.1 Estimated average requirements (MJ/d) according to body weight and physical activity level (PAL)*

Body weight (kg)	BMR† MJ/d	PAL				
		1.4	1.5	1.6	1.8	2.0
♂						
30	4.97	7.0	7.5	8.0	9.0	9.9
35	5.34	7.5	8.0	8.6	9.6	10.7
40	5.71	8.0	8.6	9.1	10.3	11.4
45	6.08	8.5	9.1	9.7	11.0	12.2
50	6.45	9.0	9.7	10.3	11.6	12.9
55	6.82	9.6	10.2	10.9	12.3	13.6
60	7.19	10.1	10.8	11.5	12.9	14.4
65	7.56	10.6	11.3	12.1	13.6	15.1
♀						
30	4.58	6.4	6.9	7.3	8.2	9.2
35	4.86	6.8	7.3	7.8	8.7	9.7
40	5.14	7.2	7.7	8.2	9.2	10.3
45	5.42	7.6	8.1	8.7	9.8	10.8
50	5.70	8.0	8.5	9.1	10.3	11.4
55	5.98	8.4	9.0	9.6	10.8	12.0
60	6.26	8.8	9.4	10.0	11.3	12.5

* Department of Health (1991). *Dietary reference values for food and nutrients for the United Kingdom*. HMSO, London.
† BMR, Basal metabolic rate calculated as per Table A4.1.

Table A6.2 Estimated average requirements (EARs) for energy of children 0–18 years*

Age	EAR MJ/d (kcal/d)	
	♂	♀
0–3 months	2.28 (545)	2.16 (515)
4–6 months	2.89 (690)	2.69 (645)
7–9 months	3.44 (825)	3.20 (765)
10–12 months	3.85 (920)	3.61 (865)
1–3 years	5.15 (1 230)	4.86 (1 165)
4–6 years	7.16 (1 715)	6.46 (1 545)
7–10 years	8.24 (1 970)	7.28 (1 740)
11–14 years	9.27 (2 220)	7.72 (1 845)
15–18 years	11.51 (2 775)	8.83 (2 110)

* Department of Health (1991). *Dietary reference values for food and nutrients for the United Kingdom.* HMSO, London.

Table A6.3 Reference nutrient intakes for protein (RNI)*

Age	Weight (kg)	RNI (g/d)
0–3 months	5.9	12.5
4–6 months	7.7	12.7
7–9 months	8.8	13.7
10–12 months	9.7	14.9
1–3 years	12.5	14.5
4–6 years	17.8	19.7
7–10 years	28.3	28.3
♂		
11–14 years	43.0	42.1
15–18 years	64.5	55.2
19–50 years	74.0	55.5
50+ years	71.0	53.3
♀		
11–14 years	43.8	41.2
15–18 years	55.5	45.4
19–50 years	60.0	45.0
50+ years	62.0	46.5
Pregnancy		
Lactation		+6.0
0–4 months		+11.0
4+ months		+8.0

* Department of Health (1991). *Dietary reference values for food and nutrients for the United Kingdom.* HMSO, London.

Table A 6.4 RNIs for vitamins*

Age	Thiamin (mg/d)	Riboflavin (mg/d)	Niacin (mg/d)[†]	Vitamin B$_6$ (mg/d)[‡]	Vitamin B$_{12}$ (µg/d)	Folate (µg/d)	Vitamin C (mg/d)	Vitamin A (µg/d)	Vitamin D
0–3 m	0.2	0.4	3	0.2	0.3	50	25	350	8.5
4–6 m	0.2	0.4	3	0.2	0.3	50	25	350	8.5
7–9 m	0.2	0.4	4	0.3	0.4	50	25	350	7
10–12 m	0.3	0.4	5	0.4	0.4	50	25	350	7
1–3 y	0.5	0.6	8	0.7	0.5	70	30	400	7
4–6 y	0.7	0.8	11	0.9	0.8	100	30	500	—
7–10 y	0.7	1.0	12	1.0	1.0	150	30	500	—
♂									
11–14 y	0.9	1.2	15	1.2	1.2	200	35	600	—
15–18 y	1.1	1.3	18	1.5	1.5	200	40	700	—
19–50 y	1.0	1.3	17	1.4	1.5	200	40	700	—
50+ y	0.9	1.3	16	1.4	1.5	200	40	700	10

♀									
11–14 y	0.7	1.1	12	1.0	1.2	200	35	600	—
15–18 y	0.8	1.1	14	1.2	1.5	200	40	600	—
19–50 y	0.8	1.1	13	1.2	1.5	200	40	600	—
50+ y	0.8	1.1	12	1.2	1.5	200	40	600	10
Pregnancy	+0.1§	+0.3	¶	¶	¶	+100	+10	+100	10
Lactation									
0–4 m	+0.2	+0.5	+2	¶	+0.5	+60	~+30	+350	10
4+ m	+0.2	+0.5	+2	¶	+0.5	+60	+30	+350	10

† Nicotinic acid equivalent.

‡ Based on protein providing 14.7 % of the EAR for energy.

§ Last semester only.

¶ No increment.

* Data from Department of Health (1991). Dietary reference values for food and nutrients from the United Kingdom. HMSO, London. Table from appendix 6.2, pp.716–17 of Thomas. B.92001). Manual of dietetic practice, 3rd edn. Blackwell science, Oxford.

Table A 6.5 RNIs for minerals*

Age	Ca (mg/d)	P (mg/d)	Mg (mg/d)	Na (mg/d)	K (mg/d)	Cl (mg/d)	Fe (mg/d)	Zn (mg/d)	Cu (mg/d)	Se (µg/d)	I (µg/d)
0–3 m	525	400	55	210	800	320	1.7	4.0	0.2	10	50
4–6 m	525	400	60	280	850	400	4.3	4.0	0.3	13	60
7–9 m	525	400	75	320	700	500	7.8	5.0	0.3	10	60
10–12 m	525	400	80	350	700	500	7.8	5.0	0.3	10	60
1–3 y	350	270	85	500	800	800	6.9	5.0	0.4	15	70
4–6 y	450	350	120	700	1100	1100	6.1	6.5	0.6	20	100
7–10y	550	450	200	1200	2000	1800	8.7	7.0	0.7	30	110
♂											
11–14 y	1000	775	280	1600	3100	2500	11.3	9.0	0.8	45	130
15–18 y	1000	775	300	1600	3500	2500	11.3	9.5	1.0	70	140
19–50 y	700	550	300	1600	3500	2500	8.7	9.5	1.2	75	140
50+ y	700	550	300	1600	3500	2500	8.7	9.5	1.2	75	140

♀										
11–14 y	800	625	280	1600	3100	2500	14.8‡	9.0	0.8	45	130
15–18 y	800	625	300	1600	3500	2500	14.8‡	7.0	1.0	60	140
19–50 y	700	550	270	1600	3500	2500	14.8‡	7.0	1.2	60	140
50+ y	700	550	270	1600	3500	2500	8.7	7.0	1.2	60	140
Pregnancy ‡	‡	‡	‡	‡	‡	‡	‡	‡	‡	‡	‡
Lactation										
0–4 m	+550	+440	+50	‡	‡	‡	‡	+6.0	+0.3	+15	‡
4+ m	+550	+440	+50								

‡ No increment.

‡ Supplements required if menstrual losses are high.

* Data from Department of Health (1991). *Dietary reference Values for food and nutrients from the United Kingdom*. HMSO, London. Table from appendix 6.2, pp. 716–17 of Thomas, B. (2001). *Manual of dietetic practice*, 3rd edn. Blackwell Science, Oxford.

Nutritional composition of common foods

Protein exchanges

Table A7.1 Foods containing approximately 6 g protein

	Weight (g)	Description
Meat—cooked, e.g. lean beef, lamb, pork	25	1 small slice
Sausage—cooked	40	1 large sausage
Poultry—cooked	25	1 small slice
Fish—cooked or tinned	40	1 tablespoon
Fish fingers—cooked	45	2 fingers
Egg	50	1 average hen's egg
Cheese e.g. Cheddar	25	Matchbox-sized piece
Milk—full fat, semi-or skimmed	200	Average glass ($^1/_3$ pt)
Milk powder—skimmed	15	4 teaspoons
Yogurt	125	Small pot
Pulses—cooked e.g. lentils	100	3 tablespoons
Nuts, e.g almonds, peanuts	25	15–25 nuts
Hummus	100	3 tablespoons

Table A7.2 Foods containing approximately 2 g protein

	Weight (g)	Description
Bread—white / wholegrain	25	1 large thin slice
Potato—boiled	125	2 x size of hen's egg
Potato—mashed	110	2 scoops
Chips	50	8 large
Rice—boiled	75	1½ tablespoons
Pasta—boiled	50	1 tablespoon
Breakfast cereal—cornflake type	25	small average portion
Breakfast cereal—wheat bisk type	20	1 bisk
Biscuits, e.g. plain digestive	30	2 biscuits
Cream crackers	20	4 crackers
Cake—plain sponge	25	½ small average slice
Ice cream—plain	50	1 small scoop
Baked beans	40	1 tablespoon

Table A7.3 Foods containing little protein per typical portion

	Protein content*		
Butter	0.6	Apples, pineapple	0.4
Margarine	Trace	Pear	0.3
Cooking oil	Trace	Melon	0.6
Sugar	0.5	Apple juice	0.1
Golden syrup	0.3	Cranberry juice	Trace
Jam, honey	0.5	Boiled sweets	Trace
Marmalade	0.1	Peppermints	0.5
Carrots, boiled	0.6	Cola, lemonade	Trace
Celery, cucumber, lettuce	0.5–0.8	Tea, infusion	0.1
Swede, boiled	0.3	Coffee, infusion	0.2

*g/100 g food.

Carbohydrate exchanges

Table A7.3 Foods containing approximately 10 g carbohydrate

	Weight (g)	Description
Wholemeal bread	25	1 thin slice/large loaf
White bread	20	1 thin slice/small loaf
Potatoes—boiled	60	1 size of hen's egg
Potatoes—mashed	60	1 scoop
Potatoes—roast	40	1 very small
Sweet potato—boiled	50	1 size of hen's egg
Rice—boiled, brown, white	30	¾ tablespoon
Pasta—boiled, e.g. spaghetti, macaroni	50	1 tablespoon
Pulses, e.g. lentils	60	2 tablespoons
Peas—frozen	100	3 tablespoons
Parsnip—boiled	80	1 medium
Sweetcorn—boiled	50	2 tablespoons
Thick soup, e.g. tinned vegetable	100	1 small tin
Thin soup, e.g. minestrone	250	1 standard mug
Sausages	100	2 large sausages
Beefburger, economy	100	1 economy burger
Beefburger, 100% meat = no CHO	—	—
Fish fingers	60	2 fish fingers
Breakfast cereals, e.g. branflakes	15	2 tablespoons
Breakfast cereals, e.g. wheat bisk type	20	1 bisk
Muesli, no added sugar	15	¾ tablespoon
Porridge—made with water	125	small average portion
Biscuits—plain digestive	15	1 digestive
Apple, pear	100	1 medium
Orange	120	1 small
Banana	45	½ small banana
Melon—galia, honeydew	200	1 medium slice
Pineapple, fresh	100	1 large slice
Grapes	70	15 large grapes
Orange juice—no added sugar	110	½ average glass
Apple juice—no added sugar	100	½ average glass
Cranberry juice	70	⅓ average glass
Milk—full fat, semi or skimmed	200	1 average glass
Yogurt—low fat, fruit	70	½ small pot
Yogurt—low fat, plain	135	1 small pot
Ice cream—plain dairy, vanilla	50	1 small scoop
Lemonade	170	1 small glass
Lucozade®	60	⅓ average glass
Cola	90	½ average glass
Beer—best bitter	450	¾ pint glass
Lager—premium	400	¾ pint glass
Wine—medium white	330	2½ small wine glasses
Wine—red contains 0.2 g CHO/100 ml	—	—
Crisps	20	¾ small packet
Peanuts—dry roasted	100	1 large packet

Table A7.4 Examples of household measures of foods used commonly in the UK*

Food group	Household measure	Quantity
Cereals and starchy foods	1 tablespoon of breakfast cereal	6 g
	1 medium portion breakfast cereal	40 g
	1 medium bowl porridge	200 g
	1 biscuit Weetabix	20 g
	1 medium slice of bread	35 g
	1 bread roll	50 g
	½ French stick	125 g
	4 dessertspoons of rice/cooked pasta	60 g
	2 egg-sized boiled potatoes	60 g
	1 medium plate of chips	100 g
	1 average jacket potato with skin	180 g
	1 croissant/brioche	50 g
	1 chapatti	55 g
	1 crumpet	40 g
	1 papadum grilled	10 g
	1 naan bread	160 g
Fruit	1 medium apple (without core)	100 g
	1 medium banana (no skin)	100 g
	½ avocado (flesh only)	75 g
	1 cherry (no stone)	10 g
	1 medium clementine/mandarin orange	60 g
	1 apricot (without stone)	65 g
	1 slice melon (without skin)	180 g
	1 medium tomato	85 g
	1 medium pear	170 g
	1 medium nectarine/peach (without stone)	110 g
	1 medium kiwi (without skin)	60 g
	1 grape	5 g
	½ grapefruit (flesh only)	80 g
	1 medium plum (without stone)	55 g
	1 glass of fruit juice	200 ml
Vegetables	1 average portion of boiled cabbage, cauliflower, Brussels sprouts, courgettes, mixed vegetables, or spinach	90 g
	1 medium boiled carrot	45 g
	1 slice cucumber	6 g
	1 spring onion	20 g
	1 average onion	90 g
	1 average portion of peas	65 g
	1 average tomato	85 g
	1 tablespoon sweet corn	30 g
	1 broccoli spear	45 g
Dairy products	1 glass of milk	200 ml
	1 pint of milk	585 ml
	1 pot of yogurt	125 g
	Hard cheese (small matchbox size)	30 g
	Cottage cheese—small pot	112 g

Table A7.4 (cont.)

Food group	Household measure	Quantity
Protein sources	2–3 thin slices of beef, pork, lamb	90 g
	1 medium burger	105 g
	1 rasher bacon	25 g
	1 medium chicken portion	150 g
	1 rump or fillet steak (5 oz)	115 g
	1 medium slice of ham	50 g
	2 hot dog sausages	70 g
	1 medium piece of fish	120 g
	2 sardines (tinned)	40 g
	4 fish fingers	120 g
	1 average portion tuna in a sandwich	45 g
	1 hen's egg	50 g
	1 omelette/1 portion scrambled egg	120 g
	Average portion of beans and lentils	120 g
	I small tin of baked beans	170 g
	1 handful of nuts	40 g
Fats and fat-rich	1 teaspoon of butter/margarine	5 g
	1 tablespoon of oil	11 ml
	1 packet of crisps	28 g
Sweet foods	1 sugar cube	5 g
	1 sachet of sugar	10 g
	2 squares of chocolate	5 g
	1 dessertspoon of jam	30 g
	1 sweet biscuit	20 g
	1 vanilla slice	110 g
	1 slice of chocolate cake/sponge cake	65 g
	1 slice of apple pie	115 g
	1 jam doughnut	75 g
	1 slice fruit cake	70 g
	1 jam tart	24 g
	1 scone	48 g
	1 hot chocolate	18 g cocoa powder
Drinks	1 small glass	150 ml
	1 medium glass	200 ml
	1 can of fizzy drink, e.g. CocaCola, Fanta.	330 ml
	1 average glass of wine	
	1 average bottle of wine	125 ml
	1 measure of spirits	750 ml
	1 mug	23 ml
		250 ml
Composite meals	1 medium pizza	300 g
	1 slice of quiche/flan	120 g
	1 average portion of stew/curry	330 g
	1 average portion of lasagne or cannelloni	450 g
	1 individual steak and kidney pie	200 g
	1 average portion of cottage/shepherds pie	300 g
Spoon sizes	1 teaspoonful	~5 ml
	1 dessertspoonful	~10 ml
	1 tablespoonful	~15 ml

*Further information: Crawley, H. (1990). *Food portion sizes*, MAFF publication. HMSO, London.

Useful contacts

Manufacturers' contact details

The manufacturers of nutritional products referred to in this book can be contacted via details below. As both products and manufacturers are subject to change, readers are advised to check the latest issue of the *British National Formulary* for the most current information.

Abbott Laboratories Ltd
Abbott House
Norden Road, Maidenhead
Berks SL6 4XE
Telephone 01628 773355

Alembic Products Ltd
River Lane
Saltney, Chester
Cheshire CH4 8RQ
Telephone 01244 680147

Complan Foods
Trafalgar House
11 Waterloo Place
London SW1Y 4AU
Telephone 0845 6003170

Fresenius Kabi Ltd
Hampton Court, Tudor Road
Manor Park, Runcorn
Cheshire WA7 1UF
Telephone 01928 594200

HJ Heinz Company Ltd
South Building,
Hayes Park
Hayes, UB4 8AL
Telephone 020 85737757

KoRa Healthcare Ltd
Frans Maas House
Swords Business Park, Swords
Co Dublin, Ireland
Telephone 00 353 1890 0406

Vitaflo Ltd
11 Century Building
Brunswick Business Park
Liverpool L3 4BL
Telephone 0151 709902

Mead Johnson Nutritionals
Uxbridge Business Park
Sanderson Road
Uxbridge UB8 1DH
Telephone 00800 88342568

Nestlé Clinical Nutrition
St George's House
Park Lane, Croydon
Surrey CR9 1NR
Telephone 020 86675130

Novartis Consumer Health
Wimblehurst Road
Horsham
West Sussex RH12 5AB
Telephone 01403 210211

Nutricia Clinical Care
White Horse Business Park
Trowbridge
Wilts BA14 0XQ
Telephone 01225 711688

SHS International Ltd
100 Wavertree Boulevard
Wavertree Technology Park
Liverpool L7 9PT
Telephone 0151 2288161

SMA Nutrition
Wyeth Pharmaceuticals
Huntercombe Lane South
Taplow, Maidenhead
Berks SL6 0PH
Telephone 01628 604377

Websites

International bodies

American Dietetic Association www.eatright.org
Arbor Nutrition guide www.arborcom.com
EU: Diet, Physical Activity and Health—EU Platform for Action www.europa.eu.int/comm/health/ph_determinants/life_style/nutrition/platform/platform_en.htm
European Federation of the Association of Dietitians www.efad.org
Food & Agriculture Organization www.fao.org
Institute of Medicine, USA www.iom.edu
International Agency for Research on Cancer www-dep.iarc.fr
International Obesity Task Force www.iotf.org
National Institute of Health (USA) Office of Dietary Supplements www.ods.od.nih.gov
United Nations Standing Committee on Nutrition www.unsystem.org/scn/
United States Department of Agriculture—MyPyramid www.mypyramid.gov
United States Department of Health & Human Services, Center for Disease Control www.cdc.gov
World Cancer Research Fund www.wcrf-uk.org
World Health Organisation
Headquarters www.who.int
European office www.euro.who.int

UK bodies

Cancer Research UK www.cancerresearchuk.org/
Consensus Action of Salt Health www.actiononsalt.org.uk
Core (formerly Digestive Disorders Foundation) www.digestivedisorders.org.uk/
Cystic Fibrosis Trust www.cftrust.org.uk/
Age Concern www.ageconcern.org.uk
Association for the Study of Obesity www.aso.org.uk
Bandolier (independent evidence-based healthcare) www.jr2.ox.ac.uk/bandolier
Better Hospital Food www.betterhospitalfood.com
British Association for Parenteral and Enteral Nutrition www.bapen.org.uk
British Dietetic Association www.bda.uk.org
British Heart Foundation www.bhf.org.uk/
British HIV Association www.bhiva.org
British Liver Trust www.britishlivertrust.org.uk/
British Medical Association www.bma.org.uk
British National Formulary www.bnf.org/bnf/
British Nutrition Foundation www.nutrition.org.uk/
British Society of Gastroenterologists www.bsg.org.uk
Caroline Walker Trust www.cwt.org.uk
Child Growth Foundation (growth charts) www.childgrowthfoundation.org

Clinical national guidelines www.sign.ac.uk
Cochrane reviews www.york.ac.uk/inst/crd/cochlib.htm
Coeliac UK www.coeliac.co.uk
Department of Health www.dh.gov.uk
Diabetes UK www.diabetes.org.uk
Dietitians in Sports and Exercise Nutrition www.disen.org/
Dietitians Working in Obesity Management www.domuk.org/
Dose Adjustment for Normal Eating www.dafne.uk.com
European Dialysis & Transplant Nurses Association & European Renal
Care Association www.edtna-erca.org
FareShare charity (redistributes surplus food for homeless)
www.fareshare.org.uk
The Food Commission www.foodcomm.org.uk
Food in Later Life www.foodinlaterlife.org
Food in schools programme www.teachernet.gov.uk;
www.wiredforhealth.gov.uk
Food Standards Agency www.food.gov.uk; www.eatwell.gov.uk;
www.salt.gov.uk
FSA Expert Group on Vitamins and Minerals Report: Safe Upper Levels
for Vitamins and Minerals www.food.gov.uk/multimedia/pdfs/
vitmin2003.pdf
General Medical Council www.gmc-uk.org
Health Professions Council www.hpc-uk.org
Heart UK www.heartuk.org.uk/
Hospital Caterers Association www.hospitalcaterers.org/
Infant feeding www.babyfriendly.org.uk/commun.asp#plan;
www.breastfeeding.nhs.uk; www.nctpregnancyandbabycare.com;
www.surestart.gov.uk www.laleche.org.uk; www.bliss.org.uk
(feeding pre-term infants)
Institute of Food Research www.ifr.ac.uk/
International Diabetes Federation www.idf.org/home/
Joint Health Claims Initiative www.jhci.co.uk
Kidney Patient Guide www.kidneypatientguide.org.uk/
Leatherhead Food Research Association www.lfra.co.uk/
MRC Human Nutrition Research www.mrc-hnr.cam.ac.uk/
National Advisory Group (INVOLVE) (supporting active public involve-
ment in NHS) www.invo.org.uk
National Heart Forum www.heartforum.org.uk/
National Institute for Clinical Excellence www.nice.org.uk
National Kidney Foundation www.kidney.org
National Osteoporosis Society www.nos.org.uk/
National Statistics Office www.statistics.gov.uk
NHS 5aday Programme www.5aday.nhs.uk
The Nutrition Society www.nutritionsociety.org.uk.
Office for National Statistics www.statistics.gov.uk
Oxford University Press www.oup.com
Patient literature www.publications.dh.gov.uk
Prader–Willi Syndrome Association www.pwsa.co.uk/
Prodigy www.prodigy.nhs.uk
The Refugee Council www.refugeecouncil.org.uk

The Royal Society of Medicine www.roysocmed.ac.uk/
The Royal College of Paediatrics and Child Health www.rcpch.ac.uk
Rowett Research Institute www.rowett.ac.uk/
The Scientific Advisory Committee on Nutrition www.sacn.gov.uk
School meals guidelines
www.dfes.gov.uk/consultations/conDetails.cfm?consultationId=1319
Scottish Intercollegiate Guidelines Network (SIGN) www.sign.ac.uk
Scottish Nutrition and Diet Resources Initiative www.sndri.gcal.ac.uk/
Slimming World® www.slimming-world.co.uk
Society of Health Education and Health Promotion Specialists
www.hj-web.co.uk/sheps/
Sustain: The alliance for better food and farming www.sustainweb.org
Walking the Way to Health Initiative www.whi.org.uk
Weight Watchers® www.weightwatchers.co.uk
Weight Wise campaign www.bdaweightwise.com/bda/

The National Statistics Socio-Economic Classification (UK)

Since 2001, the National Statistics Socio-economic Classification (NS-SEC) is used for official statistics and surveys.[1] It replaces social class based on occupation and socio-economic groups. The information required to create the NS-SEC is occupation (coded to the Standard Occupational Classification 2000) and details of employment status (whether an employer, self-employed, or employee; whether a supervisor; number of employees at the workplace). There are 8 classes, the first of which can be subdivided.

The National Statistics Socio-economic Classification Analytic Classes*

1 Higher managerial and professional occupations
  - 1.1 Large employers and higher managerial occupations
  - 1.2 Higher professional occupations
2 Lower managerial and professional occupations
3 Intermediate occupations
4 Small employers and own account workers
5 Lower supervisory and technical occupations
6 Semi-routine occupations
7 Routine occupations
8 Never worked and long-term unemployed

*For complete coverage, the 3 categories of students, occupations not stated or inadequately described, and not classifiable for other reasons are added as 'Not classified'.

A simpler, self-coded version of the NS-SEC has been developed with 5 classes for use in postal surveys or where detailed occupation information is not needed.

Simpler National Statistics Socio-economic Classification Analytic Classes

1 Higher managerial and professional occupations
2 Intermediate occupations
3 Small employers and own account workers
4 Lower supervisory and technical occupations
5 Semi-routine and routine occupations

[1] Further information: http://www.statistics.gov.uk/methods_quality/ns_sec/default.asp

Bibliography and further reading

1. Barasi, M.E. (2003). *Human nutrition*, 2nd edn. Hodder Arnold, London.

2. Baxter, K. (2005). *Stockley's drug interactions*, 7th edn. Pharmaceutical Press, London.

3. Bender, D.A. (2003). *Nutritional biochemistry of vitamins*, 2nd edn. Cambridge University Press, Cambridge.

4. Bender, A.E. and Bender, D.A. (1995). *Oxford dictionary of food and nutrition*. Oxford University Press, Oxford.

5. Bendich, A. and Deckelbaum, R.J. (2001). *Primary and secondary preventive nutrition*, 1st edn. Humana press, Totowa, New Jersey.

6. Bowman, B.A. and Russell, R.M. (2001). *Present knowledge in nutrition*, 8th edn. ILSI Press, Washington, DC.

7. Costain, L. (2003). *Diet trials: how to succeed at dieting*. BBC, London.

8. Council of Europe (2002). *Food and nutritional care in hospitals: how to prevent undernutrition*. Council of Europe Publishing, Strasbourg.

9. Department of Health (1991). *Dietary reference values for food and nutrients for the United Kingdom*. Her Majesty's Stationery Office, London.

10. Expert Group on Vitamins and Minerals (2003). *Safe upper levels for vitamins and minerals*. Food Standards Agency, London.

11. Food Standards Agency (2002). *McCance and Widdowson's the composition of food*, 6th summary edn. Royal Society of Chemistry, Cambridge.

12. Gariballa, S. (2004). *Nutrition and stroke*. Blackwell Publishing, Oxford.

13. Garrow, J.S., James, W.P.T., and Ralph, A. (2000) *Human nutrition and dietetics*, 10th edn. Churchill Livingstone, Edinburgh.

14. Geissler, C. and Powers, H. (2005). *Human nutrition and dietetics*, 11th edn. Churchill Livingstone, Edinburgh.

15. Gibney, M.J., Lenore, A., and Margetts, B. (2004). *Public health nutrition*, 1st edn. Blackwell Publishing, Oxford.

16. Gibney, M.J., Macdonald, I., and Roche, H.M. (2003). *Nutrition and metabolism*, 1st edn. Blackwell Publishing, Oxford.

17. Gibney, M.J., Vorster, H.H., and Kok, F.J. (2002). *Introduction to human nutrition*, 1st edn. Blackwell Publishing, Oxford.

18. Gibson, R.S. (2005). *Principles of nutritional assessment*, 2nd edn. Oxford University Press, Oxford.

19. Hark, L. and Morrison, G. (2003). *Medical nutrition and disease: a case based approach*, 3rd edn. Blackwell Publishing, Oxford.

20. Heber, D., Blackburn, G.L., and Go, V.L.W. (1999). *Nutritional oncology*. Academic Press, San Diego.

21. Henderson, L. and Gregory, J. (2002). *The National Diet and Nutrition Survey: adults aged 19 to 64 years.* Vol. 1. *Types and quantities of foods consumed.* HMSO, London.

22. Henderson, L., Gregory, J., and Irving, K. (2003). *The National Diet and Nutrition Survey: adults aged 19 to 64 years.* Vol. 2. *Energy, protein, carbohydrate, fat and alcohol intakes.* HMSO, London.

23. Henderson, L., Irving, K., and Gregory, J. (2003). *The National Diet and Nutrition Survey: adults aged 19 to 64 years.* Vol. 3. *Vitamin and mineral intake and urinary analytes.* HMSO, London.

24. Heyward, V.H. and Stolarczyk, L.M. (1996). *Applied body composition assessment.* Human Kinetics, Champaign, Illinois.

25. Hoare, J. and Henderson, L. (2004). *The National Diet and Nutrition Survey: adults aged 19 to 64 years.* Vol. 5. *Summary report.* HMSO, London.

26. Insel, P., Turner, R.E., and Ross, D. (2001). *Nutrition,* 1st edn. Jones and Bartlett Publishers, Sudbury, Massachusetts.

27. Mann, J., and Truswell, A.S. (2004). *Essentials of human nutrition,* 2nd edn. Oxford University Press, Oxford.

28. Margetts, B.M. and Nelson, M. (1997). *Design concepts in nutritional epidemiology.* Oxford University Press, Oxford.

29. McCallum, P.D. and Polisena, C.G. (2000). *The clinical guide to oncology nutrition.* American Dietetic Association, Chicago.

30. Ministry of Agriculture, Fisheries and Food (1999). *1997 Total diet study—aluminium, arsenic, cadmium, chromium, copper, lead, mercury, nickel, selenium, tin and zinc,* Food Surveillance Information Sheet 191, MAFF. HMSO, London.

31. Naidoo, J. and Wills, J. (2000). *Health promotion: foundations for practice,* 2nd edn. Baillière Tindall, London.

32. Östman, J., Britton, M., and Jonsson, E. (Eds.) (2004). *Treating and preventing obesity 1: an evidence-based review.* Wiley-VCH, Weinheim.

33. Payne, J.J., Grimble, G.K., and Silk, D.B.A. (2001). *Artificial nutrition support in clinical practice.* Greenwich Medical Media Ltd, London.

34. Pencheon, D., Guest, C., Melzer, D., and Muir Gray, J.A. (2001). *Oxford handbook of public health practice,* 1st edn. Oxford University Press, Oxford.

35. Reilly, C. (2004). *The nutritional trace metals.* Blackwell Publishing, Oxford.

36. Roche, A.F., Heymesfield, S.B., and Lohman, T. (1996). *Human body composition.* Human Kinetics Champaign, Illinois.

37. Royal Pharmaceutical Society of Great Britain (2005). *British national formulary,* 50th edn. British Medical Association and Royal Pharmaceutical Association of Great Britain, London. (www.BNF.org.uk)

38. Ruston, D., Hoare, J., Henderson, L., and Gregory, J. (2004). *The National Diet and Nutrition Survey: adults aged 19 to 64 years*. Vol. 4. *Nutritional status (anthropometry and blood analytes), blood pressure and physical activity*. HMSO, London.

39. Shaw, V. and Lawson, M. (2001). *Clinical paediatric dietetics*, 2nd edn. Blackwell Science, Oxford.

40. Simon, C., Everitt, H., Birtwistle, J., and Stevenson, B. (2002). *Oxford handbook of general practice*, 1st edn. Oxford University Press, Oxford.

41. Stanner, S. (2005). *Cardiovascular disease: diet, nutrition and emerging risk factors*. Blackwell Publishing Ltd, Oxford.

42. Stratton, R.J., Green, C.J., and Elia, M. (2003). *Disease-related malnutrition: an evidence-based approach to treatment*. CABI Publishing, Wallingford.

43. Thomas, B. (2001). *Manual of dietetic practice*, 3rd edn. Blackwell Science, Oxford.

44. Thorgood, M. and Coombes, Y. (2000). *Evaluating health promotion: practice and methods*, 2nd edn. Oxford University Press, Oxford.

45. Todorovic, T.E. and Micklewright, A. (2004). *A pocket guide to clinical nutrition*, 3rd edn. British Dietetic Association, Birmingham.

50. Webster-Gandy, J. (2006). *Understanding food and nutrition*, Family Doctor Books, Poole.

Index